Transdisciplinary Perioperative Care in Colorectal Surgery

Kok-Yang Tan
Editor

Transdisciplinary Perioperative Care in Colorectal Surgery

An Integrative Approach

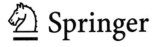

Editor
Kok-Yang Tan
Department of Surgery
Khoo Teck Puat Hospital
Singapore

ISBN 978-3-662-44019-3   ISBN 978-3-662-44020-9   (eBook)
DOI 10.1007/978-3-662-44020-9
Springer Heidelberg New York Dordrecht London

Library of Congress Control Number: 2014951514

© Springer-Verlag Berlin Heidelberg 2015
This work is subject to copyright. All rights are reserved by the Publisher, whether the whole or part of the material is concerned, specifically the rights of translation, reprinting, reuse of illustrations, recitation, broadcasting, reproduction on microfilms or in any other physical way, and transmission or information storage and retrieval, electronic adaptation, computer software, or by similar or dissimilar methodology now known or hereafter developed. Exempted from this legal reservation are brief excerpts in connection with reviews or scholarly analysis or material supplied specifically for the purpose of being entered and executed on a computer system, for exclusive use by the purchaser of the work. Duplication of this publication or parts thereof is permitted only under the provisions of the Copyright Law of the Publisher's location, in its current version, and permission for use must always be obtained from Springer. Permissions for use may be obtained through RightsLink at the Copyright Clearance Center. Violations are liable to prosecution under the respective Copyright Law.
The use of general descriptive names, registered names, trademarks, service marks, etc. in this publication does not imply, even in the absence of a specific statement, that such names are exempt from the relevant protective laws and regulations and therefore free for general use.
While the advice and information in this book are believed to be true and accurate at the date of publication, neither the authors nor the editors nor the publisher can accept any legal responsibility for any errors or omissions that may be made. The publisher makes no warranty, express or implied, with respect to the material contained herein.

Printed on acid-free paper

Springer is part of Springer Science+Business Media (www.springer.com)

Preface

The field of colorectal surgery has undergone tremendous developments in recent decades. Not only have there been exciting developments in surgical techniques rendering surgery less invasive, but there are also new perspectives and insights into improving perioperative management, and new outcome measures have been defined. At the same time, more complex patients are challenging the limits of surgical technique and perioperative care. This immense potential for excellent outcomes in colorectal surgery, however, needs to be reconciled with the need for coordinated multifaceted care, yet recognizing that resources are limited.

There is, thus, a pressing need for us to streamline our processes and heighten our clinical productivity in colorectal surgery. To facilitate the delivery of top-quality seamless surgical care to our patients, there has to be constant improvement and minimizing of wastages. The different components of health care have to be integrated in a transdisciplinary fashion. There needs to be excellent communication and collaboration with constant attention to detail and precision. This should be done in an environment of constant learning, research, and innovation.

This book discusses in depth the integration of care in colorectal surgery in a transdisciplinary fashion. After the provision of pertinent background information, the complexities of current management in colorectal surgery are discussed, followed by a description of transdisciplinary care. Subsequent chapters focus on a range of issues associated with the surgical and perioperative care of colorectal surgery, with an emphasis on how the multiple facets of care can be integrated through a transdisciplinary approach. Each chapter provides helpful take-home messages in bullet point form, and numerous informative figures and tables are also included. The authors are surgeons, physicians, anesthetists, oncologists, and nursing and allied health professionals with extensive experience in the field.

Singapore   Kok-Yang Tan

Contents

1 Current Challenges of Surgical Care and the Transdisciplinary Model 1
Junice Wong and Kok-Yang Tan

2 Integrative Transdisciplinary Care of Elderly Surgical Patients 13
Kok-Yang Tan

3 Transdisciplinary Nursing 29
Phyllis Xiu-Zhuang Tan, Marc W.J. Ong, and Kok-Yang Tan

4 Transdisciplinary Management of Perioperative Nutrition 41
Yee-Lee Cheah, George Chee-Hong Toh, Jian-Wei Heng, and Eric Wei-Long Wee

5 Enhanced Recovery 77
Edward Ratnasingham Shanthakumar and Geraldine Pei-Chin Cheong

6 The Role of a Pharmacist in a Transdisciplinary Geriatric Surgery Team 93
Doreen Su-Yin Tan and Adeline Hsiao-Huey Wee

7 Prehabilitation and Rehabilitation in Colorectal Surgery 103
Sharon Cheng-Kuan Lim, Melissa Zhi-Yan Heng, and Gregory Heng

8 Integrative Approach to Laparoscopic Surgery for Colorectal Cancer 119
Fumio Konishi, Takayoshi Yoshida, Yusuke Komekami, and Chunyong Lee

9 Team-Based Integrative Care for Recurrent and Locally Advanced Rectal Cancer Surgery 131
Min-Hoe Chew

10 Multimodal Approach to Familial Colorectal Cancer 139
Sarah Jane Walton and Sue Clark

11 Transdisciplinary Fecal Incontinence Management.............. 157
Surendra Kumar Mantoo and Paul Antoine Lehur

12 Integrating Science and Technology to Proctology.............. 173
Frederick H. Koh and Ker-Kan Tan

13 Transdisciplinary Management in Geriatric Oncology.......... 189
Sung W. Sun, Koshy Alexander, and Beatriz Korc-Grodzicki

14 Metastatic Colon and Rectal Cancer: Role of Multidisciplinary Team-Based Management.................................. 199
Dedrick Kok-Hong Chan, Tian-Zhi Lim, and Ker-Kan Tan

15 Transdisciplinary Stoma Care 227
Yu-Jing Ong, Choo-Eng Ong, Lay-Choo Chee,
and Gregory K.E. Heng

16 Healing and Psychosocial Issues Surrounding Surgery.......... 247
Mary Rockwood Lane and Michael Samuels

Index 259

Current Challenges of Surgical Care and the Transdisciplinary Model

1

Junice Wong and Kok-Yang Tan

> **Take-Home Pearls**
> - The delivery of comprehensive surgical care is becoming more challenging owing to developments in surgical options, information available, patient, and social factors.
> - Management of surgical patients requires well-coordinated subspecialty and allied healthcare.
> - Multidisciplinary care is insufficient in delivering the level of care required.
> - Transdisciplinary care seeks to build upon and improve on the existing model of multidisciplinary care.
> - Implementation of transdisciplinary care requires changes on an administrative, organisational, and individual standpoint.

1.1 Introduction

The delivery of surgical care has become increasingly complex especially in recent years. There have been massive developments in surgical options all with more complex decision-making processes, and thus there is a need for healthcare individuals to delve deeper into their areas of expertise resulting in subspecialisation. There is also an increasing dependence on other subspecialists with other domain expertise in the care of a single patient. Yet there is an overwhelming need for every patient to be considered as a "whole" and not just in terms of organ systems or

J. Wong • K.-Y. Tan (✉)
Geriatric Surgery Service, Department of Surgery, Alexandra Health,
Khoo Teck Puat Hospital, Singapore, Singapore
e-mail: kokyangtan@gmail.com

© Springer-Verlag Berlin Heidelberg 2015

K.-Y. Tan (ed.), *Transdisciplinary Perioperative Care in Colorectal Surgery: An Integrative Approach*, DOI 10.1007/978-3-662-44020-9_1

specific pathologies. There is now a discrepancy between the comprehensive care that every patient wants and the ability of a single healthcare professional to deliver that comprehensive care.

Globally, we are seeing the rise of what has been termed the "silver tsunami". This is where an increasingly ageing population poses issues not only in terms of workforce economics but also on healthcare demands. This change in the population means that the patient population that the surgical team manages will become even more challenging. There are many other factors that have to be considered if one aspires to deliver comprehensive care. As such, it is essential for hospitals and healthcare professionals to relook the way we manage surgical patients, with a special emphasis on the complexities of their socioeconomic, functional, and health status. In this chapter, we will explore the factors challenging the delivery of comprehensive surgical care and discuss how we can reorganise to deliver more comprehensive care.

1.2 The Complexities of Current Surgical Management

1.2.1 The Abundance of Information Available

There is increasing research on the management of individual diseases and the development of new technologies and techniques. For instance, there are now minimally invasive options for colonic resections (e.g., "traditional" laparoscopy, robotic-assisted surgery, single-incision laparoscopy), each touted to be beneficial in one way or another. The amount of literature available online is vastly increasing. A quick search on PubMed for "colorectal cancer" churns out more than 160,000 articles. New evidence and trials for chemotherapeutic and targeted therapies are ever emerging – each more promising than the last. Critical appraisal of this ever-increasing information is important. Many of these studies are on different patient cohorts and the outcome measures and definitions of complications may be very variable. Even attempts at systematic reviews and meta-analyses may result in biased conclusions due to methodological flaws. Even implementation of practices based on randomised controlled trials needs to be considered with care based on local conditions and expertise. Thus interpretation of the information may be complex. This gives rise to a dazzling, and often confusing, load of information that even clinicians struggle to digest.

All these mean that the art and science of decision making is not so straightforward anymore. When deciding on which options to offer patients, very often the focus is on providing "evidence-based" treatment. This could mean the most radical surgery to reduce tumour burden or the newest targeted therapy. With each specialty and allied care professional having well-meaning "best-evidence" opinions, the individual patient as a whole can get overwhelmed. There is an added danger that "evidence-based" treatment options are not individualised to each particular patient and the big picture is missed.

1.2.2 The Changing Profile of Patients

Physically, people are living longer, often with other chronic medical problems in tow. Treatment of a disease, while taken on by a particular specialist, will necessarily have bearing on the treatment of other comorbidities. Polypharmacy remains a valid concern for many of these patients, some of which are clueless about their medical conditions. Elderly patients' predisposition to the "geriatric giants" of falls, cognitive impairment, incontinence, immobility adds to the increased demands of care. This makes the medical management of elderly patients much more challenging.

Patients and their families' mind-sets, too, have changed with the times. With information (erroneous or not) easily available online and in books, many would have their own perceived ideas of what treatment they expect or the type of recovery they will experience. In addition to that, there is a huge array of religious/traditional/homoeopathic remedies that seem equally, if not more, attractive than modern medicine.

No longer are physicians seen as the sole or main decision maker pertaining to treatment, but now the preferences of patients and their family members have to be taken into account. We have to recognise that patients themselves are important stakeholders in their treatment. As such there is an important need for patients to be able to analyse their own situations and be part of the decision-making process. On the other hand, family dynamics play an important part as well in certain cultures. There may be situations where different members of the family and/or the patient have differing views trying to stake a claim in the decision-making process, thus leading to more confusion.

1.2.3 The Changing Profile of Society

In many societies, there will also be strains to the social framework as it struggles to support the sick and elderly. Families are more compact with less offspring and less reliance on extended families and relatives. The so-called Sandwich Generation are tasked with raising their families while looking after their elderly parents as well. This is taxing not just financially, but also in terms of time and effort.

What this means is that pre-hospitalisation and post-discharge care is not a given. Part and parcel of ensuring good outcomes for the sick is optimisation of health and function preoperatively and dedicated rehabilitation after the acute phase of illness/surgery. Hence, holistic care of surgical patients is not limited to just the duration which they spend in hospital, but extends to their care in the community and at home. There is a need to integrate care not only horizontally across the different disciplines taking care of the patient during the hospital stay but also vertically taking into consideration the needs at the level of primary care and home care.

1.2.4 The Complexities of Healthcare Infrastructure

With the constraints within households as described, hospitals and society as a whole have to take on a larger burden of care. Rehabilitative hospitals are often oversubscribed with long waiting times; applications for voluntary nursing homes and hospices can be a long and tedious affair. The transient nature of the care provided for in hospitals predisposes to a breakdown in continuity of care between home/hospital/step-down facilities. Physicians and surgeons keen to discharge patients to free up much-needed hospital beds may overlook other issues such as caregiver training and home modification.

1.3 The Problem with Multidisciplinary Care

Currently, the introduction of multidisciplinary teams in oncological as well as chronic disease models has also increased in many developed countries (e.g., the United Kingdom, Europe, the United States, Australia). This has developed in part as recognition that disease management is a complex process that involves separate subspecialties and professional groups. As highlighted by Taylor et al., however, much of available evidence still focuses more on individual decision-making process rather than overall organisational decisions (Taylor et al. 2010).

1.3.1 The Pitfalls of Multidisciplinary Care

The need for highly specialised knowledge and skill can become a problem when it is not paralleled by the knowledge and skills on how to work effectively together. The intention of bringing together different specialists and allied health professionals in a multidisciplinary model, while good, has several potential pitfalls. These pitfalls are a result of a lack of collaboration and coordination between the different groups involved and can be analogous to an architect (the surgeon or primary physician) tasked to build a house for a client (the patient). The client may have a desired outcome that needs to be communicated to the architect, which in turn sets off a chain of duties that need to be done by various other groups of people or "specialists" (e.g., contractors, electricians, bricklayers, etc.). The process of house building may be set back for various reasons, resulting in an undesirable outcome for the client.

1.3.1.1 Pitfall #1: Failure in Shared Vision and Goal

Firstly, there should be a shared vision and goal. When building a house, what the client has in mind may be different from what the architect perceives. Unless the vision is communicated clearly and in terms that both sides can understand, there is a risk that the final result will reflect the architect's rather than the client's desires. There needs to be an exchange of ideas such that any unrealistic expectations brought forth by the client can be addressed swiftly and tampered accordingly. It is also the responsibility of the architect to ensure this vision is then understood by the other groups of "specialists" such that there is seamless execution of the plan.

1 Current Challenges of Surgical Care and the Transdisciplinary Model

In the establishment of the surgical plan for major colorectal surgery, the possibility of the patient and surgical team not having a common goal and vision is real. An elderly patient may be willing to undergo major surgery because he/she may want to preserve his/her autonomy and independence from the complications of the pathology and he/she may not be very particular about long-term survival. A surgeon on the other hand may be obsessed with performing the most radical cancer operation so as to ensure the best long-term survival; in doing so certain risks may be taken. When the goal of the patient and the surgeon differs, surgical decision making suffers.

This problem is further confounded by team members also not identifying a common goal set. The anaesthetist may share the same goal with the surgeon and be convinced to push the limits of anaesthetic care to accommodate this radical operation. The cardiologist then suggests that this same elderly patient undergo heart surgery just so that he/she can subsequently withstand this radical cancer operation and more events spiral into place. All this time, the medical social worker understood that this was not what the patient asked for but did not think that there was an alternative.

Another patient may be adamant that he/she does not wish to have a stoma, insisting on a riskier operation despite his/her multiple poorly controlled comorbidities and frailty. He/she does not understand the complexities of a low rectal anastomosis and its accompanying poorer bowel function. The surgeon insists on a stoma and performs it. He/she then instructs the nurse to take care of the stoma on this same patient who is unable to accept the stoma and refuses to learn how to manage it. The goal of making the patient understand the situation and come to terms with accepting the stoma is completely missed.

1.3.1.2 Pitfall #2: Failure in Planning and Coordination

Secondly, despite a common vision and goal, there may be a failure in planning and coordination. Timing is essential in house building. Each preceding step needs to be in place before progression can take place. Foundations need to be laid before the building is erected, if not the house is bound to fail. Prior to laying bricks, the window and door frames need to be ready to ensure a good fit and to prevent revision of work.

Similarly, before embarking on major surgery for elderly patients with diminished reserves and limited resources, a good "foundation" would entail preoperative planning to optimise their functional status and build up their nutrition. Counselling and preparing them to use postoperative tools would ensure a better "fit" into the rehabilitative plan once surgery has taken place.

1.3.1.3 Pitfall #3: Failure of Members of the Team to Communicate Effectively

Prior to casting the floor slab, it is imperative that the plumber lays the pipes in the ground as sewer is discharged, usually, via gravity flow. Similarly, floor traps, openings in floors, etc., must be coordinated and installed. At this stage there are no walls to guide the tradesmen. Hence, the precise locations of fixtures and walls have to be communicated to the plumber very clearly. Any error will result in hacking and abortive works. Depending on the construction and finish of the walls, the laying of cables must be coordinated in advance. Positions of power points on walls or floors must be planned and communicated effectively to the electrician in advance so that the cables are installed within the cavity of the brick walls and can be pulled out at the precise location of the power outlet.

In a fast-paced multidisciplinary approach, individuals may still easily be working in silos only concentrating on their area of expertise. Different members of the team may visit the patient at different times and note their inputs in the case notes. Without proper communication lines laid, some of these inputs may inadvertently be missed or misinterpreted. A geriatric physician may have seen a patient and noted that there may be early signs of cognitive impairment; however, this subtle finding was not clearly communicated to the surgeon and anaesthetist. As such the latter two doctors involved in the care then failed to recognise the increase risk of postoperative cognitive dysfunction and delirium. The nurse in charge then did not institute any measures to reduce the risk of delirium and this resulted in the patient sustaining a fall in the early postoperative period.

Good communication is thus crucial in determining a holistic care plan for the patient.

1.3.1.4   Pitfall #4: Failure of Members of the Team to Understand What the Other Is Doing

The role of the painter needs to be understood. Should painting commence too early, some remaining works (e.g., power points) may not be completed and "touching up" may then be required. This is not prudent as the paint may not match even after a week and is conspicuous. If the painter comes on too late, the carpet or polished timber floor may need protection and any spills or stains may damage the floor finish.

A surgeon is convinced of the benefits of incentive spirometry during the perioperative period and insists that this is the standard of care for all the patients. The physiotherapists however have other ideas. Some patients are just not suitable for incentive spirometry; they are unable to learn the proper use of the incentive spirometer and thus do not derive the benefits of the device. The physiotherapists also have other innovative methods of encouraging adequate lung expansion in the perioperative period. In this situation, if the surgeon had understood the processes of pulmonary rehabilitation that the physiotherapists undertake, he/she may have become more acceptable of other methods.

1.3.1.5   Pitfall #5: Failure in Completion and Follow-Through

Lastly, there may be a failure in completion and follow-through. Specific individuals may have embarked on the project of house building, only to see different groups drop out at different times. For example, the contractor may run into financial issues leading to the hiring of a new contractor midway through the project. This may lead not only to delays but also weaken the shared vision formed from the beginning.

Similarly, patients may be seen by an anaesthetist preoperatively and counselled on epidural analgesia, but intra-operatively another team takes over and decides on another modality. A third anaesthetist may see the patient postoperatively to adjust the pain medications required. Although each modality is a justifiable means of analgesia, but from the patient standpoint, it can be confusing and undesirable.

1.4 Transdisciplinary Care: What Is It?

Given the limitations of multidisciplinary care as illustrated earlier, transdisciplinary care seeks to build on the benefits of multidisciplinary care and essentially take it to the next level of collaboration.

The concept of transdisciplinary care has been previously described in several settings such as in early childhood intervention, as well as in the context of a local colorectal geriatric surgical service by Tan and Tan (2013).

1.4.1 The Difference Between Interdisciplinary, Multidisciplinary, and Transdisciplinary Care

While the multidisciplinary model involves brief communication with each member contributing an assessment after applying a discipline-specific skill set, there is little discussion between team members at any point in the process except to share conclusions (see Fig. 1.1).

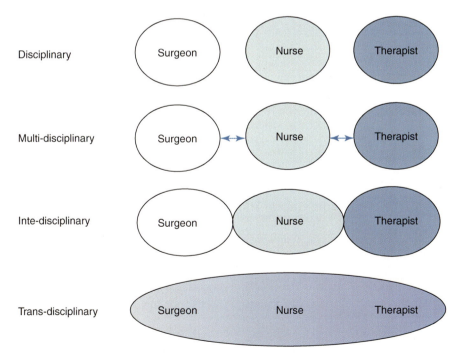

Fig. 1.1 The evolution from disciplinary to transdisciplinary (Adapted from Colón et al. (2008))

The interdisciplinary model acknowledges the overlap in knowledge of the different team members and facilitates horizontal communication at many points in the process of evaluating and treating a patient.

The transdisciplinary model of care takes collaboration to a higher level, incorporating ongoing cross-disciplinary education and regulated overlapping roles (Nandiwada and Dang-Vu 2010). This model also includes the patient/family members as part of the team (Ruddy and Rhee 2005). By institutionalising frequent communication and by regulating team members' overlapping roles, this collaboration prevents fragmentation and duplication of services along disciplinary lines.

Transdisciplinary healthcare involves reaching into the spaces between the disciplines to create positive health outcomes through collaboration. This is likened to a multiplayer sports team where each has their own role and responsibilities, and implicit trust is required, together with practice, to get the best outcome. In this case, the outcome is improved health and quality of life for patients with multiple comorbidities and extenuating social circumstances.

Rather than having each specialty work only within its realm of expertise with communication limited to brief meetings or short notes in patient progress notes, transdisciplinary care seeks to be integrative. As described by King et al. (2009), transdisciplinary care seeks to share roles across discipline boundaries to encourage increased communication and collaboration within the team. Implementation of a shared care plan is the goal, with the patient at the centre of it.

The traditional barriers of hierarchy and protocol-based red tape are dispensed with and free exchange of communication is encouraged.

As highlighted by Andre Vyt, interprofessional teamwork exists when not only appropriate referrals are made but when there is a joint contribution in setting up care and treatment plans (Vyt 2008). In a transdisciplinary approach, the knowledge of each other's working methods and competencies has reached such a high level and the shared care planning runs so smoothly that it is difficult for outsiders to identify immediately which team member has which profession. However transdisciplinary does not simply refer to a confusion of dissolution of professional identities; rather, it points out the intensity of shared goal setting, the commonality of a shared reference framework, and the swift interplay between the team members.

1.4.2 The Fundamentals of Transdisciplinary Care

Reilly (2001) put forth the following premises as fundamental in transdisciplinary care, and this is further illustrated by Tan and Tan (2013) (Fig. 1.2):

Role extension – Involves the need for constant improvement within one's own specialty such that one has security in one's own role and responsibility. This helps to resolve turf issues and boundaries.

Role enrichment – Seeks to increase one's knowledge outside of one's discipline and thus acquire the knowledge from other disciplines within the team. This is

1 Current Challenges of Surgical Care and the Transdisciplinary Model

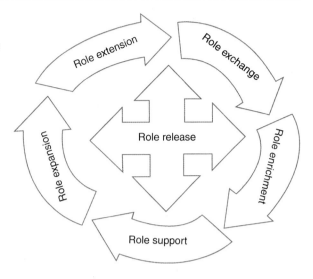

Fig. 1.2 The interactions between the different aspects of transdisciplinary care are a continuous interlinking one as illustrated by Fig 1.2 (Adapted from King 2009)

achieved by a commitment to collaborative work and excellent communication between team members.

Role expansion – Via intensive, ongoing interaction and learning between team members, role expansion is achieved whereby each member of the team begins to pick up the skills and knowledge of the other disciplines.

Role release – Possibly the most crucial element of transdisciplinary care is the concept of role release. This involves members of the team being willing to give up and release their own unique interventions and being willing to allow other team members to be able to take up their role.

Role support – This allows a blurring of the boundaries of the traditional multidisciplinary roles and requires the ongoing willingness of each team member both to trust each other and to support each other (Fig. 1.2).

1.4.3 Implementation of Transdisciplinary Care

To achieve effective interprofessional collaboration, there are some necessary ingredients:

- Interprofessional competencies
- Management and administration that promotes interdisciplinary consultation
- A shared goal
- Efficient communication and information management

Interprofessional competency refers to the blanket skill set needed for effective collaboration with other members – it includes the harmonisation of one's own ideas with that of others, cooperation in care planning, analysis of problems, and communication with other professionals. There needs to be an understanding of each team member's competencies and working methods, the structure of healthcare facilities, system processes, and goals. They also need to be able to analyse complex situations and formulate an opinion and defend it in a group setting.

Effective leadership that promotes a culture of openness and communication needs to be coupled with team members that complement each other's expertise. There should be mutual respect and understanding of the competencies, roles, and contributions of the other professionals without any prejudice or stereotypes. They should search for a common goal and agree upon clear end points.

Healthcare professionals are rarely at the same place at the same time. Organising meetings involving all the team members is difficult and costly and often does not take place in a timely manner for each individual patient.

In this aspect, modern technology and communication tools are helpful. Smart phones, emails, and even online group circles can facilitate rapid exchange of information. Data sheets and progress charts may be uploaded for members to access. Great care however has to be taken in ensuring patient confidentiality during this process. Furthermore, there is no substitute for a good and convivial working relationship between team members that only personal contact can bring about.

Formal meetings should be well prepared with availability of documents and key persons, clear direction from the leader regarding problems, and analysis of an intervention strategy. A system of documentation and proper follow-up after meetings is essential as well.

Conclusion

It has become clear that the traditional model of multidisciplinary care is insufficient in providing optimal, comprehensive healthcare for patients with complex needs, including elderly patients. Transdisciplinary care should herald a new standard of care that would not only improve clinical outcomes but further develop our existing healthcare as a cohesive team. The assets of a well-functioning interprofessional collaboration have been shown to both improve the care effectiveness for persons with chronic diseases and also lead to a higher degree of work satisfaction in healthcare workers.

References

Colón W et al (2008) Chemical biology at the US National Science Foundation. Nat Chem Biol 4:511–514

King G et al (2009) The application of a transdisciplinary model for early intervention services. Infants Young Child 22(3):211–223

Nandiwada DR, Dang-Vu C (2010) Transdisciplinary health care education: training team players. J Health Care Poor Underserved 21:26–34

Reilly C (2001) Transdisciplinary approach: an atypical strategy for improving outcomes in rehabilitative and long-term acute care settings. Rehabil Nurs 26(6):216–220, 244

Ruddy G, Rhee K-S (2005) Transdisciplinary teams in primary care for the underserved: a literature review. J Health Care Poor Underserved 5(16):248–256

Tan KY, Tan PXZ (2013) Transdisciplinary care for elderly surgical patients. In: Colorectal cancer in the elderly. Springer, Berlin/Heidelberg

Taylor C et al (2010) Multidisciplinary team working in cancer: what is the evidence? Br Med J 340:c951

Vyt A (2008) Interprofessional and transdisciplinary teamwork in health care. Diabetes Metab Res Rev 24(Suppl 1):S106–S109

Integrative Transdisciplinary Care of Elderly Surgical Patients

2

Kok-Yang Tan

Take-Home Pearls
- Elderly surgical patients are complex with numerous facets to be managed.
- Holistic management demands an understanding of normal physiology, geriatric syndromes, nutrition, ADLs and psychosocial issues and how they interact with each other.

2.1 Complexities of the Elderly Patient

The approach to an elderly cancer surgery patient cannot be similar to that of a younger patient. While age alone has been shown to be not an independent predictor of poorer outcomes in some studies, elderly patients do come with more "baggage". The team managing an elderly patient has to often grapple with more issues than just the cancer pathology. Altered physiology and reduced functional reserves giving rise to the phenotype of frailty, co-morbidities and reduced abilities in activities of daily living exist in varying degrees and interplay with each other in elderly patients. Making sense of the complexities of each patient is mandatory for optimal management. With this comes the need for the understanding of the physiology of ageing and development of reduced functional reserves.

The process of ageing is accompanied by changes to the physiology of the body. While at a younger age, the physiological reserves of the different organ systems are bountiful, in an older person, these reserves may become depleted. In a younger person, normal homeostasis can be achieved without using any of these

---

K.-Y. Tan
Geriatric Surgery Service, Department of Surgery, Khoo Teck Puat Hospital,
Alexandra Health, Singapore, Singapore
e-mail: kokyangtan@gmail.com

© Springer-Verlag Berlin Heidelberg 2015
K.-Y. Tan (ed.), *Transdisciplinary Perioperative Care in Colorectal Surgery:
An Integrative Approach*, DOI 10.1007/978-3-662-44020-9_2

physiological reserves. On the other hand, an elderly person often depends on their physiological reserves to maintain homeostasis. These reserves are further depleted by competing co-morbidities. It should however be noted that biological ageing and accumulation of co-morbidities are separate processes but these two processes are not mutually exclusive and are interwoven together in a complex manner. As such, the ability to withstand acute illness and surgical stress is significantly reduced. In these situations, the elderly body may not be able to cope with the increased demands, and rapid decompensation occurs. The degree to which functional reserves are depleted is very heterogeneous, and a clear distinction should be made between biological ageing and chronological ageing.

This chapter explores the different facets of the elderly surgical patient that need to be addressed before optimal management can be achieved and suggests how care needs to be integrated in order to provide the multifaceted care that is demanded by an elderly surgical patient.

2.1.1 Physiological Changes in the Elderly

2.1.1.1 Changes to the Heart

The heart is perhaps one of the key organs that demonstrate both biological ageing and accumulation of disease in the elderly. It is well documented that an ageing heart has a reduction in the number of myocytes and an increase in the collagen content. This leads to reduced ventricular compliance that is often further aggravated by stiffening of outflow tracts (Rosenthal and Kavic 2004). The overall effect is that while there is maintenance of resting cardiac output, maximal capacity is reduced with ageing. There may also be changes to the autonomic tissue of the heart leading to an increased risk of arrhythmia and altered homeostatic balance of the heart function. Cardiac disease is also the most common co-morbidity in the elderly, and cardiac complications are most often associated with poorer outcomes (Tan et al. 2006).

2.1.1.2 Changes to the Respiratory Function

Ageing changes to the respiratory system include the decline in chest wall compliance secondary to structural changes of kyphosis, contractures of the intercostal muscles and calcification of costal cartilage (Christmas et al. 2006). In the lung parenchyma, there is loss of elasticity and collapse of small airways (Campbell 2000). These changes contribute to decreased functional residual capacity and residual volume and increased dead space. Furthermore, autonomic changes also result in a reduced response to hypercarbia and hypoxia (Campbell 2000). There may also be reduction in the natural protective mechanisms of the respiratory tract (Marik 2001). These factors lead to the increased susceptibility to pneumonia, aspiration and other pulmonary complications.

2.1.1.3 Changes to the Renal Function

By the age of 75, a person can lose about one third to half of their original nephron function. This functional decline of renal tubules makes dehydration a particular problem as the capacity to compensate for non-renal losses is reduced (Rosenthal and Kavic 2004). There is also a reduced ability to maintain fluid and electrolyte homeostasis. This is often further confounded by the medications that the elderly are taking. These renal changes need to be considered in the pharmacology for elderly patients. Altered renal and hepatic drug metabolisms place the elderly patient at a higher risk of developing drug toxicities. Renal function may also be adversely affected by physiological changes to the voiding function with an increased prevalence of difficulty in voiding or urinary retention.

2.1.1.4 Changes to the Digestive System
The entire digestive system can be affected by ageing. Changes include changes to the nature and amounts of the secretions, changes in the autonomic system resulting in decreased peristalsis and reduction in gastric motility. Intestinal bacterial overgrowth may then occur. This is further aggravated by the altered ability to produce saliva and masticate, leading to a reduced choice of food. Nutritional absorption is thus affected.

It is thus not surprising that protein-energy malnutrition may quickly develop in the elderly when faced with stress (Lipschitz 2000).

2.1.1.5 Changes in the Nervous System
A steady loss of functional neurons starts to occur as early as the age of 25. With ageing, there is a slower response to stimuli, changes in the perception of the senses and also an increased risk of insomnia, irritability, memory loss and visual-motor deficits. The prevalence of dementia also increases with age. Dementia is an important entity in elderly surgical patients as it is the greatest risk factor for postoperative delirium which occurs in between 15 and 53 % of postoperative cases (Demeure and Fain 2006).

2.1.1.6 Changes to the Integumentary System
The skin loses elasticity and subcutaneous fat as a person ages. The small blood vessels under the skin also become more fragile. Injury secondary to shearing forces or pressure occurs more frequently; bruising is more common. The skin in the elderly is also more frequently dry owing to reduced oil and sweat production, coupled with reduced nutrient blood supply to the skin; wound infections are more common. Reduced vascular circulation and loss of subcutaneous tissue also predispose hypothermia in the elderly.

It is important to note that these changes occur in a very heterogeneous fashion in the elderly patient. The changes in the different organ systems occur at different paces and are confounded by co-morbidities and other environmental issues. While it is important to understand these changes, it is more important to individualise management strategies based on the unique assessment of the functional status of these systems in each elderly surgical patient.

2.1.2 Frailty and Geriatric Syndromes

The use of the clinical paradigm of frailty in the assessment of elderly patients is increasingly being recognised. There are still some controversies surrounding the definition and applications of the syndrome of frailty. There is consensus however that the core features include impairments in multiple, interrelated systems, resulting in a reduced ability to tolerate stressors (Bergman et al. 2007). A very easily conceptualised physical phenotype of the syndrome of frailty is one that uses the criteria in Linda Fried's proposed definition (Fried et al. 2001). The criteria include assessment of weight loss, physical exhaustion, physical activity level, grip strength and walking speed. The details of the use of these criteria are detailed in a later chapter. Others authors however suggest that the operational use of frailty in clinical assessment goes beyond the physical description suggested by Fried and must include cognitive, functional and social assessment as well. It is interesting to note that frailty need not exist in persons with multiple co-morbidities; conversely some older persons with little or no disease show the classic signs of frailty (Fried et al. 2001). As such, frailty provides a totally new dimension as a tool that quantifies the vulnerability of elderly patients to stressors including surgery. And this may be independent of the co-morbidities of the same patient. This may explain why elderly patients deemed to have been optimised for surgery through traditional clinical and biochemical markers may still have poor outcomes (Makary et al. 2010). A recent study on elderly surgical patients showed precisely this concept (Tan et al. 2012). After optimisation based on traditional clinical and biochemical markers, while a high co-morbidity index score was not associated with a higher risk of postoperative morbidity, patients who were frail had a nearly four times higher risk. The phenotype of decreased resilience to surgical insult may in part be due to altered physiological systems, inflammatory state and immune function in frail patients (Walston et al. 2002; Leng et al. 2004).

The importance of assessment of geriatric parameters in a patient undergoing major surgery is increasingly being recognised. These geriatric parameters have been associated with not only poorer short-term outcomes (Ganai et al. 2007; Robinson et al. 2009) but also with an increased risk of delayed discharge and postoperative institutionalisation (Robinson et al. 2009; Makary et al. 2010).

2.1.3 Nutritional Aspects

While malnutrition is not inevitable in the process of ageing, there are many changes in the ageing body that makes an elderly person vulnerable to malnutrition. The main cause of undernutrition in the elderly is decreased food intake.

2.1.3.1 Poor Appetite
Poor appetite, or anorexia, is a major cause of decreased food intake and malnutrition in the elderly. Low physical activity, pain, social isolation and a number of diseases such as malignancies, depression or dementia may all lead to poor appetite. This is further confounded by impaired taste and smell. This impairment may lead to reduced enjoyment of food. Often, this is further exacerbated by disease and drugs. The prevalence of atrophic gastritis has been shown to rise with age, and

atrophic gastritis is a proven cause of malabsorption. An example of medication side effect is that of a 79-year-old lady that was severely bothered by a bitter taste in her mouth and was unable to eat anything. She had complained of this symptom to a few physicians with no solution. However, a pharmacist subsequently scrutinised the onset of this symptom and discovered that it was the clarithromycin, given to eradicate *Helicobacter pylori* infection, that caused the symptoms. Her symptoms disappeared after cessation of the medication.

2.1.3.2 Poor Dentition in the Elderly

The percentage of edentulism increases with age. The number of teeth left also declines steadily with age. Loss of teeth is associated with a reduced ability to masticate food. Absence of the posterior tooth pairs is associated with a reduced variety of food consumed. Even full denture wearers have a poorer diet compared with dentate people. The inability to maintain adequate oral health may also have a negative impact of food chewing and intake.

2.1.4 Activities of Daily Living

Activities of daily living (ADLs) refer to the basic tasks of everyday life. Persons of any age can experience problems in performing ADLs; however, the elderly population are particularly vulnerable to this problem. Disability increases exponentially with advancing age. While the ability to do ADLs and the presence of co-morbidities are not mutually exclusive, some elderly persons with no co-morbidities may have significant disability and vice versa.

2.1.4.1 Basic Activities of Daily Living

A significant number of elderly persons face difficulties in basic activities of daily living. These include activities that involve personal hygiene and grooming, feeding, dressing, toileting and bladder and bowel control. Basic physical mobility functions may also be compromised such as the ability to transfer from bed to chair, ambulation and climbing stairs. Over the years, different clinical tools have evolved in the measurement of ADLs. These scales include the Katz ADL scale and the Barthel scale which had subsequently been modified (this scale will be discussed in a later chapter). These tools not only provide a way to quantify the disability in a very heterogeneous elderly population but also allow some differentiation of the interventions needed to care for these persons. Disability in basic ADLs will likely result in the need for a rather involved carer.

2.1.4.2 Instrumental Activities of Daily Living

While basic ADLs are useful in measuring the functional disability in the home setting, they fail to address all the activities that are required for independent living in the community. Many elderly persons may be able to perform the basic activities in their own homes; however, they may struggle to perform activities that include marketing, preparing a meal, housework, laundry, taking care of personal finances and taking medications. All these activities affect independent living and are particularly relevant in the setting of a postsurgical patient. The ability and need for an elderly individual to perform instrumental ADLs are dictated by his or her living arrangement and social support. An elderly individual living in an institution may not need to perform cooking or housework, while another who stays at home may have the inability to cook due to the presence of a younger wife cooking for him.

2.1.4.3 Cognitive Impairment

Cognitive impairment may affect the ADL status of an elderly. However, it should be noted that cognitive impairment and ADLs are separate domains. Elderly individuals who have cognitive impairment need not necessarily have a poor ADL status. As such, assessing ADLs alone in elderly patients may inadvertently miss individuals with cognitive impairment.

2.1.4.4 Activities of Daily Living in Elderly Surgical Patients

Cohort studies on elderly surgical patients have shown that patients with poor presurgical ADL status are more vulnerable to surgical complications. These patients are also likely to have significant deterioration in their functional status after surgery if not adequately rehabilitated (Tan et al. 2006). Thus, special attention has to be paid to this aspect during the perioperative period to avoid the need for the eventual use of long-term care services. ADLs and functional outcomes in elderly surgical patients have also been ignored by many surgeons. This was recently highlighted when a literature search on surgical outcomes in elderly patients found a paucity of data on the functional outcomes in elderly patients after surgery (Chee and Tan 2010).

2.1.5 Psychosocial Aspects

The continued well-being of an elderly individual does not hinge purely on health but also on the other aspects including the personal finances, social networking and social contribution. Social exclusion and isolation together with retirement stresses and notion of impending death can lead to the poor well-being of the elderly. Concomitant psychological issues including depression further deepen this problem. These aspects are further addressed in other chapters.

The complexities of an elderly surgical patient go beyond just the co-morbidities.

The normal physiology of ageing, geriatric syndromes, nutritional issues, activities of daily living and psychosocial issues all have to be taken into consideration when managing such a patient.

2.2 Transdisciplinary Approach in Elderly Surgical Patients

Having understood the complexities of an elderly surgical patient, it is then not difficult to understand the need for coordinated multifaceted care for these patients. The truth is that many modern institutions offer the resources to provide

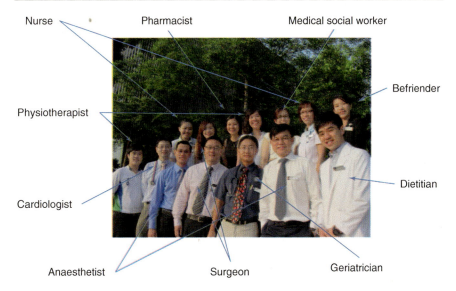

Fig. 2.1 Khoo Teck Puat Hospital Transdisciplinary Geriatric Surgery Team

this multifaceted care through the availability of multiple disciplines in clinical medicine and allied health. The availability of multidisciplinary care has often been presumed to be the final frontier of delivering optimal care to an elderly surgical patient. But is multidisciplinary care really the final frontier? When there is a surgical patient who has multiple co-morbidities, the primary surgeon will refer the patient to the dietitian and the cardiac specialist before the surgery. After the surgery, the physiotherapist will get involved in the rehabilitation, and upon discharge, a pharmacist will dispense medications to the patient. This is multidisciplinary care, but there are potential pitfalls to this model of care. The pitfalls have already been described in Chap. 1. Our unit advocates a transdisciplinary approach towards management of geriatric surgical patients. This transdisciplinary approach represents a higher evolution of the multidisciplinary approach. The key components in this transdisciplinary approach are described in the following section.

2.2.1 Key Components of Khoo Teck Puat Hospital Geriatric Surgery Service Integrative Transdisciplinary Model of Care

With the above-mentioned pitfalls of multidisciplinary care in mind, the Khoo Teck Puat Hospital Geriatric Surgery Service modelled the care of elderly surgical patients using a transdisciplinary approach (Fig. 2.1). The concept of transdisciplinary approach as an evolution of multidisciplinary care is not new. The biggest champions of this model are nurses. It is however only very recently that this model of care has been found to be useful in providing more holistic, coordinated and

Twice per week home visits during prehabilitation

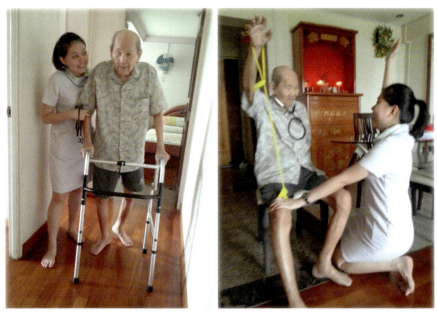

Fig. 2.2 Patient involvement and active engagement in the prehabilitation process before surgery

seamless care for surgical patients. The key components of the transdisciplinary model of care for elderly surgical patients are as follows:

2.2.1.1 Patient Involvement in the Team

In this model, the patient is actively involved in the entire process. The patient is actively educated through multimedia tools on the pathology of their disease. This is followed by a stepwise consenting process for the proposed surgical procedure. Options for other viable options are discussed in a team-based fashion. The patient is then engaged actively in the process of prehabilitation (Fig. 2.2) and, after the operation, is empowered to perform activities of living early and also with the process of rehabilitation (Fig. 2.3). The patient is considered an essential component of the team. Through processes of education and engagement, compliance with the care plan is heightened.

2.2.1.2 Early Goal-Setting Identifiable to the Team

This component involved the identification of the key goals for the treatment of the patient. These goals are identifiable to the patient and family members and also to the entire team. These goals have to be individualised to the patient and should not be forced on the patient. Team members may discuss about the validity of these goals at initial assessment but have to be aligned once there is consensus.

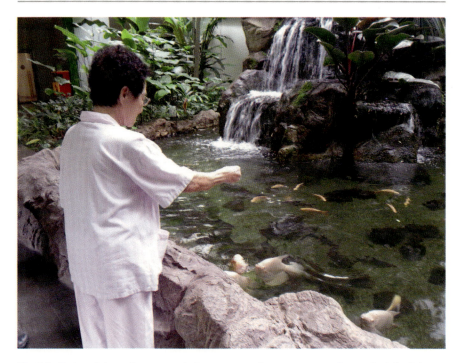

Fig. 2.3 Patient 4 days after surgery being empowered to go to our gardens to feed the fishes as part of the process of building confidence to return home for independent living

2.2.1.3 Enhanced Coordination

The coordination of care is crucial to the delivery of seamless care to surgical patients. As such, the nurse clinicians on the team play a central role in providing oversight of the total care of each patient. Input from each element of the team is tracked by the coordinating nurse, and at the same time, targets are set with regard to the timing within which the intervention is to be performed. Patients who need to undergo prehabilitation have target milestones set and the date for surgery set. This is followed by coordination of inputs from the dietitian and physiotherapist not only in the inpatient setting but also in the outpatient setting and in patients' homes (Fig. 2.4).

Completed interventions are documented such that other members of the team are aware.

2.2.1.4 Heightened Communication

This is performed through formal meetings, frequent ad hoc discussions among team members, communications sheets in the case notes and the use of multimedia technology. Although this heightened communication is useful in the enhancement of care, patient confidentiality cannot be compromised and measures are put in place to ensure that this standard is upheld.

Fig. 2.4 Home visits to help patients stay compliant to treatment strategies and medications

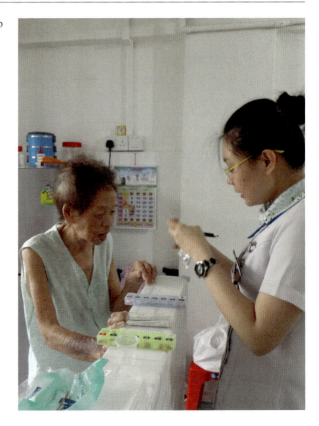

2.2.1.5 Role Enhancements

The enhancement of the roles of the individuals in this team-based care in the implementation of transdisciplinary care includes role extension, role enrichment, role expansion, role release and role support. Role extension demands a constant learning attitude towards attaining knowledge of one's discipline and in doing so become secure with one's own role in the system. This is followed by role enrichment which involves acquiring knowledge and understanding of other disciplines and then role expansion as one then starts to educate other members of the team about one's own expertise. Only with these can role release and support occur, breaking the boundaries of traditional disciplines, and individuals can then exert an effect in a transdisciplinary fashion.

2.2.1.6 Start to Finish

The team's involvement in the surgical patient is from start to finish. The same individuals are present at the initial diagnosis and assessment, follow through consenting and prehabilitation, see the patient through surgery and are there for the rehabilitation, tackling problems with the patient as they arise. Care does not stop with discharge but continues into outpatients and the community (Fig. 2.5). Only through this process can the team truly build rapport with the patient and truly understand the difficulties faced by the patient during this whole process.

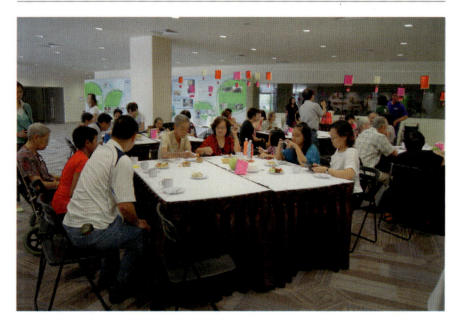

Fig. 2.5 Gathering of postsurgical patients to ensure that they continue to have the ability for independence and social integration

2.3 Integrative Decision-Making and Care Planning for Elderly Surgical Patients

Integrative care of an elderly surgical patient starts with proper surgical decision-making. The decision-making process is team-based and stepwise. It is critical to understand that decision-making in these elderly patients needs to take into full consideration the goals and concerns of the patient. Thus, engagement of the patient into this decision-making process through education and consultation on management approach is vital. In a recent study on the type of information patients desired before undergoing visceral surgery, more than 64 % of patients were keen to participate in medical decision-making with regard to management of surgical complications and management in the intensive care unit (Uldry et al. 2013). It is not appropriate to concentrate on the immediate perioperative period as 30-day mortality and morbidity may not clearly define good outcomes for elderly surgical patients. Functional recovery and independence are likely more important (Chee and Tan 2010). Furthermore another recent study from the Netherlands warned that a significant number of patients die within a year after curative colorectal surgery, and this data should impact our decisions in offering surgery (Gooiker et al. 2012).

The team should take into consideration clinical findings including co-morbidity index and frailty, together with aspects of nutrition, functional status and psychosocial problems in the decision-making process. These can only be assessed through a team-based approach with different members of the team providing expertise in the assessment process. A more holistic picture of the patient can then be painted to aid in the decision-making process. The integration of geriatric assessment techniques have been shown to improve perioperative outcomes (Cheema et al. 2011).

Engagement of the family is important in this whole process, especially in certain cultures. The importance of the family was elegantly summarised in a Taiwanese study where surgical patients were found to perceive the importance of the family through maintaining family well-being, being useful as information broker and also as an advocate for the patient (Lin et al. 2013).

Surgical decision-making also involves team-based discussions on what to do, when to do and how to go about achieving the targets set for a particular patient. All members of the team including the anaesthetist, physicians and nurses must have an aligned vision for the patient. This then culminates in a stepwise consenting process that has been described in a previous book (Tan 2013).

Perioperative care planning also demands an integrative approach. Prehabilitation has to be linked seamlessly to immediate perioperative care and then to rehabilitation. At different stages, the components of care involved may be different. Prehabilitation involves education, nutritional preparation and mobility training together with muscle training. Immediate perioperative interventions involve planning for the conduct of the surgery, surgical techniques, prophylactic measures, anticipatory measures including lines and tubes and also pain relief measures. Rehabilitation on the other hand concentrates on functional recovery. Nonetheless, common targets need to be visualised, and interventions by every member of the team must be able to be coordinated with the plans of other members. Integrated decision-making involving members of the team thus becomes vital.

2.4 Integrating Prehabilitation, Rehabilitation and Nursing Care

Integration of care can be described through the description of the care of a patient managed by the Geriatric Surgery Service: Mdm GKK. Mdm GKK was 82 years old with diabetes, previous stroke, hypertension and hyperlipidaemia. She had undergone abdomino-perineal resection more than 10 years ago. She has had ongoing back pain with some resultant functional decline in recent months but with greater decline in the last 3 weeks. She was subsequently found to be anaemic with a metachronous ascending colon cancer. Mdm GKK stays alone in a one-room rented flat but has been independent thus far and hopes to continue to be independent without being a burden to her extended family members. Mdm GKK was assessed to likely benefit from cancer resection as she had good function previously and the recent decline is likely disease related and can potentially be reversed by removal of the disease. She was also found to be not frail. Nonetheless, her issues were complex, and she required multifaceted perioperative care which was delivered in a transdisciplinary fashion. Figure 2.6 describes the issues that were identified surrounding her surgical management. The roles and actions of the different players of the transdisciplinary team in the care plan for Mdm GKK are then shown in Fig. 2.7. For Mdm GKK, it was essential to develop a care plan from start to

2 Integrative Transdisciplinary Care of Elderly Surgical Patients

Issues identified	Players	Integration processes
Colon tumour	Surgeon Nurses Anaesthetist	• Establish diagnosis. • Risk stratification. • Educate patient on disease pathology. • Family conference with patient and family. • Explore individualized treatment goals. • Discuss treatment options in relation to individual goals and risk stratification. • Pre-operative education to manage expectation and improve peri-op engagement. • Surgical, anaesthesia and analgesia planning.
Back pain from recent fall sec to postural giddiness and iron deficiency anaemia. Functional decline sec to limited mobility from back pain	Geriatrician Anaesthetist Cardiologist Orthopaedics Physiotherapist Pharmacist Dietitian Nurses	• Optimization of medical condition and review of medications to correct postural hypotension and electrolytes imbalance. • Blood transfusion to correct anaemia that can attribute to giddiness. • Exclusion of orthopaedics related injury causing back pain from recent fall. • Pain management for back pain to improve compliance and engagement in prehabilitative exercises. • Nutritional optimization with consideration for anaemia, hypoalbuminemia and risk of malnutrition due to poor social support and limited mobility. • Reinforcement of management plans with indication explained through education for better compliance.

Risk for post	Geriatrician
	Nurses
	Surgeon
	Anaesthetist
	Pharmacist
	Physiotherapist
	Dietitian
		• Identification of risk factors and implementation of preventive measures.
		  1. Impaired mobility from surgical and back pain
		  2. Pre-op medications for management of back pain (Morphine, Tramadol and Gabapentin)
		  3. Iron deficiency anaemia
		    (Decreased oxygen capacity in view of low hb).
		  4. Electrolytes imbalance
		    (Potassium OA: 2.8mmol/L, Na: 131).

Social support 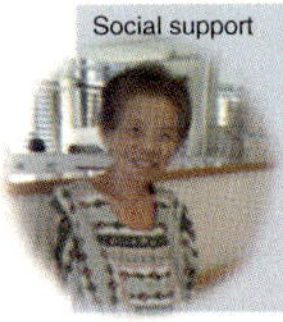	MSW
	Physiotherapist
	Nurses
	Dietitian
		• Stays alone in one room rented flat.
		• In view of acute functional decline and lack of caregiver support, referred for prehabilitation at community hospital.
		• Discharge plans explored before surgery.:
		    • Continued rehabilitation after operation or
		    • Home with home-based rehabilitation by nurses and allied health members with meal delivery support during early post operative period.
		Pre-emptive referral to community hospital made to minimise length of hospital stay.

Fig. 2.6 Issues identified in Mdm GKK and the players and interventions involved

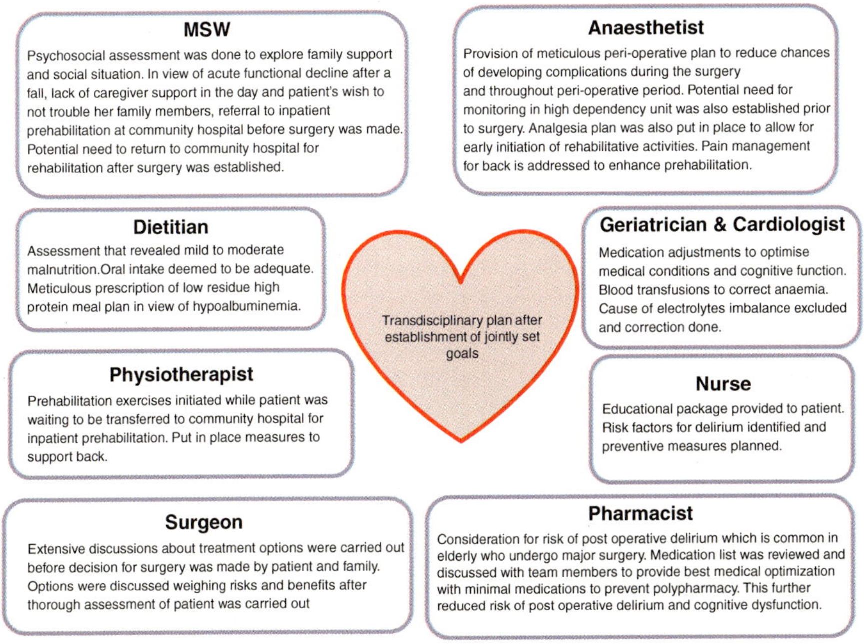

MSW
Psychosocial assessment was done to explore family support and social situation. In view of acute functional decline after a fall, lack of caregiver support in the day and patient's wish to not trouble her family members, referral to inpatient prehabilitation at community hospital before surgery was made. Potential need to return to community hospital for rehabilitation after surgery was established.

Anaesthetist
Provision of meticulous peri-operative plan to reduce chances of developing complications during the surgery and throughout peri-operative period. Potential need for monitoring in high dependency unit was also established prior to surgery. Analgesia plan was also put in place to allow for early initiation of rehabilitative activities. Pain management for back is addressed to enhance prehabilitation.

Dietitian
Assessment that revealed mild to moderate malnutrition. Oral intake deemed to be adequate. Meticulous prescription of low residue high protein meal plan in view of hypoalbuminemia.

Geriatrician & Cardiologist
Medication adjustments to optimise medical conditions and cognitive function. Blood transfusions to correct anaemia. Cause of electrolytes imbalance excluded and correction done.

Transdisciplinary plan after establishment of jointly set goals

Physiotherapist
Prehabilitation exercises initiated while patient was waiting to be transferred to community hospital for inpatient prehabilitation. Put in place measures to support back.

Nurse
Educational package provided to patient. Risk factors for delirium identified and preventive measures planned.

Surgeon
Extensive discussions about treatment options were carried out before decision for surgery was made by patient and family. Options were discussed weighing risks and benefits after thorough assessment of patient was carried out

Pharmacist
Consideration for risk of post operative delirium which is common in elderly who undergo major surgery. Medication list was reviewed and discussed with team members to provide best medical optimization with minimal medications to prevent polypharmacy. This further reduced risk of post operative delirium and cognitive dysfunction.

Fig. 2.7 Transdisciplinary care plan for Mdm GKK

finish starting with prehabilitation and nutritional optimisation, following through with meticulous surgery after medical optimisation, early development of a rehabilitation plan and anticipation of possible medical and social issues in the perioperative period. Mdm GKK returned to her premorbid functional status within 6 weeks after surgery, and home visits were made to ensure that she remained well.

Conclusion

Geriatric surgical patients are complex and demand multifaceted care which can only be delivered optimally in a collaborative transdisciplinary fashion.

References

Bergman H, Ferrucci L et al (2007) Frailty: an emerging research and clinical paradigm–issues and controversies. J Gerontol A Biol Sci Med Sci 62(7):731–737

Campbell E (2000) Physiologic changes in respiratory function. In: Zenilman ME, Rosenthal RA, Katlic MR (eds) Principles and practice in geriatric surgery. Springer, New York

Chee J, Tan KY (2010) Outcome studies on older patients undergoing surgery are missing the mark. J Am Geriatr Soc 58(11):2238–2240

Cheema FN, Abraham NS et al (2011) Novel approaches to perioperative assessment and intervention may improve long-term outcomes after colorectal cancer resection in older adults. Ann Surg 253(5):867–874

Christmas C, Makary MA et al (2006) Medical considerations in older surgical patients. J Am Coll Surg 203(5):746–751

Demeure MJ, Fain MJ (2006) The elderly surgical patient and postoperative delirium. J Am Coll Surg 203(5):752–757

Fried LP, Tangen CM et al (2001) Frailty in older adults: evidence for a phenotype. J Gerontol A Biol Sci Med Sci 56(3):M146–M156

Ganai S, Lee KF et al (2007) Adverse outcomes of geriatric patients undergoing abdominal surgery who are at high risk for delirium. Arch Surg 142(11):1072–1078

Gooiker GA, Dekker JW et al (2012) Risk factors for excess mortality in the first year after curative surgery for colorectal cancer. Ann Surg Oncol 19(8):2428–2434

Leng SX, Cappola AR et al (2004) Serum levels of insulin-like growth factor-I (IGF-I) and dehydroepiandrosterone sulfate (DHEA-S), and their relationships with serum interleukin-6, in the geriatric syndrome of frailty. Aging Clin Exp Res 16(2):153–157

Lin ML, Pang MC et al (2013) Family as a whole: elective surgery patients' perception of the meaning of family involvement in decision making. J Clin Nurs 22(1–2):271–278

Lipschitz D (2000) Nutrition. In: Leipzig R, Cassel CK, Cohen HJ (eds) Geriatric medicine: an evidence-based approach. Springer, New York. pp 1009–1021

Makary MA, Segev DL et al (2010) Frailty as a predictor of surgical outcomes in older patients. J Am Coll Surg 210(6):901–908

Marik PE (2001) Aspiration pneumonitis and aspiration pneumonia. N Engl J Med 344(9):665–671

Robinson TN, Eiseman B et al (2009) Redefining geriatric preoperative assessment using frailty, disability and co-morbidity. Ann Surg 250(3):449–455

Rosenthal RA, Kavic SM (2004) Assessment and management of the geriatric patient. Crit Care Med 32(4 Suppl):S92–S105

Tan K-Y (ed) (2013) Colorectal cancer in the elderly. Springer, Berlin/Heidelberg

Tan KY, Chen CM et al (2006) Which octogenarians do poorly after major open abdominal surgery in our Asian population? World J Surg 30(4):547–552

Tan KY, Kawamura YJ et al (2012) Assessment for frailty is useful for predicting morbidity in elderly patients undergoing colorectal cancer resection whose comorbidities are already optimized. Am J Surg 204(2):139–43

Uldry E, Schafer M et al (2013) Patients' preferences on information and involvement in decision making for gastrointestinal surgery. World J Surg 37(9):2162–71

Walston J, McBurnie MA et al (2002) Frailty and activation of the inflammation and coagulation systems with and without clinical comorbidities: results from the Cardiovascular Health Study. Arch Intern Med 162(20):2333–2341

Transdisciplinary Nursing

3

Phyllis Xiu-Zhuang Tan, Marc W.J. Ong, and Kok-Yang Tan

Take Home Pearls

- Surgical management is becoming more complex, demanding more coordinated and multifaceted care.
- There are inherent pitfalls in the current multidisciplinary nursing model.
- The transdisciplinary model of nursing addresses some of these pitfalls but demands enhancements of the roles of nurses.
- There is evidence to show that transdisciplinary nursing reduces nursing errors.

3.1 Introduction

The elderly constitute an increasing portion of the developed world's population and have become one of the high-risk patient populations faced by the surgeon. Elderly patients are frail, functionally dependent and coupled with multiple complex comorbidities; they pose increasing challenges in surgical management and demand multifaceted care (Tan and Chua 2013). This has to be delivered through an effective interdisciplinary team approach in which nurses play an integral contributory role (Tan and Chua 2013).

P.X.-Z. Tan (✉)
Department of Nursing Administration, Khoo Teck Puat Hospital, Singapore, Singapore
e-mail: phyllistanxz@gmail.com

M.W.J. Ong
Department of Surgery, Khoo Teck Puat Hospital, Singapore, Singapore

K.-Y. Tan
Department of Surgery, Khoo Teck Puat Hospital, Singapore, Singapore

Geriatric Surgery Service, Khoo Teck Puat Hospital, Singapore, Singapore
e-mail: kokyangtan@gmail.com

© Springer-Verlag Berlin Heidelberg 2015
K.-Y. Tan (ed.), *Transdisciplinary Perioperative Care in Colorectal Surgery:
An Integrative Approach*, DOI 10.1007/978-3-662-44020-9_3

Nursing for hospitalised patients is based on a three-shift rotation per day to provide seamless and dedicated care throughout the duration of their stay. For the patients admitted to the surgical unit, the surgeons and various allied health members review them over only short periods each day. Nurses are therefore integral in ensuring that the nursing care aspect and safety of patients are not overlooked in the absence of the primary surgical team. In a complex elderly surgical patient who demands multifaceted care, the constant changing of nursing shifts and inconsistent allocation of nursing staff may give rise to episodic and fragmented care. This may potentially result in a compromised post-operative recovery process. For care to be effectively delivered to this group of vulnerable elderly, it is essential to adopt an approach that is holistic with a high level of communication and coordination (Tan 2013).

In this chapter, we will discuss two models of nursing care: firstly, multidisciplinary nursing which is adapted by most of the local hospitals and, secondly, transdisciplinary nursing which is an evolution from the former.

3.2 Multidisciplinary Nursing

Similar to multidisciplinary team-based approach where individual medical specialists and allied health members provide opinions based on their expertise separately, multidisciplinary nursing can also give rise to uncoordinated and fragmented care. In multidisciplinary nursing, the elderly patient often lacks ownership from the nursing staff. Nursing staff of varied specialised training often work in silo with respect to care for the patient and provide input only related to their field of specialty.

For instance, an elderly patient with cardiac failure, diabetes mellitus and renal impairment who needs surgical resection for colorectal cancer may be seen by various nurse specialists.

The general ward nurse assigned to look after this patient during his/her shift may only encounter this patient once throughout the patient's stay. He/She will see to the routine and basic nursing needs but due to the constant changing of nursing shifts, multiple nurses may be involved in the patient's care. The stoma nurse then sees this patient to perform stoma siting before surgery and impart knowledge on stoma management to him/her. The nurses from the diabetic, renal and cardiac teams subsequently review the patient to provide the necessary education with intent to optimise the physiological status of the respective organs preoperatively. The wound nurse may be called on board to review the surgical wound that has developed an infection. The pain management nurse specialist then ensures that pain is well managed post-operatively. Hence pre- and post-operative counselling delivered through this multidisciplinary nursing approach is often carried out in a one-off manner by a myriad of nursing staff and may ultimately result in poor compliance and efficacy.

Nurse specialists in the multidisciplinary approach are often termed as an 'I'-shaped personnel as described by Tim Brown in the book *Change by Design* to be specialists who have depth of knowledge in their area of specialty but lacking the disposition for collaboration across disciplines (Brown 2009). Post-operative review by specialist nurses in the multidisciplinary nursing team is done on an ad hoc basis when deemed necessary by the surgeon or attending ward nurse who is assigned to look after the elderly patient during his/her shift.

Communication in multidisciplinary nursing can also be challenging. The thought processes of the surgical team may not be effectively communicated to the individual nurse specialist. For instance, the surgeon who is planning for surgery of the large intestine may prefer nutrition to be optimised with low-residue diet to enhance bowel clearance later as part of surgical planning. The diabetic nurse involved may then encourage the patient to increase dietary fibre in attempt to reduce carbohydrate intake and optimise glycaemic control. This may result in a confused patient, who, given the conflicting information, decides to manage his/her own health possibly in a counterproductive manner. The random allocation of ward nurses results in a lack of consistent care that may inadvertently compromise communication among team members. The multidisciplinary nursing approach is thus vulnerable to care that is less wholesome and holistic.

An example of fragmented multidisciplinary care is 75-year-old, retired Mr. Tan E. K. who underwent emergency exploratory laparotomy for perforated bowel. He had part of his large intestine resected and stoma created for faecal diversion. He stays in a simple three-room flat with his elderly wife and has no children. With limited education, Mr. Tan and his wife only understand simple Mandarin and dialects. His predicament is challenged further by financial constraints.

During his stay in the hospital, Mr. Tan was looked after by different ward nurses who were randomly assigned. Four days prior to his discharge from the hospital, a newly graduated ward nurse (Nurse A) noticed there was faecal leakage from the stoma appliance and had seek help from her senior (Nurse B). Nurse B rendered the necessary stoma care to Mr. Tan and, while doing so, taught him on some basics of emptying the stoma pouch when it is filled with effluent. This was communicated to Nurse A, who misinterpreted this information as completion of caregiver training for stoma care to his wife instead. This false message was perpetuated among the different nurses who subsequently were involved in the care of Mr. Tan till the day he was discharged, resulting in his wife never receiving any training at all.

Mr. Tan was also noted to have superficial wound infection from his surgical incision for which help from the wound nurse was sought. Given the impression that caregiver training on stoma care had been completed, she provided the appropriate wound management plans. Stoma care was hence neglected once again.

On his discharge day, another randomly assigned ward nurse (Nurse C) on duty performed wound care as advised by the wound nurse prior to discharge. Mr. Tan was also referred to the outpatient service for wound care. He was subsequently discharged from the ward without prescription of stoma appliances. Nurse C assumed that stoma appliances had been ordered by the wound/stoma nurse which is the practice in her institution after the completion of caregiver training. Both Mr. Tan and his wife had the impression that stoma appliance was also meant to be changed at the outpatient setting and, hence, did not make further enquiries.

It was unfortunate that Mr. Tan encountered leakage from his stoma appliance on the following day after his discharge from the hospital. The stoma effluent had contaminated his wound dressing. In a state of fear and anxiety, the already financially constrained Mr. Tan returned to the hospital's emergency department, incurring additional but potentially avoidable costs. The stoma nurse was referred at the emergency department to provide the appropriate teaching and intervention for both his stoma and wound.

The Swiss Cheese model of accident causation is clearly evident in the above scenario. The care of Mr. Tan could have been better coordinated if nurses were not working in silo in respect to their area of specialty. The care across or beyond one's boundary could have potentially avoided the inconveniences Mr. Tan and his family experienced after discharge from the hospital. For instance, the wound nurse could have expressed her concern regarding the patient's understanding of stoma care and addressed it accordingly instead of focusing solely on the aspect of wound care. The multiple ward nurses who took care of Mr. Tan wrongly assumed that caregiver training was appropriately administered but not once was it confirmed and verified. This could be avoided by revising with the patient upon discharge to ascertain whether he fully comprehends all aspects of his care at home.

The fragmentation and poor coordination of care through multiple nurses in this model may further introduce fear and apprehension in the elderly post-surgical patient if all aspects of his care in the recovery stage are not addressed comprehensively.

3.3 Transdisciplinary Nursing

Transdisciplinary approach is a product of evolution from multidisciplinary to a more integrated, collaborative and less compartmentalised model (Tan and Chua 2013). It involves reaching into the spaces between the disciplines and specialties to create positive health outcomes through collaborative efforts (Nandiwada and Dang-Vu 2010). An approach that dispenses hierarchy coupled with constant communication among team members, this model aims to provide the most holistic care to the elderly surgical patients, taking their physiological, physical, psychosocial and socioeconomic factors into consideration.

The transdisciplinary nursing model transforms 'I'-shaped individuals into 'T'-shaped nurse specialists where the vertical stroke of the 'T' represents the depth of skill that contributes to the creative process and the horizontal stroke represents disposition of the collaborative effort across disciplines (Brown 2009). The target in this model of care is not in each person doing their individual job well but by working together in a more integrated fashion that brings about a higher sense of purpose in achieving the goals of the geriatric surgical patient. These goals are often associated with returning them to their premorbid functional state after major surgery and preserving their quality of life.

Besides her specialised knowledge, the 'T'-shaped transdisciplinary nurse is also one that possesses the attributes that contribute to the horizontal stroke of the 'T'.

The Director of Nursing from Alexandra Health, Khoo Teck Puat Hospital (Singapore), describes the 'T'-shaped nurse with horizontal stroke as one who fulfils the competencies in practice-based learning and improvement, interpersonal and communication skills, patient care as well as system-based practices. Reilly (2001) explained role extension, role enrichment, role expansion, role release and role support as requirements of transdisciplinary model of care.

In the transdisciplinary nursing model of care, nursing staff has the capability to:

1. Acquire knowledge of one's discipline constantly and attain security in one's role and responsibility, thus able to extend one's role to resolve turf issues (Reilly 2001).
2. Seek continuous improvement in oneself beyond the formal education of one's profession. Role enrichment involves acquiring of knowledge and understanding of other disciplines in the team through excellent communication and collaboration (Tan and Tan 2013).
3. Expand role by performing skills of other team players at appropriate timings to enhance the benefits for the elderly patient who is recovering from major surgery. Role expansion can be better demonstrated through enrichment that aims to improve the knowledge of other team members on one's expertise through meetings or in-service sessions.
4. Apply knowledge and thought processes that are associated with other members in the transdisciplinary team (i.e. medical specialists, allied health members and nurse specialists). Role release can be effected by one team member with consultation from other members (Rainforth 1997; Shelden and Rush 2001). It is through feedback and encouragement from other team members that role support is incorporated for the betterment of each member.
5. Communicate and collaborate effectively among patients, families and the healthcare team to align and achieve the goals established together with the elderly surgical patient.

3.4 The Transdisciplinary Nurse

In Alexandra Health (Singapore) where transdisciplinary model of care was first introduced for elderly patients undergoing major colorectal resections, the Geriatric Surgery Service consists of dedicated medical specialists, allied health members and nurse clinicians. The nurse clinician coordinates the team and takes on the ownership of the elderly surgical patients focusing primarily on nursing perspective, i.e. directing proper nursing care to junior nurses on nursing issues. She is the consistent nurse in a nursing team which can comprise of randomly assigned nurses and sees the patients daily through the perioperative period together with members of the geriatric surgery team. This nurse also acts as the bridge that links the communication gap between patients and families, nursing staff and members of the transdisciplinary team.

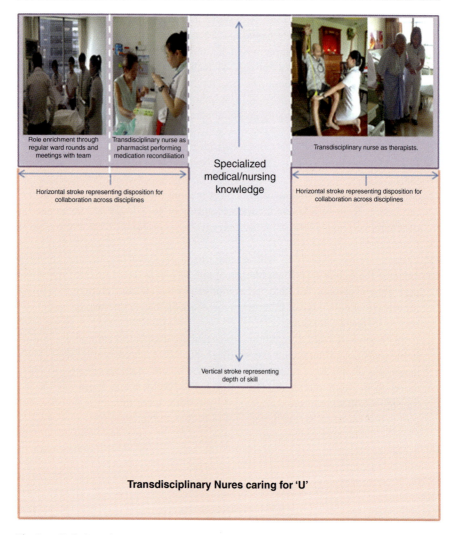

Fig. 3.1 Holistic patient-centred care formulated by 'T'-shaped transdisciplinary nurse and 'U' that is referred to as 'You', the geriatric surgical patient

Members of the transdisciplinary Geriatric Surgery Service conduct regular meetings as a platform for the requirements of this model described by Reilly (2001) to be incorporated. Practice-based learning and improvement was feasible through discussions on cases managed by the team. Interpersonal and communication skill had allowed effective role enrichment, release and support among team members. Through this platform, the transdisciplinary nurse was able to establish the horizontal stroke of the 'T' that represents the disposition and collaboration across disciplines as illustrated in Fig. 3.1.

3 Transdisciplinary Nursing

Table 3.1 Preoperative role of the nurse in transdisciplinary nursing

Preoperative transdisciplinary nursing	
Risk stratification	Preoperative assessment to stratify the risks of patient and direct who in the team can optimise for his/her operation
Goal setting	Goals jointly set with patient and communicated to all team members
Planning	Pre- and post-operative optimisation plan will be made with considerations above. This is done through effective communication and collaboration with all members of the Geriatric Surgery Service. Means of communication with the patient and family will be established in the planning phase with considerations for cognitive and intellectual status of individual patients as well as limitations from physiological changes related to the ageing process
Education	Educational package will be provided after the surgeon's consultation for psychological preparation. Personalised prehabilitation plans established with patient and team members during the planning phase as well as measures to prevent post-operative delirium will be reinforced during the education process to allow better patient engagement during the perioperative period

The team recognised that achieving exemplary surgical and functional outcome for elderly patients involves not only rehabilitation during early post-operative days but a period of prehabilitation is crucial to optimise their nutritional, functional and physiological state before major surgery. The transdisciplinary nurse works collaboratively with allied health members to visit elderly surgical patients who satisfy criteria for home-based optimisation regime during prehabilitation and rehabilitation phases. She would take on the role as physiotherapist and assist the patients with strengthening exercises to enhance their functional recovery to baseline following major surgery. This nurse also plays the role as dietitian and reviews the oral intake and nutritional status with plans established together with the team's dietitian. The role as pharmacist is also undertaken by the same nurse during home visits to ensure that the physiological health of the elderly surgical patients is effectively optimised through medication compliance.

Tables 3.1 and 3.2 further illustrate the perioperative role of the nurse in transdisciplinary nursing.

3.4.1 Case Study

Mdm. Tan S. N. is an 84-year-old lady with a background history of hypertension and hyperlipidaemia. She is widowed with two children and stays with her son who works as lecturer in the university. Family is extremely supportive. She is independent in managing her own activities of daily living and is community ambulant without aid. Mdm. Tan was diagnosed with cancer of the colon. Both patient and family were extensively spoken to by the surgeon together with the nurse specialist on her disease process as well as exploration of treatment goals and options. Benefits and risks of various treatment options were discussed bearing in mind the risk stratification for the patient.

Table 3.2 Post-operative role of the nurse in transdisciplinary nursing

Post-operative transdisciplinary nursing	
Nursing care	Constant post-operative reviews with focus on the following:
	Communication and supervision of junior nurses to manage nursing care and goals that are in line with goals established with the transdisciplinary geriatric surgery members
	Clinical assessment of patient between team reviews to detect early signs of perioperative complications
	Constant updates on progress and management plans to patient, family and team members. This is to allow mutual understanding for better management of expectations during the course of recovery
	Role release and role support among team members to allow for rehabilitative activities to take place from first post-operative day
Education	Reinforcement of preoperative education to improve compliance
Discharge care	Post-discharge follow-up to ensure the well-being of patient is maintained

Although her risk profiles were unremarkable, Mdm. Tan was adamant towards refusal for surgical resection of her diseased colon. Ample time was invested to establish the rapport and trust between the nurse and patient before further counselling and reiteration of surgeon's advice could take place. Mdm. Tan eventually understood that the likelihood of having her independence robbed by the disease process would soon become a reality if surgery was not performed. The rapport established had allowed Mdm. Tan to confide her fears and worries to the trusted nurse which were predominantly loss of independence and being a burden to her family. Educational slides with video testimonies of patients with similar conditions who have had surgeries done were shown to reassure her of the high possibility of a good surgical outcome with collaboration of the transdisciplinary Geriatric Surgery Team. She eventually agreed to undergo surgery after much consideration and support received. Jointly set goals were communicated to all members of the transdisciplinary team to establish a care plan that focused on achieving the goals.

During her early post-operative days, quality nursing care was rendered to compliment the established goals which include closer monitoring and reporting of any deranged parameters, protocol-driven prevention of post-operative delirium, timely administration of oral analgesics for pain free rehabilitation, elimination of disturbances to sleep and proper communication of treatment plans to Mdm. Tan and her family. With support from the family and healthcare team, Mdm. Tan's active engagement during the perioperative period had allowed her to recover uneventfully from her major surgery. She had returned to her premorbid functional status on the day of discharge which was within a week post-operatively. A few days after her discharge from the hospital, Mdm. Tan noticed there was purulent discharge oozing from her surgical site. She could then receive treatment for the superficial wound infection from a transdisciplinary team member without having to go through the hassle of long waiting hours at the emergency department.

3 Transdisciplinary Nursing

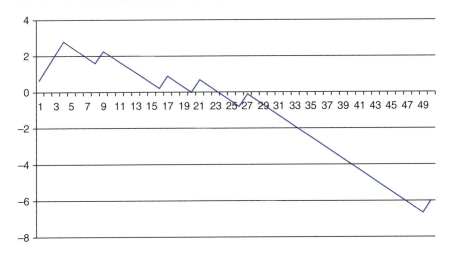

Fig. 3.2 CUSUM curve of nursing care in transdisciplinary approach

She was extremely appreciative of the effort from the transdisciplinary team for spending much time and patience that changed her mind towards surgery and the holistic care she received throughout her hospitalisation from all members of the healthcare team. She continued to do well functionally and resumed her usual daily activities without many difficulties. Mdm. Tan participates in annual gathering organised by the Geriatric Surgery Service of Alexandra Health (Singapore) for their elderly patients who underwent their surgical journey with them.

The Geriatric Surgery Service of Alexandra Health (Singapore) maintains a database that tracks the outcome of elderly patients after major colorectal surgery. Outcomes of nursing care for 130 patients above 75 years old who underwent major colorectal resection between January 2007 and March 2012 were reviewed. Nursing failures during the course of care were identified. These included inaccurate documentation, delayed recognition of deterioration, non-compliance to orders and improper discharge planning. Comparisons were made between the transdisciplinary model and traditional multidisciplinary model of care. Cumulative summation (CUSUM) methodology was used to plot sequential performance of both groups. A continuous downward slope as illustrated in Fig. 3.2 denotes sequential success, while a graph without consistent trend as shown in Fig. 3.3 denotes inconsistent nursing outcomes.

Differences in demographics, comorbidities and functional status of both groups as shown in Table 3.3 were not significant. In Table 3.4, the overall nursing failures were lower in the transdisciplinary group compared to the standard group. Results analysed as shown in Table 3.5 revealed that patients who were not managed perioperatively using the transdisciplinary approach had 5.7 times higher risk of nursing failures which were independently associated with Clavien 2 and above complications.

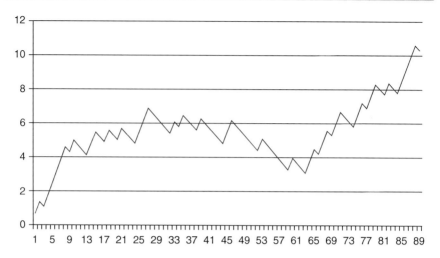

Fig. 3.3 CUSUM curve of nursing care in non-transdisciplinary group

Table 3.3 Demographics, comorbidities and functional status of both groups

		Transdisciplinary (n=41)	Non-transdisciplinary (n=89)	p value
Gender	Female	21 (51.2 %)	43 (48.3 %)	0.758
	Male	20 (48.8 %)	46 (51.7 %)	
ASA	1–2	16 (39 %)	48 (53.9 %)	0.114
	3–4	25 (61 %)	41 (46.1 %)	
Comorbidity index	Below 4	37 (90.2 %)	79 (88.8 %)	0.8
	Above 4	4 (9.8 %)	10 (11.2 %)	
Barthel's	Below 80	6 (14.6 %)	12 (13.4 %)	0.8
	Above 80	35 (85.4 %)	61 (68.5 %)	
	No data	–	16 (18.1 %)	
Urgency	Elective	31 (75.6 %)	66 (74.2 %)	0.86
	Emergency	10 (24.4 %)	23 (25.8 %)	

With the analysed results, the Geriatric Surgery Service at Alexandra Health (Singapore) concluded that transdisciplinary approach reduces nursing failures which is independently associated with morbidity.

In order for evolution to take place from multidisciplinary nursing model to transdisciplinary nursing, it is quintessential that a paradigm shift occurs from the traditional nursing practice of nurses only performing basic nursing care related to activities of daily living, while the rest of the activities pertaining to the recovery process are left to be performed by various specialists and allied health members.

Nurses form the frontline in terms of time spent with the patient when compared to surgeons, medical specialists and allied health members. Breaking the boundary to take on greater roles can create positive impact on the outcome of recovery for the

3 Transdisciplinary Nursing

Table 3.4 Multivariate analysis correlating to nursing failures

Risk outcome	Risk ratio	95 % CI	p
ASA $\geq$3	1.097	0.375–3.211	0.804
Comorbidity index $\geq$4	1.388	0.305–6.318	0.613
Barthel's index $\leq$80	1.573	0.443–5.577	0.224
Urgency (emergency)	1.524	0.438–5.302	0.150
Clavien $\geq$2	3.136	1.043–9.430	0.005
Not transdisciplinary	5.662	1.685–19.027	0.002

Table 3.5 Factors contributing to nursing failures in both groups

Types of nursing failures	Transdisciplinary ($N=41$)	Non transdisciplinary ($N=89$)
Overall nursing failure	9.8 % ($n=4$)	41.6 % ($n=37$)
Inaccurate documentation	Nil	13.5 % ($n=12$)
Delay in recognition of deterioration	2.4 % ($n=1$)	25.8 % ($n=23$)
Non compliance to orders	7.3 % ($n=3$)	18.0 % ($n=16$)
Improper discharge planning	Nil	5.6 % ($n=5$)

elderly surgical patient. In order to achieve transdisciplinary care, nursing staff must be empowered with the autonomy to perform skills or tasks at a greater level and across disciplines. The barriers of engaging oneself beyond the described responsibilities of a nurse need to be overcome before evolution can take place. The key factors to build the horizontal stroke on 'I'-shaped nurses who work in silos to transform them into 'T'-shaped transdisciplinary nurses are to equip them with the fundamentals of relevant skills, knowledge and effective communication. With this added confidence, nurses can then expand roles and undertake greater responsibilities.

One good example is collaboration with the physiotherapists to enhance the rehabilitation potential of elderly surgical patients. With various precautionary assessment tools such as fall precaution in place, nurses are often abiding by these strict measures to prevent falls among the patients. The fear of penalty associated with a fall occurrence in patients often prevents the nursing staff from engaging in activities that may expedite the recovery process of patient following major surgery. Nurses tend to leave it to the 'trained' personnel in this instance, physiotherapists, to avoid the risk of a patient falling under their watch. This routine often results in nurses neglecting an imperative aspect of patient recovery borne either due to fear of accidents occurring or due to a lack of interest in hastening the recovery process of a post-surgical patient.

If every nurse that comes on each shift participates in a common and shared rehabilitation plan, the patient would receive rehabilitative physiotherapy four times a day instead of once daily during the therapist's attendance. This alone will prevent muscle weakening or functional decline associated with prolonged confinement to bed which may inadvertently contribute to the fall risk of the patient. Other complications related to prolonged bed rest such as chest infection, deep vein thrombosis and urinary tract infection may also be avoided.

> **Conclusion**
>
> The management of a complex elderly surgical patient requires a holistic approach. Multidisciplinary nursing model should evolve to a transdisciplinary nursing model to compliment the same model of care adopted by the Geriatric Surgical Team. This will essentially involve a high level of communication and coordination among team members to deliver the highest level of care to this group of complex and vulnerable elderly surgical patients.

References

Brown T (2009) Change by design: how design thinking transforms organizations and inspires innovations. HarperCollins, New York

Nandiwada DR, Dang-Vu C (2010) Transdisciplinary health care education: training team players. J Health Care Poor Underserved 21(1):26–34

Rainforth B (1997) Analysis of physical therapy practice acts: implications for role release in educational environments. Pediatr Phys Ther 9:54–61

Reilly C (2001) Transdisciplinary approach: an atypical strategy for improving outcomes in rehabilitative and long-term acute care settings. Rehabil Nurs 26(6):216–220, 244

Shelden ML, Rush DD (2001) The ten myths about providing early intervention services in natural environments. Infants Young Child 14(1):1–13

Tan PXZ, Chua GC (2013) Nursing care of the elderly surgical patients. In: Tan KY (ed) Colorectal cancer in the elderly. Springer, Berlin/Heidelberg, pp 121–140

Tan KY, Tan PXZ (2013) Transdisciplinary care for elderly surgical patients. In: Tan KY (ed) Colorectal cancer in the elderly. Springer, Berlin/Heidelberg, pp 83–92

Transdisciplinary Management of Perioperative Nutrition

4

Yee-Lee Cheah, George Chee-Hong Toh, Jian-Wei Heng, and Eric Wei-Long Wee

Myth #1

Enteral feeding cannot be started in patients without bowel sounds or passage of flatus or stool.

Truth #1

There are no studies showing a correlation between bowel sounds or peristalsis and feeding tolerance; therefore, ESPEN does not recommend withholding enteral feeding based on bowel sounds or passage of flatus or stool (McClave et al. 2009).

Myth #2

There is no limit to the individualized modifications that can be made to the constituents of a PN bag, e.g., replacement electrolytes, extra protein, and drugs (e.g., insulin).

Y.-L. Cheah (✉)
Department of Surgery, Khoo Teck Puat Hospital, Singapore, Singapore
e-mail: cheah.yee.lee@alexandrahealth.com.sg

G.C.-H. Toh
Department of Nutrition and Dietetics, Khoo Teck Puat Hospital, Singapore, Singapore
e-mail: toh.george.ch@alexandrahealth.com.sg

J.-W. Heng
Department of Pharmacy, Khoo Teck Puat Hospital, Singapore, Singapore
e-mail: heng.jian.wei@alexandrahealth.com.sg

E.W.-L. Wee
Department of General Medicine, Gastroenterology, Khoo Teck Puat Hospital,
Singapore, Singapore
e-mail: wee.eric.wl@alexandrahealth.com.sg

© Springer-Verlag Berlin Heidelberg 2015
K.-Y. Tan (ed.), *Transdisciplinary Perioperative Care in Colorectal Surgery:
An Integrative Approach*, DOI 10.1007/978-3-662-44020-9_4

Truth #2

There are many compatibility and stability issues pertaining to PN. PN is an emulsion that may crack (if proportion of fat components and nonfat components are wrong) or precipitate (if electrolytes safety ranges are exceeded, e.g., calcium, phosphate, or various salt forms of drugs or additives interact with PN). Insulin should not be added in PN unless the patient is metabolically stable with consistent requirements of insulin doses (e.g., home PN). Always check with the compounding pharmacist in your institution.

Myth #3

PN is not expensive with current improvements in the production process; therefore, we should administer PN even if the benefit is marginal.

Truth #3

Careful deliberation, financial counselling, and engaging the patient and family are necessary when starting PN. The risks overweigh the benefits most of the time unless the patient is truly indicated (enteral access/feeding attempted and nonfeasible and severely malnourished). Average cost of 7 days of PN including cost of PICC insertion, PN bag, and lab monitoring is estimated to be SGD$2,400, and this figure excludes the cost of possible complications (e.g., infection) and increased duration of admission that may be associated with PN use.

Take-Home Pearls

- Colorectal surgical patients are at risk of malnutrition (up to 39 %).
- Malnutrition negatively affects surgical outcomes, hospital lengths of stay, and cost of hospitalization.
- All patients should be screened and appropriately diagnosed with malnutrition based on guidelines internationally developed and accepted by medical nutritional societies.
- Transdisciplinary management of nutrition therapy, via the Nutrition Support Team, is crucial for success in the treatment of malnutrition.
- At the initiation of nutrition therapy, daily requirements for calories, protein, fluid, electrolytes, trace elements, and vitamins should be calculated and monitored throughout the length of treatment.
- Routine prolonged fasting before surgery and routine nasogastric decompression after surgery should be avoided.
- Preoperative nutrition therapy, ideally enteral nutrition, is recommended in severely malnourished patients.
- Immediate resumption of oral intake in elective surgery is safe and not associated with anastomotic leak.
- In malnourished patients unable to meet requirements via oral intake alone, nutritional therapy is recommended, ideally enteral nutrition; parenteral nutrition should be reserved for patients unable to tolerate enteral nutrition.
- During the period of nutrition therapy, careful monitoring must be performed to identify and treat complications associated with each therapy.

4.1 Introduction

Colorectal surgery patients are at risk of malnutrition due to a multitude of factors including poor intake secondary to intestinal obstruction or cancer-associated anorexia, impaired absorption in inflammatory bowel disease, excessive losses from intestinal fistulas, and a marked inflammatory response in the setting of sepsis from perforated diverticulitis or tumor. The influence of malnutrition on surgical outcomes has been increasingly recognized since 1939, when Studley first reported on the association between preoperative weight loss and mortality in surgical patients (Studley 1936). Improvements in research methodology and refinement of therapeutic methods have led to the establishment of internationally accepted clinical guidelines on nutrition therapy from the European Society for Clinical Nutrition and Metabolism (ESPEN) and the American Society for Parenteral and Enteral Nutrition (ASPEN). In the era of modern colorectal surgery, optimization of the patient's nutritional status plays an important role in improving the results of surgical intervention. This chapter will provide an overview on the nutritional management of the colorectal surgery patient.

4.2 Influence of Malnutrition on Surgical Outcomes

The worldwide prevalence of malnutrition in hospitalized patients ranges from 15 to 50 % (Kondrup et al. 2003; Sorensen et al. 2008; Lim et al. 2012; Waitzberg et al. 2001), while up to 39 % of colorectal cancer patients are malnourished (Schwegler et al. 2010; Chen et al. 2011). Populations around the world are rapidly aging with a projected World Health Organization (WHO) estimate of two billion people aged 60 years and older by the year 2050 (World Health Organization 2013). This population has a significant risk of malnutrition, with reported rates of 14 % in nursing home occupants, 39 % in hospitalized patients, and 51 % in patients undergoing rehabilitation (Kaiser et al. 2010).

In addition to preexisting malnutrition, weight loss tends to occur during the course of a hospital admission; a UK study of inpatients revealed that 39 % of normal patients and 75 % of malnourished patients lost an average of 5–10 % of body weight during their hospital stay (McWhirter and Pennington 1994). Adverse hospital routines contribute to this decline; patients are frequently ordered nil by mouth prior to investigations, meals are served at predetermined times, and hospital food is often less palatable. The data on prevalence of malnutrition, however, has often been difficult to interpret and compare because of various different methods used for diagnosis and screening.

In 2012, the Academy of Nutrition and Dietetics and ASPEN released a consensus statement on a standardized set of diagnostic characteristics (previously endorsed by ASPEN and ESPEN) to be used to identify and document adult malnutrition with the aim of improving consistency in definition (White et al. 2012). Malnutrition was defined based on the etiology of the condition and broadly categorized according to the level of inflammation (Fig. 4.1). Six clinical characteristics which support the presence of malnutrition were identified; at a

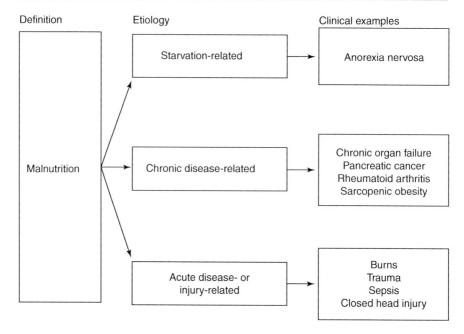

Fig. 4.1 Definition of malnutrition

minimum two out of six characteristics were required for diagnosis of adult malnutrition:

- Insufficient energy intake
- Weight loss
- Loss of muscle mass
- Loss of subcutaneous fat
- Localized or generalized fluid accumulation that may sometimes mask weight loss
- Diminished functional status as measured by handgrip strength

The influence of malnutrition on operative mortality and morbidity in general surgery (Studley 1936; Mullen et al. 1980; Gibbs et al. 1999; Stijn et al. 2013) and colorectal surgery patients (Schwegler et al. 2010; Lohsiriwat et al. 2008; Planas et al. 2007) has been extensively reported. Nutrients are crucial in the synthesis of proteins involved in the immune response to surgery and the inflammatory phase of wound healing (Haydock and Hill 1986; Scrimshaw and San Giovanni 1997; Rai et al. 2002). Malnutrition is a risk factor for overall complications, specifically nosocomial infections (Pessaux et al. 2003; Schneider et al. 2004) and impaired respiratory muscle function (Windsor and Hill 1988), leading to higher rates of surgical site infection and postoperative pneumonia.

Patients with malnutrition have significantly longer hospital stays, likely associated with an increased risk of complications and delayed recovery from such complications (Chima et al. 1997; Braunschweig et al. 2000; Middleton et al. 2001; Kyle et al. 2005; Pirlich et al. 2006; Kudsk et al. 2003b). The treatment cost of complications and the longer lengths of hospital stay in malnourished patients increase the economic burden of their hospitalization. The cost of treating a patient at risk of malnutrition is estimated to be 20–36 % higher than the average of the respective diagnosis-related group (Chima et al. 1997; Amaral et al. 2007). A study of patients in 25 Brazilian hospitals revealed a 60.5 % increase in daily expenses (US$138) for malnourished patients (Correia and Waitzberg 2003). Patients at nutritional risk were also more likely to require home health-care services or transfer to a transitional facility upon discharge.

Some groups have taken the opposite approach and analyzed the benefits of nutrition therapy on patients at risk of malnutrition. Adequate preoperative and postoperative nutrition therapy based on a standardized nutritional assessment model significantly decreased overall complications, major septic complications, and mortality in surgical patients (Mullen et al. 1980). The Veterans Affairs Total Parenteral Nutrition Cooperative Study Group demonstrated fewer noninfectious complications in the severely malnourished patients treated with perioperative total parenteral nutrition (PN) (The Veterans Affairs Total Parenteral Nutrition Cooperative Study Group 1991).

4.3   Transdisciplinary Clinical Nutrition Education and Nutrition Support Team (NST)

Despite the high occurrence and negative impact of malnutrition on clinical outcomes and hospitalization costs, the nutritional status of patients remains poorly identified and documented (Waitzberg et al. 2001; Singh et al. 2006; Gout et al. 2009). This highlights the need for a continuing education program in clinical nutrition for health-care providers, which should begin in medical and nursing schools (Acuna et al. 2008) and extend into residency and nursing training curricula.

Medical societies and quality improvement organizations have proposed structured guidelines to screen, identify, and treat malnutrition. Crucial to the successful implementation of these guidelines is the formation of nutrition support teams (Nehme 1980; Schneider 2006). The NST represents a model of transdisciplinary management where specialists from multiple disciplines combine their knowledge and expertise to achieve management decisions and outcomes superior to those obtained in isolation. An effective NST is a physician-led team of doctors, nurses, dieticians, and pharmacists who actively manage patients through daily clinical rounds using evidence-based protocols (Gales and Gales 1994). These teams are expected to interact closely with referring physicians, promote awareness, and improve the education of health-care providers in all aspects of nutrition care. The exact composition and roles of team members should be adapted to fit local demands and resources.

Successful NST practice has led to an increase in the appropriate use of PN and reduction in catheter-related complications and metabolic derangements (Nehme 1980; Gales and Gales 1994; Sriram et al. 2010). The implementation of an NST and nutritional clinical practice guidelines in a set of patients undergoing elective surgery for colorectal cancer resulted in a significant reduction in postoperative complications and hospital length of stay (Planas et al. 2007). It is important for each NST to determine performance goals or aims in terms of clinical nutrition outcomes of their patients. Regular audit of performance indicators will identify areas which require improvement or a change in clinical practice (Schneider 2006).

4.4 Clinical Pathway for Nutrition Risk Screening, Assessment, Therapy, and Monitoring

Nutrition screening is a simple process to identify patients at risk of malnutrition who will require a more thorough and detailed nutrition assessment to determine nutritional status (Kondrup et al. 2003). Many guidelines recommend screening in all cancer patients during the initial preoperation evaluation, either in the inpatient or outpatient setting. It is often challenging, however, to accurately measure nutritional status. Several markers have been explored as an indicator of nutritional status including albumin, prealbumin, and total lymphocyte counts (Elia 2000), but no single clinical or laboratory marker can be recommended as a comprehensive indicator of nutritional status. Levels of laboratory markers may be lowered during the acute phase response in inflammatory conditions making them unreliable in patients presenting with an acute colorectal problem (Fuhrman 2002).

In the 1990s, The Joint Commission mandated nutrition screening within 24 hours of admission, followed by a full nutrition assessment if found to be at nutritional risk. This guideline has since been widely adopted; however, colorectal patients who are undergoing elective procedures on the day of admission ought to be screened preoperatively in the outpatient clinic (Kudsk et al. 2003a). Nutrition screening tools should be easy to use, cost-effective, valid, reliable, and sensitive. Several nutrition screening tools have been described including the Mini Nutritional Assessment (MNA) (Vellas et al. 1999), the Malnutrition Universal Screening Tool (MUST) (Ferguson et al. 1999), and the Nutritional Risk Screening (Kondrup et al. 2003). The main limitations of these tools are the dependency on subjective parameters and clinical judgment and the variable evidence of their accuracy and reliability.

After nutrition screening, patients who are identified to be at risk of malnutrition should receive a more detailed nutritional assessment by a nutrition expert. This is a complete and systematic examination of the metabolic, nutritional, or functional variables which allows the NST to create an appropriate nutritional plan for each patient (Kondrup et al. 2003). ASPEN recommends using the Subjective Global Assessment (SGA), which is an assessment tool that consists of both the patient's history and physical assessment (Fig. 4.2). Patients are subjectively classified as A (well nourished), B (moderate malnutrition), or C (severe malnutrition) (Detsky et al. 1987). The SGA is a validated and simple assessment that predicts postoperative complications with high accuracy (Baker et al. 1982).

NUTRITIONAL ASSESSMENT FORM (SGA)
Nutrition & Dietetics Department

Ward / Bed: _____

OBJECTIVE ASSESSMENT

Weight: _____ kg   Height: _____ m

BMI: _____ kg/m²   Alb: _____ g/L (Date: _____)

Please stick Patient's Name Label within the Box

SUBJECTIVE GLOBAL ASSESSMENT

I. History

   a) <u>Weight Change</u>   Usual Body Weight = _____ kg
      Overall loss in past 6 months: _____ kg
                                _____ %   ☐ < 5% (small)
                                           ☐ < 5-10% (potentially significant)
                                           ☐ > 10% (definitely significant)

      Change in past 2 weeks: ☐ Increased
                                       ☐ No Change
                                         ☐ Decreased

   b) <u>Dietary Intake</u>
      Compare to normal   ☐ Good & No Change (1 share/meal)
                             ☐ Change: _____ weeks: ☐ Borderline (½ – ¾ share/meal)
                                                        ☐ Poor   (¼ – ½ share/meal)
                                                        ☐ Very Poor (NBM or <¼ share/meal)

   c) <u>Gastrointestinal</u>   ☐ None or < 2 weeks
      <u>Symptoms</u>   ☐ Persisted > 2 weeks   ☐ Nausea   ☐ Diarrhoea
                                                    ☐ Vomiting   ☐ Anorexia

   d) <u>Functional Ability</u>   ☐ Full Capacity
                                       ☐ Dysfunction: _____ weeks ☐ Mild to Moderate Loss of Stamina
                                                                                ☐ Chair-bound
                                                                                ☐ Bedridden

   e) <u>Metabolic Demands</u> ☐ No Stress   ☐ Low Stress   ☐ Moderate Stress   ☐ High Stress

II. Physical (refer to next page)

	Normal	Mild	Moderate	Severe
Loss of subcutaneous fat (triceps, chest)				
Muscle wasting (quadriceps, deltoids)				
Oedema (sacral, ankle)				
Ascites				

III. SGA Rating   ☐ Well Nourished   ☐ Mild to Moderate Malnutrition   ☐ Severe Malnutrition

                     * Recent dry weight gain   * > 5% dry wt loss without recent gain   * >10% dry weight loss
                     * Mild fat & muscle loss   * Decreased dietary intake   * Severe fat & muscle wasting
                     * Improved historical   * Mild fat & muscle loss   * Some oedema

Dietitian: _____

Date: _____

Fig. 4.2 Subjective Global Assessment

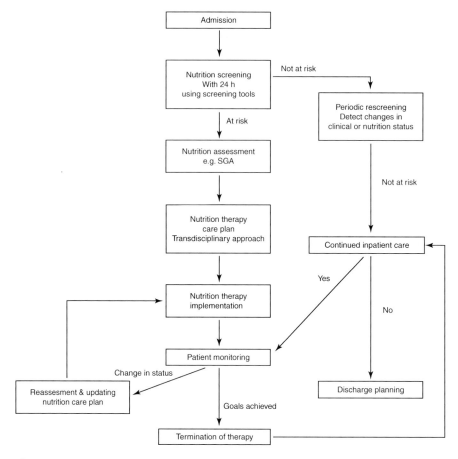

Fig. 4.3 Clinical pathway for nutrition risk screening, assessment, therapy, and monitoring

Patients assessed to be malnourished will require a nutrition therapy care plan, which should be delivered by a transdisciplinary team of nutrition experts, especially for those requiring PN. Regular reassessments of nutritional status must be conducted throughout the hospital stay to identify any changes in clinical or nutritional status, which may impact current nutrition status and therapy (Fig. 4.3).

4.5 Calculating Nutritional Requirements

The crucial element in designing a nutrition therapy care plan is the calculation of a patient's daily energy requirement. The daily requirement depends on resting energy rate, diet-induced thermogenesis, and physical activity (Manchanda 2003). The resting energy expenditure of patients after major colorectal surgery increased by 13% compared to those in healthy volunteers, with no difference in urinary

4 Transdisciplinary Management of Perioperative Nutrition

Table 4.1 Common energy expenditure equations

Equation (year)	Calculation
Harris–Benedict (1919)	Men: Wt (13.75) + Ht (5) – age (6.8) + 66
	Women: Wt (9.6) + Ht (1.8) – age (4.7) + 655
Mifflin–St Jeor (1990)	Men: Wt (10) + Ht (6.325) – age (5) + 5
	Women: Wt (10) + Ht (6.25) – age (5) – 161
Penn State (1998, 2004, 2001)	Age $\geq$ 60 with BMI $\geq$ 30 kg/m²: Mifflin (0.71) + Tmax (85) + Ve (63) – 3,085
	All others: Mifflin (0.96) + Tmax (167) + Ve (31) – 6,212

Wt weight (kg), *Ht* height (cm), *BMI* body mass index, *Tmax* maximum body temperature in the previous 24 h (degree Celsius), *Ve* minute ventilation recorded from ventilator (L/min)

nitrogen losses (Soop et al. 2004). The change in the energy expenditure of cancer patients is variable and is dependent on body composition and tumor type and stage (Elia 2005).

Indirect calorimetry represents the gold standard for measuring energy expenditure in the clinical setting. This machine, however, is often unavailable due to its high cost. Most nutrition therapists use predictive equations to estimate energy expenditure; the components of these equations usually include characteristics which influence the amount of fat-free mass including body weight, height, age, and gender. Many equations have been developed for healthy individuals (Table 4.1) and can be adjusted for sick patients using stress factors (Frankenfield et al. 2004).

ESPEN recommends the use of 25 kcal/kg ideal body weight as an approximate estimation of daily energy requirements and 30 kcal/kg ideal body weight during severe stress. ESPEN guidelines also recommend 1.2–1.5 g/kg ideal body weight/day of protein to limit nitrogen losses in surgical patients (Braga et al. 2009).

In addition to calorie and protein requirements, patients should receive daily recommended amounts of fluids, electrolytes, trace elements, and vitamins (Tables 4.2, 4.3, and 4.4) (Langley 2007; Clark 2007).

4.6 Preoperative Management of Nutrition in Colorectal Surgery

4.6.1 Immediate Preoperative Management

Routine prolonged periods of fasting before surgery should be avoided. It is now known that consuming fluids up to 2 h before general anesthesia does not increase the risk of aspiration (Jones et al. 2011). There is also a lack of evidence to show harm when this is performed in patients at risk of reflux and gastroparesis, such as those with diabetes mellitus, gastroesophageal reflux disease, and obesity (Smith et al. 2011).

In addition, providing carbohydrate calories just before surgery in the form of a carbohydrate drink has been shown to shorten the length of hospitalization, reduce

Table 4.2 Daily electrolytes requirements, etiologies, and clinical consequences of abnormalities

Electrolyte	Recommended daily intake	Abnormal levels	Causes	Clinical consequences
Sodium	1–2 mmol/kg/day	Low	Replacement of lost solute with water	Malaise
			SIADH	Delirium
			Renal failure	Seizures
			Medications	Coma
				Respiratory arrest
		High	Loss of water	Lethargy
			Iatrogenic (e.g., excessive use of hypertonic saline)	Irritability
				Seizures
				Coma
Potassium	1–2 mmol/kg/day	Low	Increased GI/GU losses	Muscle weakness
			Medications (e.g., insulin, nebulizers)	Ileus
			Carbohydrate loading	Cardiac arrhythmias
				Rhabdomyolysis
		High	Increased intake	Muscle weakness
			Reduced urinary excretion (e.g., renal failure, medications)	Paralysis
				Cardiac arrhythmias
Magnesium	4–10 mmol/day	Low	Impaired intestinal absorption	Tetany
			Increased renal excretion	Seizures
				Cardiac arrhythmias
				Sudden cardiac death
		High (rare)	Chronic kidney disease	Bradycardia
				Hypotension
				Asystole

Calcium	5–7.5 mmol/day	Low	Chronic kidney disease Hypoparathyroidism	Tetany
			Vitamin D deficiency	Hypoactive reflexes
			Alcoholism	Anxiety
			Hyperphosphatemia	Hallucinations
				Hypotension
		High	Malignancy Hyperparathyroidism	Constipation
				Muscle weakness
				Confusion
				Lethargy
Phosphate	20–40 mmol/day	Low	Increased renal elimination	Delirium
			Refeeding syndrome	Seizures
			Respiratory alkalosis	Respiratory failure
				Cardiac failure
				Cardiac arrhythmias
		High	Chronic kidney disease	Hypocalcemia
			Hypoparathyroidism	ECG changes
				Paresthesia

SIADH syndrome of inappropriate antidiuretic hormone secretion, *GI* gastrointestinal, *GU* genitourinary

Table 4.3 Daily trace element requirements, function, and clinical consequences of deficiency

Trace element	Recommended daily intake	Function	Deficiency
Chromium	10–15 mcg	Glucose and lipid metabolism	Rare
		Potentiation of insulin action Enhances tyrosine phosphorylation of the insulin receptor	Weight loss
			Neuropathy
			Impaired glucose tolerance
			Glucosuria
			Hyperlipidemia
Copper	0.3–0.5 mg	Oxidation–reduction and electron transfer reactions involving oxygen	Uncommon
		Component of metalloenzymes (used for collagen and elastin production, dopamine conversion to norepinephrine)	Defects in connective tissue
			Anemia
			Leukopenia
			Neutropenia
			Hypercholesterolemia
			Cardiac dysfunction
Manganese	60–100 mcg	Component of metalloenzymes (arginase, used for urea production; manganese superoxide dismutase, provides antioxidant function; pyruvate carboxylase, used in carbohydrate synthesis)	Rare
			Neurotoxicity
			Poor reproductive performance
			Abnormal bone and cartilage formation
			Ataxia
			Growth retardation
			Defects in carbohydrate and lipid metabolism

Selenium	20–60 mcg	Defense against oxidative stress	Keshan disease (cardiomyopathy in pediatric population)
		Regulation of thyroxine	Skeletal muscle disorders
		Regulation of the redox status of vitamin C and other molecules	
Zinc	2.5–5 mg	Component of enzymes (RNA polymerase, alkaline phosphatase)	Growth retardation
		Structural role in protein folding	Hair loss
		Lipid peroxidation	Diarrhea
		Apoptosis, cellular proliferation, and differentiation	Delayed sexual maturation and impotence
		Immune function	Eye and skin lesions
			Loss of appetite
			Delayed wound healing
Iron	8–18 mg	Oxidative metabolism	Impaired physical work performance
		Heme proteins (hemoglobin, myoglobin, cytochromes)	Mental delay
		Electron transfer	Cognitive impairment
			Hypochromic–microcytic anemia

Table 4.4 Daily vitamin requirements, function, and clinical consequences of deficiency

Vitamin	Recommended daily intake	Function	Deficiency
A	700–900 mcg	Bone growth	Night blindness
		Reproduction	Hyperkeratosis
		Cell division	Anorexia
		Immunity	Phrynoderma
		Cell differentiation	Depressed T-helper cell activity
			Impaired mucus secretion
B1 (thiamine)	1.1–1.2 mg	Coenzyme in metabolism of carbohydrates and branched-chain amino acids	Beriberi
			Wernicke's encephalopathy
			Lactic acidosis
B2 (riboflavin)	1.1–1.3 mg	Coenzyme in numerous redox reactions	Ariboflavinosis (sore throat, hyperemia, and edema of pharyngeal and oral mucous membranes, cheilosis, angular stomatitis, glossitis, seborrheic dermatitis, normochromic–normocytic anemia)
B3 (niacin)	14–16 mg	Coenzyme in numerous redox reactions	Pellagra (pigmented rash, vomiting, constipation or diarrhea, bright red tongue, neurological symptoms including depression, apathy, headache, fatigue, and loss of memory)
B5 (pantothenic acid)	5–15 mg	Component of coenzyme A Component of the fatty acid synthase complex	Extremely rare
			Irritability and restlessness
			Nausea, vomiting, and abdominal cramps
			Numbness, paresthesia, muscle cramps, staggering gait
B6 (pyridoxine)	1.3–1.7 mcg	Coenzyme in the metabolism of amino acids, glycogen, and sphingoid bases	Seborrheic dermatitis
			Microcytic anemia
			Epileptiform convulsions

B12	2.4–5 mcg	Cofactor for methionine synthase and L-methylmalonyl-CoA mutase which are essential for normal blood formation and neurologic function	Pernicious anemia
			Neurological manifestations (sensory disturbances in the extremities, motor disturbances, gait abnormality)
			Cognitive changes (loss of concentration, memory, disorientation, and frank dementia)
			Visual disturbances
			Insomnia
			Impotency
			Impaired bowel and bladder control
C (ascorbic acid)	200 mg	Antioxidant	Anorexia
		Biosynthesis of connective tissue components (collagen, elastin, fibronectin, proteoglycans, bone matrix, elastin-associated fibrillin), carnitine, and neurotransmitters	Fatigue
			Scurvy (anemia, bleeding gums, perifollicular hemorrhage, impaired wound healing)
D	2.5–15 mcg	Maintenance of normal blood levels of calcium and phosphorus	Osteomalacia
		Promotes bone mineralization	Osteoporosis
		Regulates cell growth, differentiation, immune function	
E	15 mg	Antioxidant	Neuronal degeneration
		Plays role in immune function and in DNA repair	Platelet aggregation
		Inhibits cell proliferation, platelet aggregation, and monocyte adhesion	Decreased red blood cell survival
			Hemolytic anemia
			Skeletal muscle lesions

(continued)

Table 4.4 (continued)

Vitamin	Recommended daily intake	Function	Deficiency
K	90–120 mcg	Coenzyme for synthesis of proteins involved in blood coagulation and bone metabolism	Rare
			Bleeding
Folic acid	400 mcg	Coenzymes involved in DNA synthesis, amino acid interconversions, single-carbon metabolism, methylation reactions	Hypersegmented neutrophils, macrocytic anemia
			Weakness, fatigue
			Difficulty concentrating, irritability
			Palpitations
			Shortness of breath

4 Transdisciplinary Management of Perioperative Nutrition

the loss of muscle mass, and possibly result in an earlier return of gut function (Jones et al. 2011; Noblett et al. 2006). Patients undergoing surgery in a fed state will not suffer from thirst or hunger. This reduces catabolism, maintains lean body mass, and reduces insulin resistance (Gustafsson et al. 2012; Ljungqvist and Søreide 2003). Therefore, patients undergoing colorectal surgery should continue to receive preoperative nutrition up to 2 h before the operation. This is given in the form of an oral carbohydrate drink on the day of the surgery (Smith et al. 2011). In diabetic patients, carbohydrate loading may be given with diabetic medication if necessary (Gustafsson et al. 2012; Nygren et al. 2012).

4.6.2 Preoperative Nutrition Therapy for Malnourished Patients

In the preoperative period, successful nutritional intervention aims to optimize caloric goals, improve nitrogen balance and lean body mass, and replenish depleted micronutrients in malnourished patients undergoing elective colorectal surgery. This involves the provision of fortified enteral or PN. Interventions may be divided into the provision of micro- and macronutrients, provision of immunonutrition, and reducing the period of fasting before surgery.

It may seem intuitive to optimize caloric goals and protein intake in every patient before surgery, but the benefits of delaying surgery to pursue nutritional optimization have only been shown in malnourished patients. Trials on preoperative nutrition optimization of malnourished patients have demonstrated reduced rates of surgical site infection, perioperative mortality, and length of hospitalization (Mullen et al. 1980; The Veterans Affairs Total Parenteral Nutrition Cooperative Study Group 1991; Burden et al. 2011; Bozzetti et al. 2000). ESPEN, therefore, recommends preoperative nutritional support in severely malnourished patients. Nutritional support is given for 10–14 days before the operation. Surgery may be delayed if safe to do so, in order to optimize patients for the procedure.

4.6.2.1 Enteral Nutrition (EN)
EN is always preferred to PN as the former provides nutrition to enterocytes and is physiological and associated with less electrolyte, metabolic, and infective complications. Enteral formulas have less of an economic burden, and since EN does not require intravenous access, it is more cost-effective and easier to deliver in the outpatient setting (Bozzetti et al. 2001). The majority of surgical patients will achieve their nutritional goals with the addition of fortified oral supplements. If oral intake is still poor, then EN may be advanced with the use of a nasoenteral tube.

4.6.2.2 PN
If malnourished patients are unable to tolerate EN, e.g., partial bowel obstruction or high-output enterocutaneous fistula, PN should be given to optimize their nutrition. PN is recommended if the enteral intake is less than 60 % of the requirements and the anticipated duration of PN is more than 10 days or if the patient is unable to eat for more than 7 days (Braga et al. 2009).

4.6.2.3 Combined EN and PN

There is a paucity of data on combined enteral and PN in the preoperative period. Studies have concentrated on combined therapy in the postoperative critically ill patient, and this will be discussed in the postoperative nutrition section.

4.7 Postoperative Management of Nutrition in Colorectal Surgery

4.7.1 Nasogastric Decompression

Routine nasogastric tube decompression of the stomach after elective colorectal surgery is not recommended. Multiple meta-analyses have shown an increased risk of fever, atelectasis, and pulmonary infection and no benefit in anastomotic leak rates with the routine use of a nasogastric tube postoperatively (Cheatham et al. 1995; Nelson et al. 2005).

4.7.2 Postoperative Nutrition Therapy for Malnourished Patients

4.7.2.1 EN

Immediate oral intake after recovery from anesthesia is safe in elective surgery and is not associated with an increased risk of anastomotic dehiscence (Reissman et al. 1995; Han-Geurts et al. 2007; Lewis et al. 2009). The most recent meta-analysis suggested a reduction in morbidity and mortality and decreased length of hospital stay (Lewis et al. 2009). In malnourished patients, consumption of oral nutritional supplements postoperatively was associated with a reduction in chest and wound infections. This practice also led to improvements in both physical and mental quality of life measurements 18 months after surgery (Beattie et al. 2000).

If patients at nutritional risk are unable to consume an adequate amount of supplements via the oral route, enteral therapy can be provided via feeding tubes, e.g., nasoenteral or jejunostomy tubes. The use of these tubes is well tolerated and should be attempted before switching to PN (Braga et al. 2002). Since jejunostomy tubes are inserted at the time of the colorectal procedure, preoperative identification of patients at risk is required to optimize operative planning.

Early EN (started 6 h after end of the operation) improves gut oxygenation as compared to postoperative PN (Braga et al. 2001). At the cellular level, PN is associated with villous atrophy and increased gut permeability secondary to inflammation (Zaloga 2006). High-risk surgical patients who receive EN have significantly less septic complications compared to patients on total PN (Moore et al. 1992). Similar findings were found in malnourished patients undergoing surgery for gastrointestinal cancer; postoperative EN resulted in less overall complications, specifically infectious complications (Bozzetti et al. 2001). The increase in infection rates was not attributed to the higher blood glucose concentrations found in patients receiving PN

4 Transdisciplinary Management of Perioperative Nutrition

(Kudsk et al. 2001); many of the older studies, however, did not analyze the effect of hyperglycemia on outcomes. The overall daily cost of EN is generally cheaper than PN (Bozzetti et al. 2001; Braga et al. 2001), making this form of therapy more cost-effective. Currently, most nutritional guidelines strongly recommend a preference for EN whenever the gastrointestinal tract is available for feeding.

4.7.2.2 PN

Most elective colorectal surgery patients should be able to tolerate enteral therapy if required. Routine use of PN is not recommended in well-nourished patients (The Veterans Affairs Total Parenteral Nutrition Cooperative Study Group 1991) or in those with adequate enteral intake within 7–10 days after surgery (Braga et al. 2009; McClave et al. 2009). On the other hand, examples of patients who might require PN would be those after emergency colorectal surgery with septic shock or postoperative patients who suffer from complications resulting in the inability to receive and absorb enteral feeding secondary to ileus or obstruction, enteric fistula, impaired splanchnic perfusion, or short gut syndrome. These patients may be highly catabolic due to the stress from surgery (may require multiple operations) and the inflammatory response to complications. PN is useful in this setting to avoid further deterioration in nutritional status.

4.7.2.3 Combined EN and PN

Evidence for the routine use of combined enteral and PN in surgical patients is limited. A systematic review of five relatively small studies on combination nutrition therapy in critically ill patients failed to show benefit in clinical outcomes when compared to EN alone (Dhaliwal et al. 2004), whereas a randomized controlled trial revealed reduced nosocomial infections in patients who received combined therapy (Heidegger et al. 2013). ESPEN does recommend a combination of enteral and supplementary parenteral feeding in patients who are unable to reach nutritional goals via the enteral route alone (Braga et al. 2009).

4.8 Immunonutrition

Immunonutrients are postulated to have modulating effects on the immune stress response associated with surgery, potentially reducing harm. Common examples of immunonutrients include amino acids such as arginine and glutamine, micronutrient antioxidants, omega-3 fatty acids, and nucleotides (Jones and Heyland 2008). Immunonutrients are found in the food which we consume, however, during periods of severe stress, a state of relative or absolute immunonutrient deficiency may occur. Replenishing this deficiency or supplementing increased quantities has been purported to modulate the local and systemic inflammatory response, improve metabolic control (e.g., reduce insulin resistance), and enhance immunity (Xu et al. 2009). Studies on immunonutrition are relatively young with a heterogeneous patient selection and wide variability in the specific type of immunonutrients prescribed and outcome measures.

4.8.1 Glutamine

Glutamine is an important substrate for rapidly proliferating cells such as lymphocytes and enterocytes. Low plasma glutamine levels are known to occur in the critically ill and post-surgery patients (Lloyd and Gabe 2007). Glutamine supplementation is believed to maintain the integrity of enterocytes and reduce the risk of sepsis by reducing bacterial translocation. Some clinical trials have shown that glutamine reduces the excessive production of cytokines and enhances immune function, while others have refuted the benefits by showing no change in gut mucosal inflammation, intestinal permeability, and risk of bacterial translocation (Aosasa et al. 1999; Hulsewé et al. 2004).

In the clinical setting, the administration of intravenous glutamine 5–6 days before surgery and after surgery has been shown to decrease incidence of wound infections, intra-abdominal abscesses, wound dehiscence, and duration of hospitalization (Oguz et al. 2007). A recent meta-analysis on glutamine-enriched PN versus standard PN in abdominal surgery patients confirmed that glutamine significantly reduced the length of hospitalization and infectious complications and improved nitrogen balance, but did not reduce mortality (Yue et al. 2013).

Of note, glutamine should be avoided in patients with significant renal impairment as it may aggravate azotemia, in decompensated liver disease as it may cause encephalopathy and in multi-organ failure as it may increase mortality (Vanek et al. 2011; Heyland et al. 2013). There is currently no consensus on when glutamine should be started in the surgical patient or the optimal duration for which it should be continued. Therefore, the use of glutamine at this point in time should be an individualized decision.

4.8.2 Other Types of Immunonutrition

Arginine, omega-3 fatty acids, and nucleotides are frequently studied together because of their availability as combined oral preparations. These preparations may be described as an "arginine-based immunonutrition therapy" which actually contains omega-3 fatty acids and nucleotides as well.

Arginine is a semi-essential amino acid which becomes essential during stress and tissue injury and is utilized by rapidly dividing cells such as lymphocytes and enterocytes. The provision of arginine has been shown to enhance nitrogen retention and promote protein synthesis (Stechmiller et al. 2004). Omega-3 fatty acids are derived from fish oils. Omega-3 fatty acids have an immune-modulating effect, improve ventilation time in acute lung injury, and possibly reduce mortality in critical illness (Mayer and Seeger 2008). Finally, nucleotides form the building blocks of deoxyribonucleic acid, ribonucleic acid, and other metabolic compounds. During catabolism, the synthesis of nucleotides may be inadequate requiring external supplementation.

A few meta-analyses and systematic reviews have been conducted on arginine-based immunonutrition therapies in surgical patients. These studies have shown that

4 Transdisciplinary Management of Perioperative Nutrition 61

immunonutrition therapy reduces the duration of hospitalization and infections, without reducing mortality. The benefits are seen when immunonutrition is extended from the preoperative to the postoperative period (Jones and Heyland 2008; Cerantola et al. 2011).

ESPEN currently recommends providing immunonutrition therapy comprising of arginine, omega-3 fatty acids, and nucleotides to patients undergoing abdominal surgery, from 5 to 7 days before operation till 5–7 postoperative days (Weimann et al. 2006).

4.9 A Practical Approach to EN Therapy

EN can be administered through a nasogastric, nasoduodenal, nasojejunal, or enterostomy tube (gastrostomy or jejunostomy). Gastric feeding is more physiologic and is easier to administer as it allows for a larger volume and higher osmotic load than the small intestine. Post-pyloric feeding may be used in patients at high risk of aspiration, with gastric dysmotility or gastric obstruction (Kulick and Deen 2011).

Administration of EN should be based on the patient's medical issues, nutrition status, enteral route access, and condition of the gastrointestinal tract. It can be administered by bolus, intermittent, or continuous infusion. Bolus feeding is defined as rapid administration of a bolus feed/water by syringe. The feedings may be initiated three to eight times per day with increases of 60–120 ml every 8–12 h as tolerated up to the goal volume (Bankhead et al. 2009). This technique, however, may cause "dumping" syndrome if it is delivered into the jejunum too rapidly and should therefore be avoided whenever possible. Continuous infusion, which is defined as feeding for 24 h continuously either by gravity or feeding pump, may help to prevent "dumping" in some patients (Dieticians Association of Australia Nutrition Support Interest Group Manual 2011). In practice, the continuous infusion method can be initiated at a rate of 10–40 ml/h and advanced to the goal rate by increasing 10–20 ml/h every 8–12 h as tolerated (Bankhead et al. 2009).

Many different formulas are available, through several different companies (Table 4.5). The selection of formulas should be based on the individual nutrition assessment of the patient.

4.10 A Practical Approach to PN Therapy

4.10.1 Types of PN

4.10.1.1 Central PN (CPN)
CPN is a complete, balanced formulation which comprises dextrose; amino acids; intravenous fat emulsion; electrolytes such as sodium, potassium, magnesium, calcium, and phosphorus; vitamins; and multiple trace elements such as zinc, copper, manganese, chromium, and selenium. The resultant formulation is a hyperosmolar (1,300–1,800 mOsm/l) solution that must be delivered into a large-diameter vein

Table 4.5 Enteral formulas

Type	Characteristics	Examples (all names are trademarked)
Polymeric, standard	Nutritionally complete and lactose-free	Ensure, Isocal
Polymeric, high calorie	Nutritionally complete and lactose-free	1.5 kcal/ml – Ensure Plus, Resource Plus, Fortisip
	Increase in caloric content	2.0 kcal/ml – Resource 2.0
Polymeric with fiber	Nutritionally complete and lactose-free	Jevity
	With fiber added	
Diabetic formulas	Nutritionally complete	Glucerna, Glucerna Triple Care, and Resource Diabetic
	Lower carbohydrate and higher monounsaturated fat content	
Pulmonary formulas	Nutritionally complete	Pulmocare
	Lower in carbohydrate	
	Increase in caloric content	
Renal formulas	Potassium, phosphorus, and magnesium lower than in standard formulas	High protein: Novasource Renal, Nepro
	Protein content high in the formulas recommended for patients on renal replacement therapy and low in those not on dialysis	Low protein: Suplena
Modular	Contains a single nutrient such as protein, fat, and carbohydrate	Protein: Propass, Myotein, Beneprotein
		Fat: MCT oil
		Carbohydrate: Carborie
		Fiber: Fibrebasic

such as the superior vena cava, where the high blood volume and flow rate can rapidly dilute the hypertonic PN to minimize complications associated with hypertonic infusions (Task Force for the Revision of Safe Practices for Parenteral Nutrition et al. 2004). Appropriate central line access is required for administration.

CPN infusions deliver complete nutrition in a reasonable fluid volume and may be concentrated even further for patients who require fluid restriction. CPN is considered the preferred route for patients requiring PN, particularly those with average to high caloric and protein requirements and patients with a prolonged duration of therapy including patients at nursing homes and extended health-care establishments or ambulatory patients requiring home PN.

4.10.1.2 Peripheral PN (PPN)

PPN is meant for peripheral venous infusion; the PN osmolarity is below 850 mOsm/l though it has the same composition as CPN (De Cicco et al. 1989). Large fluid volumes must be administered to provide a calorie and protein dose comparable to CPN. PPN is not ideal for patients who are at risk of fluid overload and is definitely not a suitable option for patients who have poor peripheral vein access or when the provision of calories cannot be fulfilled due to high energy requirements (Task Force for the Revision of Safe Practices for Parenteral Nutrition et al. 2004). PPN may be used to provide nutritional support to a selected group of patients with mild to moderate malnutrition and low calorie requirements or as a supplement to EN for a limited period of time, with stringent aseptic access insertion techniques and close monitoring for thrombophlebitis (Pittiruti et al. 2006).

4.10.2 Venous Access

4.10.2.1 Central Access

A central venous catheter (CVC) is a catheter whose tip lies in the distal vena cava or right atrium. Two broad categories of CVCs exist, namely, non-tunneled versus tunneled and implanted. The choice of catheter is governed primarily by the duration of PN, although the risk of infections, cost, and expertise for the care of lines are important considerations (Table 4.6) (Pittiruti et al. 2006; Ryder 2006; Radd et al. 1993; Moureau et al. 2002).

Non-tunneled CVC. This is the most common catheter used in the acute perioperative setting if the PN duration is short. Access can be obtained with a percutaneous venipuncture using a subclavian, jugular, or femoral approach. Sutures at the exit site are necessary to anchor the catheter in place with the help of a sterile dressing. Short-term non-tunneled catheters, such as the central venous pressure (CVP) lines, are often inserted in intensive care units to measure CVP or administer fluids and medications. They usually have multiple ports which can be used for PN infusion for a relatively short period of time, ranging from a few days to weeks (Pittiruti et al. 2006).

The peripherally inserted central catheter (PICC) is a common non-tunneled CVC which offers some advantages over the centrally inserted CVC, if PN is intended for the short to medium term. PICCs can last longer, up to 3 months, if proper catheter care is rendered and is a suitable option for home PN patients (Ryder 2006). Some evidence suggests that PICC use may be preferable as it is associated with fewer mechanical complications during insertion and has a lower rate of infection (De Cicco et al. 1989; Radd et al. 1993). PICC placement is usually done in an interventional radiology suite but can also be performed at the bedside and at home if trained personnel are available.

Tunneled CVC and Implanted Port. Tunneled CVCs, such as the Hickman and Broviac, or an implanted port needs to be considered if long-term PN of more than 3 months is necessary. The use of non-tunneled CVCs is discouraged in home PN patients in view of the high rates of infection, obstruction, dislocation, and venous thrombosis (Moureau et al. 2002). Implanted port access has the advantage of minimal alteration to body image and ease of self-care.

4.10.2.2 Peripheral Access

PPN can be safely administered via peripheral access using a standard peripheral cannula or midline catheter for a short period of time (Table 4.6). While peripheral

Table 4.6 Venous access for PN

Access type	Type of line	Remarks
Peripheral	Intravenous cannula	Suitable for 7–10 days
		Cannula needs to be changed every 3 days
		Easily inserted
		Easily dislodged, extravasation risk
		Suitable for peripheral PN only
		Peripheral PN associated with high volumes of fluids due to low osmolality
Central (non-tunneled)	Percutaneous central lines (jugular/subclavian/femoral veins)	Suitable for 7–10 days
		Difficult to care
		Readily available in the hospital and intensive care
		Subclavian route preferred (lowest risk of infection)
		Femoral route should be avoided (highest risk of infection and thrombosis)
		Internal jugular route is the easiest to insert
		Inexpensive
Central (non-tunneled)	Peripherally inserted central catheter (PICC)	Suitable if <1 month
		Inserted into a vein in the antecubital area or upper forearm. Extends into the superior vena cava
		Well tolerated
		Easy to care
		Few complications at placement
		Inexpensive
Central (tunneled)	Tunneled, cuffed catheters (e.g., Hickman®, Broviac®, Hohn®, or Groshong® catheters)	Suitable if >1 month
		Tunneled through subcutaneous tissue before entering the vein
		Easy to care
		Lower risk of catheter-related infection
		Expensive
Central (implanted)	Subcutaneous access device (totally implanted device) – port systems	Suitable if >1 month
		Completely implanted device under the skin
		Requires special port cannula
		Frequent needling may be uncomfortable
		Freedom of movement when not in use
		Easy to care
		Expensive

access provides the convenience of not requiring insertion of a central line, the common complication of peripheral venous thrombophlebitis dictates catheter change and rotation to a new site every 48–72 h.

4.10.3 Selecting Appropriate PN Formulations

PN administration has evolved from complicated and individual bottle infusion systems to either a simple ready-to-use multi-chamber PN bag or a customized PN admixture produced in a sterile laboratory environment (Pertkiewicz and Dudrick 2011; Rollins et al. 1990).

4.10.3.1 Ready-to-Use PN

Ready-to-use formulas are packaged in a multi-chamber bag with two or three main components separated by a seal that can be broken upon rolling or squeezing the bag. The two main components are amino acid and dextrose; the third component containing lipid can be omitted if fat-free PN is desired. The components are mixed within the closed system just before use, and compatible additives such as electrolytes, multivitamins, trace elements, and drugs can be added aseptically in compounding laboratory. After mixing, storage of these bags should be kept at 2–8 °C and be administered within 24 h. The main advantages of these bags include the ease and convenience of administration and a reduced risk of contamination during the compounding process. Alterations to the proportions of the individual nutrient components (e.g., increasing protein to meet increased catabolic demands) are impossible, and there are limits imposed on the quantity of electrolytes to ensure the stability of the mixture (Muhlebach et al. 2011).

4.10.3.2 Customized PN

Customized compounding of PN allows for adjustment of the admixture to the individual needs of the patient. This is important for long-term PN and in patients with rapidly changing metabolic requirements, e.g., reduction of the fat component in liver dysfunction or hypertriglyceridemia, increase in the amino acid component in sarcopenia, reduction of the amount of electrolytes, and restricting PN volume in patients with end-stage renal failure. Strict pharmaceutical practices should be adopted for PN compounding. Quality control standards in the compounding laboratory need to be adhered to ensure that PN preparations are physicochemically stable, sterile, and safe for administration (Muhlebach et al. 2009).

4.10.4 Understanding PN Constituents

Components in PN typically include:

1. Macronutrients (energy substrates)

   - Carbohydrate
   - Protein
   - Lipid

2. Micronutrients

- Electrolytes
- Vitamins
- Trace elements

3. Water

Depending on the type of PN formulation and compounding services available, the proportion and combinations of these constituents can be altered based on the individualized needs of the patient.

4.10.4.1 Carbohydrate

Carbohydrates should cover 50–60 % of the total energy requirements in PN as glucose is the major circulating carbohydrate fuel in the body. The most commonly used carbohydrate energy substrate is dextrose (glucose), which provides 3.4 kcal/g. It is important to note that in times of stress, the acute stress response causes markedly elevated glucose turnover, yet glucose utilization does not increase in tandem. Hence, the 24-h infusion rates of dextrose should not exceed 3–5 mg/kg/min in adult patients to avoid causing hyperglycemia (Carpentier et al. 2011).

4.10.4.2 Lipid

Lipids generally make up 25–40 % of the total infused energy, providing 9 kcal/g. Formulations containing a mixture of soybean long-chain triglycerides (LCT) together with medium-chain triglycerides (MCT) have been used in Europe for more than 20 years. Recently, olive oil, fish oil, and structured lipid preparations have been introduced and marketed for their immunomodulating properties. Studies have shown that the rapid delivery of omega-3 fatty acids to tissue cell membranes modulates important metabolic and immune reactions (Wirtitsch et al. 2007). Lipid emulsions should be reduced in moderate hypertriglyceridemia (2.0–3.5 mmol/l) and avoided in severe hypertriglyceridemia (>4.5 mmol/l).

4.10.4.3 Protein

Crystalline amino acids are used in the compounding of PN to provide protein, and they yield 4 kcal/g of energy. Amino acid solutions usually contain 13–20 amino acids including all of the essential amino acids. The usual requirement for a healthy adult is 0.8–1 g/kg/day, providing approximately 20 % of the energy requirement. During illness and convalescence, intakes of 1.5 g/kg/day in patients with adequate renal function have been shown to be beneficial (Furst et al. 2011).

4.10.4.4 Fluids and Electrolytes

A general guide to determining the volume of PN for adults with normal hydration status would be approximately 30–40 ml/kg/day. Factors such as excessive fluid losses and impaired fluid clearance should be taken into consideration. The maintenance amount of various electrolytes also needs to be calculated to ensure electrolyte balance in PN patients (Table 4.2). The negative ions, acetate and chloride, do not have standard ranges, but their proportions are adjusted accordingly to maintain normal acid–base balance. Contributions of electrolytes from the maintenance drip should also be taken into account when determining the amount of electrolytes in the PN mixture. Timely monitoring of serum electrolytes is imperative as patients tend to have varying electrolyte requirements and further adjustments may be required.

4.10.4.5 Vitamins and Trace Elements

Patients requiring nutrition support and PN might be depleted of certain vitamins and trace elements. In addition, they may have increased requirements as a result of illness and stresses. It is therefore essential to provide an adequate amount of these micronutrients (Tables 4.3 and 4.4). Commercial preparations of injectable trace elements and multivitamins, both fat- and water-soluble vitamins, can be added into PN bags during compounding.

4.11 Complications of Enteral and PN

The safety and efficacy of nutrition therapy has been markedly improved using transdisciplinary management methods, increased research, experience, and education. There are still serious complications associated with each therapy, and precautions should be taken to minimize risks and identify and treat complications early and appropriately (Table 4.7).

4.11.1 Metabolic Complications

Electrolyte abnormalities are common, and the importance of monitoring electrolytes cannot be overemphasized, especially in those who have abnormal electrolyte values at baseline. A minimum daily amount of the major electrolytes (sodium, potassium, phosphorus, magnesium, calcium) should be administered; requirements

Table 4.7 Complications of enteral and PN

Complications	Enteral	Parenteral
Metabolic	Electrolyte abnormalities	
	Refeeding syndrome	
	Overfeeding	
	Fluid overload	
	Gastrointestinal intolerance	Liver dysfunction
	Dumping syndrome	
Access- or catheter-related	Feeding tube blockage	Mechanical catheter complications
	Feeding tube malposition	Catheter-related sepsis
		Venous thrombosis/thrombophlebitis
		Separation of components

are dependent of patient's weight and baseline plasma values. Careful documentation of other sources of electrolytes and fluid intake is essential as additional intravenous fluid or water flushes and electrolytes supplementation can affect daily requirements.

Patients who are at increased risk of electrolyte derangement are those in an anabolic state, for example, patients who receive nutrition therapy after a period of malnutrition, i.e., refeeding syndrome. Refeeding syndrome is characterized by electrolyte derangements, heart failure, fluid overload, and death. Patients at risk of refeeding syndrome are identified by the presence of significant weight loss, poor oral intake for more than 1 week, or chronic malnutrition. Certain groups of patients tend to be at an increased risk: chronic alcoholics, prolonged periods of fasting, anorexia nervosa, and the elderly (Mehanna et al. 2008).

The overzealous feeding of patients at risk of refeeding syndrome may result in severe hypokalemia, hypophosphatemia, and hypomagnesemia. These abnormalities may lead to cramps, neuromuscular weakness, seizures, paresthesia, cardiac arrhythmia, and rhabdomyolysis. In the worst case scenario, death may occur from failure of ventilator muscle function or cardiac arrhythmias. In addition, thiamine deficiency may result in Wernicke's encephalopathy and heart failure.

Overfeeding or hyperalimentation refers to the provision of calories in excess of the patient's requirement. Overfeeding causes metabolic stress and increases the risk of steatohepatitis and bloodstream infections (Dissanaike et al. 2007). Chronic overfeeding which results in obesity is unlikely to occur in hospitalized patients. Acute overfeeding, however, is a potential problem and tends to occur with parenteral rather than EN. Overfeeding in EN generally results in gastrointestinal intolerance and diarrhea, necessitating a reduction of feeds delivered. In PN, overfeeding may not be recognized until the complications manifest. These include fluid retention, hyperglycemia, hypophosphatemia, hypertriglyceridemia, hyperazotemia, hypercalcemia, hypercapnea, steatohepatitis, and cholestatic liver disease (Klein et al. 1998).

In order to prevent refeeding and overfeeding patients, it is essential that a comprehensive nutritional assessment is conducted before feeding patients. Patients who might be at risk of refeeding syndrome and overfeeding should be identified with strict monitoring of glucose, electrolytes, liver function tests, and input and output with prompt correction of any abnormalities. Patients at risk of refeeding syndrome will require nutrition therapy to be initiated at smaller amounts and a slower rate of progression.

Liver dysfunction is an infrequent yet important complication of PN which commences typically after 2 weeks. Its etiology is complex and multifactorial, typically associated with the prolonged provision of excessive calories or lipids. The liver disease progresses from steatosis to steatohepatitis and cholestasis. In patients on chronic PN, liver dysfunction can result in liver fibrosis, eventual cirrhosis, and death. Therefore, the liver function test should be monitored periodically in patients who are receiving PN (Guglielmi et al. 2008).

The liver dysfunction is characterized by elevations in the serum gammaglutamyl transpeptidase, alkaline phosphatase, serum transaminase, and bilirubin. Common causes of hepatitis (e.g., drug-related hepatitis, cholestasis of sepsis, viral hepatitis, extrahepatic biliary obstruction) should be excluded before labeling a patient as having PN-related liver dysfunction.

Cessation of PN as soon as liver dysfunction is detected usually resolves the problem. This might not always be feasible; therefore, the initial management may be limited to reducing the calories and lipids provided, using cyclical parental nutrition, and administering ursodeoxycholic acid if oral intake is permitted (Lloyd and Gabe 2007; Guglielmi et al. 2008).

Enteral feeding may potentially cause specific problems, albeit less severe than those associated with parenteral feeding. Diarrhea and intolerance to enteral feeds may occur when hyperosmolar enteric formulas are given too rapidly. Even with iso-osmolar formulas, rapid feeding with boluses into the small intestine may result in abdominal discomfort, bloating, diarrhea, and hyperinsulinemic hypoglycemia (dumping syndrome). It is therefore crucial to select the appropriate formula, route, and rate of feeding to minimize these complications.

4.11.2 Access- or Catheter-Related Complications

Access- or catheter-related complications are related to the route of nutrient delivery. Complications involving nasogastric, nasojejunal, gastrostomy, and jejunostomy tubes in patients receiving EN include dislodgment, migration, or clogging. Misplacement of nasoenteric tubes into the respiratory passages can lead to aspiration and pneumonia. ASPEN recommends routine radiograph to confirm position of tubes prior to initiation of feeding (Bankhead et al. 2009). Migration of jejunal tubes proximally will result in feeds being delivered into the stomach which may result in high aspirates, vomiting, and aspiration.

Feeding tubes are prone to clogging due to the small diameter of the tubes, accumulation of formula sediment, and precipitations arising from interactions between medications and feeds within the tube. Regular water flushes are recommended to reduce the risk of clogging, usually 30 ml of water every 4 h (Bankhead et al. 2009).

Mechanical problems with intravenous access for PN include complications associated with the insertion of vascular access including:

- Pneumothorax
- Vascular injury
- Air embolism
- Cardiac arrhythmia
- Hemothorax

Serious complications post-insertion include sepsis and thrombosis. Catheter-related sepsis is an important complication which results in morbidity, prolonged hospitalization, increased costs, and an interruption to the patient's nutritional support. Infection may occur as a catheter-related bloodstream infection or an exit site infection. Catheter-related sepsis usually arises from a breach in sterility; therefore, any manipulation of the access ports (e.g., connecting a PN bag) should be performed in an aseptic manner after disinfection, and dressings at the catheter exit site should be kept dry at all times.

Although tunneled and cuffed catheters have lower risks of exit site infection as compared to non-tunneled catheters, they are at an equal risk of bloodstream infections if handled in a non-sterile manner. PN should not be administered via femoral catheters as the risks of infection and thrombosis are high. When a catheter-related infection is suspected, blood culture samples should be obtained from all lumens of the catheter and from a peripheral venipuncture. If an exit site infection is suspected (erythema with purulent discharge), then exit site swabs for microbial culture should be performed. If the catheter is confirmed to be the source of infection, it should be removed and a new catheter inserted at an alternative site (Phillips and Ponsky 2011).

Vascular access devices are foreign bodies which can trigger fibrin and thrombin accumulation resulting in thrombus formation. Occlusion may also occur from precipitates within the PN solution or from drug interactions. It is recommended that one lumen should be dedicated solely to PN. Prior to and after the administration of each bag of PN, the lumen should be flushed with saline to maintain and ensure patency (Phillips and Ponsky 2011). If a peripheral intravenous cannula is used to deliver PN, thrombophlebitis caused by the hypertonic solution and fluid extravasation are additional potential problems.

Other complications of PN arise as a result of the compounding process. As PN comprises of different nutrients, it is essential that the ingredients are mixed in a stable state. Instability leads to the separation of the individual components, especially lipids. Lipid separation results in a creamy layer ("creaming") seen at the top of the bag. Inadvertent administration of such a bag can result in fat embolism. The precipitation of calcium and phosphate salts is another stability issue. Incorrect preparation or excessive phosphate and calcium in the bag will cause precipitation and embolism when administered. Finally, all PN solutions should be sterile to prevent bacteremia and sepsis.

Conclusion

A significant number of patients with colorectal surgical problems are at risk of malnutrition, which negatively affects surgical outcomes, lengths of hospital stay, and cost of hospitalization. Nutritional risk screening in both the inpatient and outpatient setting is essential to detect patients who may benefit from further assessment and nutrition therapy. The ideal organization and management of any nutrition therapy is via an evidence-based transdisciplinary approach involving a team of physicians, nurses, dieticians, and pharmacists. Each colorectal surgeon should be aware of the risks and benefits of various nutrition therapy options available in the perioperative period in order to improve nutritional status and obtain optimal surgical outcomes.

References

Acuna K, Pires C, Santos G et al (2008) Detection of nosocomial malnutrition is improved in Amazon region by a standard clinical nutrition education program. Nutr Hosp 23:60–67

Amaral TF, Matos LC, Tavares MM et al (2007) The economic impact of disease-related malnutrition at hospital admission. Clin Nutr 26:778–784

Aosasa S, Mochizuki H, Yamamoto T et al (1999) A clinical study of the effectiveness of oral glutamine supplementation during total parenteral nutrition: influence on mesenteric mononuclear cells. J Parenter Enteral Nutr 23(Suppl 5):S41–S44

Baker JP, Detsky AS, Wesson DE et al (1982) Nutritional assessment: a comparison of clinical judgement and objective measurements. N Engl J Med 306:969–972

Bankhead R, Boullata J, Brantley S et al (2009) Enteral nutrition practice recommendations. J Parenter Enteral Nutr 33:122–167

Beattie AH, Prach AT, Baxter JP et al (2000) A randomized controlled trial evaluating the use of enteral nutritional supplements postoperatively in malnourished surgical patients. Gut 46:813–818

Bozzetti F, Gavazzi C, Miceli R et al (2000) Perioperative total parenteral nutrition in malnourished, gastrointestinal cancer patients: a randomized, clinical trial. J Parenter Enteral Nutr 24:7–14

Bozzetti F, Braga M, Gianotti L et al (2001) Postoperative enteral versus parenteral nutrition in malnourished patients with gastrointestinal cancer: a randomised controlled trial. Lancet 358:1487–1492

Braga M, Gianotti L, Gentilini O et al (2001) Early postoperative enteral nutrition improves gut oxygenation and reduces costs compared with total parenteral nutrition. Crit Care Med 29:242–248

Braga M, Gianotti L, Gentilini O et al (2002) Feeding the gut early after digestive surgery: results of a nine-year experience. Clin Nutr 21:59–65

Braga M, Ljungqvist O, Soeters P et al (2009) ESPEN guidelines on parenteral nutrition: surgery. Clin Nutr 28:378–386

Braunschweig C, Gomez S, Sheean PM (2000) Impact of declines in nutritional status on outcomes in adult patients hospitalized for more than 7 days. J Am Diet Assoc 100:1316–1322

Burden ST, Hill J, Shaffer JL, Campbell M, Todd C (2011) An unblinded randomised controlled trial of preoperative oral supplements in colorectal cancer patients. J Hum Nutr Diet 24:441–448

Carpentier YA, Sobotka L, Soeters P (2011) Substrates used in parenteral and enteral nutrition: carbohydrates. In: Lubos S, Simon PA, Alastair F et al (eds) Basics in clinical nutrition, 4th edn. Galen, Prague, pp 252–257

Cerantola Y, Hübner M, Grass F, Demartines N, Schäfer M (2011) Immunonutrition in gastrointestinal surgery. Br J Surg 98:37–48

Cheatham ML, Chapman WC, Key SP et al (1995) A meta-analysis of selective versus routine nasogastric decompression after elective laparotomy. Ann Surg 221:469–478

Chen Y, Liu BL, Shang B et al (2011) Nutrition support in surgical patients with colorectal cancer. World J Gastroenterol 17(13):1779–1786

Chima CS, Barco K, Dewitt MLA et al (1997) Relationship of nutritional status to length of stay, hospital costs, and discharge status of patients hospitalized in the medicine service. J Am Diet Assoc 97:975–978

Clark SF (2007) Vitamins and trace elements. In: Gottschlich MM (ed) The A.S.P.E.N. nutrition support core curriculum: a case-based approach —the adult patient, 1st edn. American Society for Parenteral and Enteral Nutrition, Maryland, pp 129–159

Correia MITD, Waitzberg DL (2003) The impact of malnutrition on morbidity, mortality, length of hospital stay and costs evaluated through a multivariate model analysis. Clin Nutr 22:235–239

De Cicco M, Panarello G, Chiaradia V et al (1989) Source and route of microbial colonization of parenteral nutrition catheters. Lancet 2:1258–1261

Detsky AS, McLaughlin JR, Baker JP et al (1987) What is subjective global assessment of nutritional status? J Parenter Enteral Nutr 11:8–13

Dhaliwal R, Jurewitsch B, Harrietha D et al (2004) Combined enteral and parenteral nutrition in critically ill patients: harmful or beneficial? A systematic review of the evidence. Intensive Care Med 30:1666–1671

Dieticians Association of Australia Nutrition Support Interest Group Manual (2011) Enteral nutrition manual for adults in health care facilities. Available at: http://daa.asn.au/wp-content/uploads/2011/11/Enteral-nutrition-manual-Oct-2011.pdf. Accessed 8 Aug 2013

Dissanaike S, Shelton M, Warner K et al (2007) The risk for bloodstream infections is associated with increased parenteral caloric intake in patients receiving parenteral nutrition. Crit Care 11:R114

Elia M (2000) Guidelines for detection and management of malnutrition. A report by the Malnutrition Advisory Group. The British Association for Parenteral and Enteral Nutrition, Maidenhead

Elia M (2005) Insights into energy requirements in disease. Public Health Nutr 8(7a):1037–1052

Ferguson M, Capra S, Bauer J et al (1999) Development of a valid and reliable malnutrition screening tool for adult acute hospital patients. Nutrition 15(6):458–464

Frankenfield DC, Smith JS, Cooney RN (2004) Validation of two approaches to predicting resting metabolic rate in critically ill patients. J Parenter Enteral Nutr 28:259–264

Fuhrman MP (2002) The albumin-nutrition connection: separating myth from fact. Nutrition 18:199–200

Furst P, Deutz NEP, Boirie Y et al (2011) Substrates used in parenteral and enteral nutrition: protein and amino acids. In: Lubos S, Simon PA, Alastair F et al (eds) Basics in clinical nutrition, 4th edn. Galen, Prague, pp 262–268

Gales BJ, Gales MJ (1994) Nutritional support teams: a review of comparative trials. Ann Pharmacother 28:227–235

Gibbs J, Cull W, Henderson W et al (1999) Preoperative serum albumin level as a predictor of operative mortality and morbidity. Arch Surg 134:36–42

Gout BS, Barker LA, Crowe TC (2009) Malnutrition identification, diagnosis and dietetic referrals: Are we doing a good enough job? Nutr Diet 66:206–211

Guglielmi FW, Regano N, Mazzuoli S et al (2008) Cholestasis induced by total parenteral nutrition. Clin Liver Dis 12:97–110

Gustafsson UO, Scott MJ, Schwenk W, Enhanced Recovery After Surgery Society et al (2012) Guidelines for perioperative care in elective colonic surgery: Enhanced Recovery After Surgery (ERAS®) Society recommendations. Clin Nutr 31:783–800

Han-Geurts IJM, Hop WCJ, Kok NFM et al (2007) Randomized clinical trial of the impact of early enteral feeding on postoperative ileus and recovery. Br J Surg 94:555–561

Haydock DA, Hill GL (1986) Impaired wound healing in surgical patients with varying degrees of malnutrition. J Parenter Enteral Nutr 10:550–554

Heidegger CP, Berger MM, Graf S et al (2013) Optimisation of energy provision with supplemental parenteral nutrition in critically ill patients: a randomised controlled clinical trial. Lancet 381:385–393

Heyland D, Muscedere J, Wischmeyer PE, Canadian Critical Care Trials Group et al (2013) A randomized trial of glutamine and antioxidants in critically ill patients. N Engl J Med 368:1489–1497

Hulsewé KW, van Acker BA, Hameeteman W et al (2004) Does glutamine-enriched parenteral nutrition really affect intestinal morphology and gut permeability? Clin Nutr 23:1217–1225

Jones NE, Heyland DK (2008) Pharmaconutrition: a new emerging paradigm. Curr Opin Gastroenterol 24:215–222

Jones C, Badger SA, Hannon R (2011) The role of carbohydrate drinks in pre-operative nutrition for elective colorectal surgery. Ann R Coll Surg Engl 93(7):504–507

Kaiser MJ, Bauer JM, Ramsch C et al (2010) Frequency of malnutrition in older adults: a multinational perspective using the mini nutritional assessment. J Am Geriatr Soc 58:1734–1738

Klein CJ, Stanek GS, Wiles CE 3rd (1998) Overfeeding macronutrients to critically ill adults: metabolic complications. J Am Diet Assoc 98:795–806

Kondrup J, Allison SP, Elia M et al (2003) ESPEN guidelines for nutrition screening 2002. Clin Nutr 22(4):415–421

Kudsk KA, Lauderkind A, Hanna MK (2001) Most infectious complications in parenterally fed trauma patients are not due to elevated blood glucose levels. J Parenter Enteral Nutr 25:174–179

Kudsk KA, Tolley EA, DeWitt RC et al (2003a) Preoperative albumin and surgical site identify surgical risk for major postoperative complications. JPEN J Parenter Enteral Nutr 27(1):1–9

Kudsk KA, Reddy SK, Sacks GS et al (2003b) Joint Commission for Accreditation of Health Care Organizations guidelines: too late to intervene for nutritionally at-risk surgical patients. J Parenter Enteral Nutr 27(4):288–290

Kulick D, Deen D (2011) Specialized nutrition support. Am Fam Physician 83:173–183

Kyle UG, Pirlich M, Lochs H et al (2005) Increased length of hospital stay in underweight and overweight patients at hospital admission: a controlled population study. Clin Nutr 24:133–142

Langley G (2007) Fluid, electrolytes, and acid-base disorders. In: Gottschlich MM (ed) The A.S.P.E.N. nutrition support core curriculum: a case-based approach —the adult patient, 1st edn. American Society for Parenteral and Enteral Nutrition, Maryland, pp 104–128

Lewis SJ, Andersen HK, Thomas S (2009) Early enteral nutrition within 24 h of intestinal surgery versus later commencement of feeding: a systematic review and meta-analysis. J Gastrointest Surg 13:569–575

Lim SL, Ong KCB, Chan YH et al (2012) Malnutrition and its impact on cost of hospitalization, length of stay, readmission and 3-year mortality. Clin Nutr 31:345–350

Ljungqvist O, Søreide E (2003) Preoperative fasting. Br J Surg 90:400–406

Lloyd DA, Gabe SM (2007) Managing liver dysfunction in parenteral nutrition. Proc Nutr Soc 66(4):530–538

Lohsiriwat V, Lohsiriwat D, Boonnuch W et al (2008) Pre-operative hypoalbuminemia is a major risk factor for postoperative complications following rectal cancer surgery. World J Gastroenterol 14:1248–1251

Manchanda SK (2003) Energy needs of the body. In: Talwar GP, Srivastavaby LM (eds) Textbook of biochemistry and human biology, 3rd edn. Prentice Hall of India Private Limited, New Delhi, p 472

Mayer K, Seeger W (2008) Fish oil in critical illness. Curr Opin Clin Nutr Metab Care 11:121–127

McClave SA, Martindale RG, Vanek VW et al (2009) Guidelines for the provision and assessment of nutrition support therapy in the adult critically ill patient: Society of Critical Care Medicine (SCCM) and American Society for Parenteral and Enteral Nutrition (ASPEN). J Parenter Enteral Nutr 33:277–316

McWhirter JP, Pennington CR (1994) Incidence and recognition of malnutrition in hospital. BMJ 308:945–948

Mehanna HM, Moledina J, Travis J (2008) Refeeding syndrome: what it is, and how to prevent and treat it. BMJ 336:1495–1498

Middleton MH, Nazarenko G, Nivison-Smith I et al (2001) Prevalence of malnutrition and 12-month incidence of mortality in two Sydney teaching hospitals. Intern Med J 31:455–461

Mirtallo J, Canada T, Johnson D, Task Force for the Revision of Safe Practices for Parenteral Nutrition et al (2004) Safe practices for parenteral nutrition. J Parenter Enteral Nutr 28(Suppl):S38–S70

Moore FA, Feliciano DV, Andrassy RJ et al (1992) Early enteral feeding, compared with parenteral, reduces postoperative septic complications. Ann Surg 216:172–183

Moureau N, Poole S, Murdock MA et al (2002) Central venous catheters in home infusion care: outcomes analysis in 50,470 patients. J Vasc Interv Radiol 13:1009–1016

Muhlebach S, Franken C, Stanga Z et al (2009) Practical handling of AIO admixtures – guidelines on parenteral nutrition. Ger Med Sci 7:Doc18. doi:10.3205/000077

Muhlebach S, Driscoll DF, Hardy G (2011) Pharmaceutical aspects of parenteral nutrition support. In: Lubos S, Simon PA, Alastair F et al (eds) Basics in clinical nutrition, 4th edn. Galen, Prague, pp 373–384

Mullen JL, Buzby GP, Matthews DC et al (1980) Reduction of operative morbidity and mortality by combined preoperative and postoperative nutritional support. Ann Surg 192:604–613

Nehme AE (1980) Nutritional support of the hospitalized patient, the team concept. JAMA · 243:1906–1908

Nelson R, Tse B, Edwards S (2005) Systematic review of prophylactic nasogastric decompression after abdominal operations. Br J Surg 92:673–680

Noblett SE, Watson DS, Huong H, Davison B, Hainsworth PJ, Horgan AF (2006) Pre-operative oral carbohydrate loading in colorectal surgery: a randomized controlled trial. Colorectal Dis 8(7):563–569

Nygren J, Thacker J, Carli F, Enhanced Recovery After Surgery Society et al (2012) Guidelines for perioperative care in elective rectal/pelvic surgery: Enhanced Recovery After Surgery (ERAS®) Society recommendations. Clin Nutr 31:801–816

Oguz M, Kerem M, Bedirli A et al (2007) L-alanin-L-glutamine supplementation improves the outcome after colorectal surgery for cancer. Colorectal Dis 9:515–520

Pertkiewicz M, Dudrick SJ (2011) Different systems for parenteral nutrition (AIO vs. MB). In: Lubos S, Simon PA, Alastair F et al (eds) Basics in clinical nutrition, 4th edn. Galen, Prague, pp 370–372

Pessaux P, Msika S, Atalla D et al (2003) Risk factors for postoperative infectious complications in non-colorectal abdominal surgery. Arch Surg 138:314–324

Phillips MS, Ponsky JL (2011) Overview of enteral and parenteral feeding access techniques: principles and practice. Surg Clin North Am 91:897–911

Pirlich M, Schutz T, Norman K et al (2006) The German hospital malnutrition study. Clin Nutr 25:563–572

Pittiruti M, Hamilton H, Biffi R et al (2006) ESPEN guidelines on parenteral nutrition: central venous catheters (access, care, diagnosis and therapy of complications). Clin Nutr 28:365–377

Planas M, Penalva A, Burgos R et al (2007) Guidelines for colorectal cancer: effects on nutritional intervention. Clin Nutr 26:691–697

Radd I, Davis S, Becker M et al (1993) Low infection rate and long durability of nontunneled silastic catheters. A safe cost-effective alternative for long-term venous access. Arch Intern Med 153:1791–1796

Rai J, Gill SS, Kumar BR (2002) The influence of preoperative nutritional status in wound healing after replacement arthroplasty. Orthopedics 25:417–421

Reissman P, Teoh TA, Cohen SM et al (1995) Is early oral feeding safe after elective colorectal surgery? A prospective randomized trial. Ann Surg 222:73–77

Rollins CJ, Elsberry VA, Pollack KA et al (1990) Three-in-one parenteral nutrition: a safe and economical method of nutritional support for infants. J Parenter Enteral Nutr 14:290–294

Ryder M (2006) Evidence-based practice in the management of vascular access devices for home parenteral nutrition therapy. J Parenter Enteral Nutr 30(Suppl):S82–S93

Schneider PJ (2006) Nutrition support teams: an evidence-based practice. Nutr Clin Pract 21:62–67

Schneider SM, Veyres P, Pivot X et al (2004) Malnutrition is an independent factor associated with nosocomial infections. Br J Nutr 92:105–111

Schwegler I, von Holzen A, Gutzwiller JP et al (2010) Nutritional risk is a clinical predictor of postoperative mortality and morbidity in surgery for colorectal cancer. Br J Surg 97:92–97

Scrimshaw NS, San Giovanni JP (1997) Synergism of nutrition, infection and immunity: an overview. Am J Clin Nutr 66(Suppl):464S–477S

Singh H, Watt K, Veitch R et al (2006) Malnutrition is prevalent in hospitalized medical patients: are housestaff identifying the malnourished patient? Nutrition 22:350–354

Smith I, Kranke P, Murat I, Smith A, O'Sullivan G, Søreide E, Spies C, in't Veld B, European Society of Anaesthesiology (2011) Perioperative fasting in adults and children: guidelines from the European Society of Anaesthesiology. Eur J Anaesthesiol 28(8):556–569

Soop M, Carlson GL, Hopkinson J, Clarke S, Thorell A, Nygren J, Ljungvist O (2004) Randomized clinical trial of the effects of immediate enteral nutrition on metabolic responses to major colorectal surgery in an enhanced recovery protocol. Br J Surg 91(9):1138–1145

Sorensen JM, Kondrup J, Prokopowicz J et al (2008) EuroOOPS: an internation, multicentre study to implement nutritional risk screening and evaluate clinical outcome. Clin Nutr 27:340–349

Sriram K, Cyriac T, Fogg LF (2010) Effect of nutritional support team restructuring on the use of parenteral nutrition. Nutrition 26:735–739

Stechmiller JK, Childress B, Porter T (2004) Arginine immunonutrition in critically ill patients: a clinical dilemma. Am J Crit Care 13:17–23

4 Transdisciplinary Management of Perioperative Nutrition

Stijn MFM, Korkic-Halilovic I, Bakker MSM et al (2013) Preoperative nutrition status and postoperative outcome in elderly general surgery patients: a systematic review. J Parenter Enteral Nutr 37:37–43

Studley HO (1936) Percentage of weight loss: a basic indicator of surgical risk in patients with chronic peptic ulcer. JAMA 106(6):458–460

The Veterans Affairs Total Parenteral Nutrition Cooperative Study Group (1991) Perioperative total parenteral nutrition in surgical patients. N Engl J Med 325:525–532

Vanek VW, Matarese LE, Robinson M, Novel Nutrient Task Force, Parenteral Glutamine Workgroup, American Society for Parenteral and Enteral Nutrition (A.S.P.E.N.) Board of Directors et al (2011) A.S.P.E.N. position paper: parenteral nutrition glutamine supplementation. Nutr Clin Pract 26:479–494

Vellas B, Guigoz Y, Garry PJ et al (1999) The Mini Nutritional Assessment (MNA) and its use in grading the nutritional state of elderly patients. Nutrition 15:116–122

Waitzberg DL, Caiaffa WT, Correia MITD (2001) Hospital malnutrition: the Brazilian national survey (IBRANUTRI): a study of 4000 patients. Nutrition 17:573–580

Weimann A, Braga M, Harsanyi L, Laviano A, Ljungqvist O, Soeters P et al (2006) ESPEN guidelines on enteral nutrition: surgery including organ transplantation. Clin Nutr 25:224–244

White JV, Guenter P, Jensen G et al (2012) Consensus statement of the Academy of Nutrition and Dietetics/American Society for Parenteral and Enteral Nutrition: characteristics recommended for the identification and documentation of adult malnutrition (undernutrition). J Acad Nutr Diet 112:730–738

Windsor JA, Hill GL (1988) Risk factors for postoperative pneumonia. The importance of protein depletion. Ann Surg 208:209–214

Wirtitsch M, Wessner B, Spittler A et al (2007) Effect of different lipid emulsions on the immunological function in humans: a systematic review with meta-analysis. Clin Nutr 26:302–313

World Health Organization. Ageing and life course. http://www.who.int/ageing/en. Accessed 15 Aug 2013

Xu J, Yunshi Z, Li R (2009) Immunonutrition in surgical patients. Curr Drug Targets 10(8):771–777

Yue C, Tian W, Wang W et al (2013) The impact of perioperative glutamine-supplemented parenteral nutrition on outcomes of patients undergoing abdominal surgery: a meta-analysis of randomized clinical trials. Am Surg 79:506–513

Zaloga GP (2006) Parenteral nutrition in adult inpatients with functioning gastrointestinal tracts: assessment of outcomes. Lancet 367:1101–1111

Enhanced Recovery

5

Edward Ratnasingham Shanthakumar
and Geraldine Pei-Chin Cheong

Take-Home Pearls

- Enhanced recovery program refers to a multidisciplinary and evidence-based approach to the perioperative management of patients undergoing surgery.
- The elements in the enhanced recovery protocol, divided into the pre-, intra-, postoperative and surgical factors, aim to reduce stress and improve recovery.
- A dedicated multidisciplinary team consisting of doctors, nurses and allied health personnel is the key to the success of the enhanced recovery program.

5.1 Introduction

Enhanced recovery program or "fast-track pathways" refers to a multidisciplinary and evidence-based approach to the perioperative management of patients undergoing surgery. Enhanced recovery program aims to achieve better patient outcomes and quicker recovery after surgery. The program also ensures that the patients are active participants in their own recovery process, and evidence-based treatments are given to them in the right time. This may result in benefits to both staff and patients.

Colorectal surgery is considered to be high-risk surgery especially because most of the patients are elderly with comorbidities. The indications for surgery in patients with colorectal disease are diverticular disease, inflammatory bowel disease, colonic cancer, ischaemic colitis, iatrogenic perforation or injury and volvulus. Since the introduction of the enhanced recovery program in elective procedures, it has been shown that length of hospital stay can be reduced along with reduction

---

E.R. Shanthakumar (✉)
Department of Anaesthesia, Khoo Teck Puat Hospital, Singapore, Singapore
e-mail: reshanthakumar@gmail.com

G.P.-C. Cheong
Department of Anaesthesia, Khoo Teck Puat Hospital, Singapore, Singapore

© Springer-Verlag Berlin Heidelberg 2015
K.-Y. Tan (ed.), *Transdisciplinary Perioperative Care in Colorectal Surgery:*
An Integrative Approach, DOI 10.1007/978-3-662-44020-9_5

in complications. It is also shown that the rates of readmissions are not increased (Kelliher et al. 2011). Some of the conditions mentioned may lead to emergency colorectal surgery where elements of enhanced recovery program may influence the outcomes as well.

The term "surgical stress response" describes the phenomenon of widespread changes in organ function mediated by the body's immunological, metabolic and endocrine reactions. Excessive stress response may cause a hypermetabolic state leading to an increased incidence of infective and noninfective complications involving major organ systems. In the 1990s, Henrik Kehlet proposed that a multimodal approach comprising preoperative, intraoperative, surgical and postoperative elements may help reduce the stress response. The hope was that stress-free anaesthesia and surgery would lead to quicker recovery with reduced morbidity and mortality (Kehlet 1997).

Enhanced recovery programs based on this approach were first developed for colorectal and intestinal surgery. Other surgical specialties subsequently developed their own pathways to improve outcomes after surgery.

Enhanced recovery programs generally include about 20 components or interventions during the perioperative period, requiring the active participation of a multidisciplinary team and the patient. The cornerstone for the success of this multimodal approach is the cooperation and enthusiasm of a multidisciplinary team of nurses, physiotherapists, pharmacists, dietitians, anaesthetists, physicians and surgeons (Fig. 5.1).

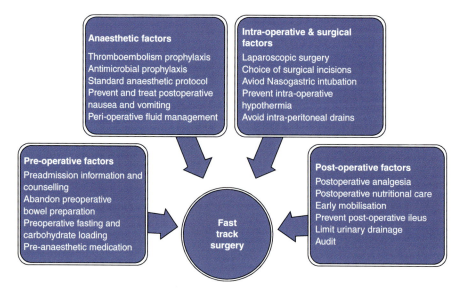

Fig. 5.1 Fast-track surgery pathways include various components divided into preoperative, anaesthetic, intraoperative and postoperative factors (Donohoe et al. 2011) (With permission from Elsevier Limited)

5.2 Preoperative Factors

5.2.1 Preoperative Evaluation and Optimization

The majority of patients undergoing colorectal surgical procedures may be elderly having significant comorbidities. It is important to optimize their condition by treating heart failure, diabetes mellitus, chronic obstructive pulmonary disease and renal disease. A preoperative assessment clinic managed by trained nurses and/or anaesthesiologists help to detect these comorbidities. Depending on the severity, the patients can then be referred to the cardiologists and other physicians for their optimization of their medical comorbidities.

Cardiopulmonary exercise testing, tests of frailty and functional capacity may help to identify patients who may need higher level of care perioperatively. Although pulmonary rehabilitation before lung resection has been proven valuable in certain groups of high-risk patients, studies of prehabilitation, in general, have produced equivocal results to date (Killewich 2006).

It may be speculative to presume that an attempt to improve nutritional status, better use of drugs and use of preoperative and postoperative physiotherapy to improve the grade of frailty would improve outcome at this stage. However, one may suspect that with the help of dietitians, pharmacists and physiotherapists in a multidisciplinary approach, prehabilitation might show benefit in well-defined patient groups. Examples of such patient groups are patients found to have poor anaerobic threshold on cardiopulmonary exercise testing or patients who are positive for being frail.

In our centre, the patients are assessed and started on a prehabilitation program by the physiotherapists with the aim of improving their frailty status. Their family members are also actively involved so that the patients can continue their prescribed exercises back in the community. For those who do not have caregivers at home, they are transferred to a rehabilitation hospital where collaborative rehabilitation plan is drawn out and instituted.

5.2.2 Preoperative Counselling

Explicit information regarding various aspects of the preoperative management, intraoperative surgical and anaesthetic procedures and postoperative recovery is given to the patients. This enables better recovery and improved pain relief postoperatively. Being well-informed, knowing what to expect and understanding how they can contribute to their recovery by mobilizing and feeding early appear to reduce the anxiety and stress related to surgery.

Interactive discussions between the patient and nurse facilitator with the aid of an information booklet can help elicit the patient's expectations and clarify queries about the procedure and recovery process. Patients who may need psychological assessment and therapy, especially those devastated by the diagnosis of a malignancy, can also be referred. Medical social workers can also be engaged to help out those in need of financial and social support.

5.2.3 Bowel Preparation

Bowel preparation causes dehydration and electrolyte imbalances (Holte et al. 2004) which may increase the risk of cardiac arrhythmias and diminished organ perfusion. Well-conducted RCTs have shown that bowel preparation is of no benefit and may even increase the incidence of anastomotic leaks and delay intestinal recovery. It is recommended that it should not be used unless there is a definitive need for it (e.g. intraoperative colonoscopy, total mesorectal excisions or ultra-low rectal tumour resections).

Whether or not bowel preparation is used, the decision should be communicated between the surgical team and anaesthesia team as the subsequent intraoperative electrolyte and fluid management may need to be altered.

5.2.4 Preoperative Fasting and Carbohydrate Loading

It was standard practice to fast patients for more than 6 h before surgery to prevent aspiration of gastric contents but a Cochrane review based on 22 RCTs has shown that it is safe for patients to have clear fluids up to 2 h before induction of anaesthesia. It is also recommended by various national anaesthesia societies that 6 h fasting for solids is adequate (Apfelbaum et al. 1999).

Carbohydrate drinks on the day before surgery and up to 2 h before surgery reduce thirst, provide calories to the patients, and reduce catabolism and the breakdown of body proteins. It has also been shown to reduce postoperative insulin resistance and hyperglycaemia facilitating an anabolic state to benefit from postoperative nutrition, hence allowing accelerated recovery and shorter hospital stay (Noblett et al. 2006).

In most uncomplicated patients, a standard dose of carbohydrate drinks can be given according to protocol. However, certain groups of patients such as those with diabetes mellitus may need a change in the concentration and dose of the carbohydrate drinks to ensure their blood glucose control remains stable. These require specialized expertise from the dietitians and pharmacists.

5.3 Anaesthetic Factors

5.3.1 Thromboembolism Prophylaxis

Both unfractionated heparin and low-molecular-weight heparins are equally effective in preventing deep vein thrombosis, pulmonary embolism and mortality. LMWH is preferred due to its convenient once-a-day dosing and reduced incidence of heparin-induced thrombocytopaenia. In patients who may have epidurals for analgesia, particular attention needs to be given to the timing of the heparin dose. It is advised that the epidural catheter should not be inserted or removed within 12 h of heparin use. In situations where heparin is contraindicated, other forms of prophylaxis such as dextrans, thromboembolism-deterrent stockings and calf compressors should be considered (Koch et al. 1997).

5.3.2 Antimicrobial Prophylaxis

It is recommended that intravenous antibiotics to cover aerobic and anaerobic organisms be given about 60 min before skin incision (Song and Gelnny 1998). There are also some suggestions that antibiotics given closer to the time of the incision may provide adequate protection. A second-generation cephalosporin and metronidazole are adequate. If surgery is prolonged, a second dose of antibiotic should be given.

It may be useful to consult the microbiologist about the specific microbiogram of the institution so that the prophylactic antibiotics may be targeted at the common organisms and their sensitivities.

5.3.3 Anaesthetic Management

The use of pre-anaesthetic medication may prolong sedation after surgery; hence they are avoided. Patients who are extremely anxious may have anxiolytics which have short half-life and no active metabolites.

The recommendation is to use short-acting drugs in either total intravenous anaesthetic or inhalational anaesthetic techniques. Drugs which may be suitable are propofol, remifentanil, sevoflurane and desflurane. Morphine and other long-acting opioids may delay recovery of intestinal motility; hence they are better avoided. Mid-thoracic epidurals may offer some advantages especially in open colorectal surgery as it may reduce the amounts of anaesthetic drugs, reduce the stress response, provide better analgesia perioperatively and potentiate immunological functions (Ahlers et al 2008). However, epidural analgesia has not been shown to improve postoperative outcome in laparoscopic surgery.

The role of the anaesthesiologists has evolved to encompass not only intraoperative anaesthetic management but also preoperative and postoperative considerations. The anaesthetic technique should be chosen after communication with the surgeons and patients, keeping in mind their effects on postoperative outcomes. It is more effective if the anaesthetic team begin their point of contact with the patient way before the day of the surgery so that perioperative plans can be suitably discussed.

5.3.4 Prevention of PONV

Some patients may feel postoperative nausea and vomiting (PONV) more stressful than the pain after surgery. The risk factors for PONV are female, nonsmoking status, motion sickness or previous PONV and use of long-acting opioids for pain control (Apfel et al. 2002). Patients who are at risk may be given prophylactic intravenous dexamethasone up to 8 mg, which was also shown to be associated with significantly lower interleukin-6 and interleukin-3 in peritoneal fluid and reduced early postoperative fatigue (Zargar-Shoshtari et al. 2009). Serotonin receptor antagonists such as ondansetron are better given near the end of surgery. Patients who are at high risk of PONV are recommended to have total intravenous anaesthesia with propofol and remifentanil. A small dose of droperidol and metoclopramide may be given in addition to the above-mentioned.

5.3.5 Perioperative Fluid Management

Traditionally the amount of intravenous fluids given perioperatively was much more than that of the actual loss. Patients appeared to gain about 3–4 kg in weight in the perioperative period. This approach can cause oedema affecting tissue oxygenation, delay the return of gastrointestinal function, impair wound and anastomotic healing and eventually lead to prolonged hospital stay (Brandstrup et al. 2003).

Goal-directed haemodynamic management using volume-, flow- or pressure-based goals has been used. It was thought that avoidance of hypovolaemia and maximum oxygen delivery to tissues and organs would be achieved with this approach. Fluids were given to achieve near maximal stroke volume by targeting maximal flow using a trans-oesophageal Doppler ultrasound probe. At times the fluid balance was positive with this approach.

Targeting zero fluid balance by calculating amount of fluid lost and replacing with the same amount of fluid and maintaining body weight is the restricted approach (Brandstrup et al. 2012). This is based on the hypothesis that excess fluids may cause interstitial oedema leading to cardiac and pulmonary complications and reduce tissue healing. It appears that maintaining adequate blood pressure is equally important as maintaining cardiac output to reduce the incidence of anastomotic leak. If the patient's blood pressure is low due to epidural analgesia, it is better treated with vasopressors instead of the traditional approach of fluid loading.

Dehydration can be avoided in the preoperative period by allowing clear oral fluids up to 2 h preoperatively and avoidance of bowel preparation. Postoperative fluid therapy should take into account maintenance requirements, sensible and insensible losses as well as pathophysiological changes causing fluid shift associated with bowel surgery. The best way to limit postoperative fluid intake is to stop intravenous fluids and return to oral fluids at the earliest.

Fluid management in the postoperative period is usually more difficult as fluid status and deficits are difficult to quantify without sophisticated tools like those used intraoperatively. Blood pressure readings and urine output monitoring are often poor surrogate measures of actual tissue perfusion. Often numerous doctors, including surgical team doctors, acute pain service team and junior doctors on duty at night, are involved in the management in the ward. A conscious team effort and awareness about avoiding fluid overload should be emphasized during the ward rounds and training.

5.4 Intraoperative Factors

5.4.1 Surgical Factors

By causing smaller area of injury, laparoscopic surgery may be considered to cause less stress response. Meta-analyses confirmed that significant improvements in short term outcomes are achievable by laparoscopic-assisted surgery as a single intervention. However, the advent of laparoscopic surgery and fast-track protocols coincided with each other and hence there is not enough evidence to show that laparoscopic-assisted surgery when compared to open surgery within an enhanced recovery program will shorten recovery time and reduce length of hospital stay (Tjandra and Chan 2006).

Incisions may be vertical, transverse or curved when open surgery is performed. Even though some RCTs suggest transverse or curved incisions lead to less pulmonary complications and pain, others have found no advantages (Grantcharov and Rosenberg 2001). A Cochrane review of RCTs showed that complication rates and recovery times were not different from vertical midline incisions. It appears that the size and direction of incisions made by surgeons depend on the anticipated difficulty from factors such as scan findings and previous scars.

5.4.2 Avoidance of Nasogastric Tubes

Patients who do not have nasogastric tubes for decompression of the stomach appear to have lower incidence of pneumonia, fever and atelectasis. A Cochrane review and meta-analysis confirmed this by finding that patients, whose stomachs were not decompressed, had earlier return of bowel function (Nelson et al. 2007). At times significant amount of air may enter the stomach at induction of anaesthesia prior to intubation, compromising surgical approach. If this happens, the stomach may be decompressed with a nasogastric tube intraoperatively. It is advised that this be removed before emergence from anaesthesia.

5.4.3 Prevention of Intraoperative Hypothermia

Anaesthesia-related factors and heat loss from exposed organs lead to hypothermia during surgery. Postoperative cardiac complications and coagulation abnormalities are aggravated by hypothermia. Hypothermia can also cause systemic changes such as exaggerated stress response and suppression of immune function. It is recommended that the temperature of the patient is maintained above 35 °C by using warmed fluid and external warming.

5.4.4 Avoidance of Intraperitoneal Drains

Drainage of peritoneal cavity was previously considered to be useful in preventing or detecting anastomotic leak early. But a meta-analysis has not shown that this is true. There may be some benefit if peritoneal drainage is performed in patients with very low anterior resections (Karliczek et al. 2006).

5.5 Postoperative Factors

5.5.1 Prevention of Postoperative Ileus

A key element of enhanced recovery is the prevention of postoperative ileus. It is a common cause of delayed recovery and discharge from hospital. Prokinetic agents have not been proven to be effective. In addition, some have been shown to have adverse effects on cardiac conduction.

Mid-thoracic epidural, through the effect on the sympathetic nervous system, improves intestinal motility compared to intravenous patient-controlled analgesia using opioids (Marret et al. 2007). Plasma electrolytes, particularly potassium concentrations, can influence intestinal motility. Fluid overloading is to be avoided in the perioperative period as it has been shown to impair intestinal motility. By reducing the amount of bowel handling, the laparoscopic approach leads to faster return of bowel function.

5.5.2 Postoperative Analgesia

In enhanced recovery, the main aim is to provide adequate analgesia with minimum amount of opioids. Inadequate analgesia leads to delayed mobilization, decreased appetite and prolonged ileus. For open surgery mid-thoracic epidural is recommended because it reduces stress response and provides optimal analgesia. For laparoscopic surgery and open surgery with smaller incisions, there are other recommended opioid-sparing techniques using local anaesthetic drugs (Moiniche et al. 1998).

Techniques available and found to be beneficial are transversus abdominis plane block (continuous or single injection); pre-peritoneal catheters inserted by surgeons at the end of surgery, before closing the abdomen; and intrathecal and wound infusions of local anaesthetics. Systemic analgesia techniques are patient-controlled analgesia using opioids and lidocaine infusions. The best chance of achieving minimal stress response is attained by optimal pain control using any of the combinations of multimodal analgesia taking into account the patients' pain threshold, associated medical conditions, allergies and possible side effects. Paracetamol regularly up to 4 g/day and NSAIDS (in patients with no contraindications) may be added as part of multimodal analgesia.

A dedicated acute pain team comprising of a specialized pain nurse and anaesthesiologist can review the patients in the ward daily to ensure their analgesia is

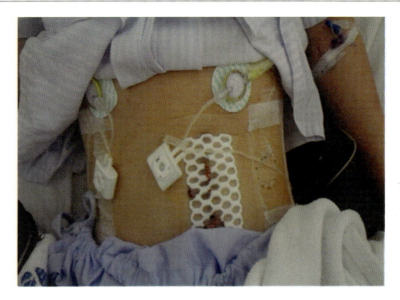

Fig. 5.2 Bilateral transversus abdominis plane block with catheters inserted for continuous infusion via elastomeric pumps for a patient who underwent open right hemicolectomy

adequate without any excessive side effects. As the acute pain round often provides a snapshot review of the patient's pain control, it may not be truly reflective of his/her pain during specific stimulus like ambulation. Timely feedback from the surgeons, nurses and physiotherapists can then ensure prompt troubleshooting and enhancement of the analgesia (Fig. 5.2).

5.5.3 Postoperative Nutritional Care

RCTs have shown that keeping patients nil-by-mouth has no advantage over early enteral or oral feeding postoperatively. Contrary to previous thinking, enteral nutrition does not seem to increase the incidence of anastomotic dehiscence. Presence of food/nutrition in the gastrointestinal tract appears to be the best prokinetic agent especially when it is known that some prokinetic agents may have deleterious side effects. Early enteral feeds have advantages such as improved healing of anastomosis, preservation of gut barrier functions, positive nitrogen balance and reduced incidence of infections. Provision of calories reduces muscle and visceral protein breakdown (Patel et al. 2012). There may be a higher chance of bloating, impaired pulmonary function and delayed mobilization when patients are fed early. Early mobilization and upright position in bed may help to circumvent this.

Patients who are malnourished and whose nutritional status preoperatively was not known benefit by oral nutritional supplements for 8 weeks. This appears to improve nutritional status, protein balance and quality of life (Beattie et al. 2000).

Oral intake should be encouraged from the day of surgery along with oral nutritional supplements until normal food intake is possible.

5.5.4 Early Mobilization

Early mobilization improves gut function. Bed rest postoperatively results in insulin resistance, breakdown of muscles, decreased muscle strength, worsened pulmonary function and poorer tissue oxygenation. There is also an increased risk of thromboembolism. Effective pain relief is the key adjuvant which facilitates early mobilization. Ambulatory thoracic epidural analgesia especially in open surgery is probably the best way to achieve this. Other techniques such as transversus abdominis plane catheters, pre-peritoneal catheters and paravertebral catheters may also be considered.

A scheduled care plan that has been discussed with the patient at the preoperative visit and agreed upon may help to motivate patients to participate actively during physiotherapy and mobilization. Patients are encouraged to sit out for 2 h on day of surgery and 6 h or more per day until discharge. Urinary catheters and abdominal drains can restrict mobility and should be removed at the earliest possible time.

Some centres encourage patients to mobilize by modifying the hospital environment such as having a separate dining and television room in the ward. These centres engage the help of healthcare attendants in the ward to help these patients mobilize while preventing unnecessary falls. The healthcare attendants, nurses and physiotherapists also need to communicate well to ensure the rehabilitation milestones for each individual patient are appropriate (Figs. 5.3 and 5.4).

5.5.5 Audit

A Cochrane review comprising 188 studies has revealed that audit and feedback can be effective in improving professional practice (Jemtvedt et al. 2006). When a new protocol is implemented, it is vital to study what is the compliance rate, what may be the reasons why compliance is poor and how successful it is in achieving the desired goals. The main goals in enhanced recovery are reduced length of hospital stay, postoperative complications, readmissions rates, mortality and expedited recovery of function back to the patients' premorbid status. It may also be prudent to consider patient satisfaction with the whole journey as an important factor.

5.6 Does Enhanced Recovery Work?

The success or failure of enhanced recovery should not only be defined in terms pertaining to the clinicians, nurses, bed management unit and hospital accountants. Ultimately, the patients' perspectives in the quality of care and recovery

5 Enhanced Recovery   87

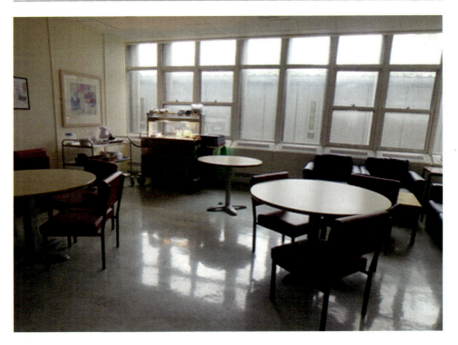

Fig. 5.3 The use of a dining area in the colorectal ward of St Mark's Hospital to encourage patients to mobilize after the surgery

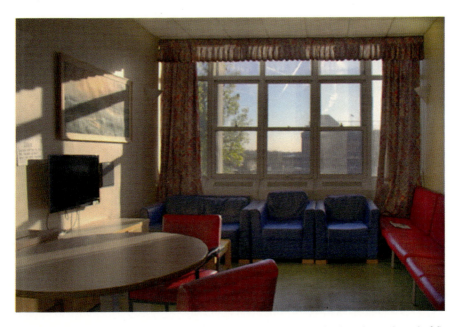

Fig. 5.4 The day room containing a television and reading material in the colorectal ward of St Mark's Hospital to encourage patient to mobilize

may also need to be measured. Success and failure may be measured broadly in these ways:

1. Outcomes such as length of hospital stay
2. Functional recovery
3. Patient satisfaction
4. Compliance with the enhanced recovery protocol

Colorectal surgery was associated with complication rates of 15–20 % and mean postoperative inpatient stays of 6–11 days. A systematic review has found that enhanced recovery protocols in colorectal surgery have a role in reducing postoperative morbidity and result in accelerated recovery. However they failed to find from the available evidence that these protocols reduce hospital readmissions or mortality (Rawlinson et al. 2011). A prospective RCT of multimodal perioperative management protocol in patients undergoing elective colorectal resection for cancer provides good evidence that a multimodal recovery program can significantly shorten hospital stay. There also appears to be faster return of function without concomitant increase in complications (Khan et al. 2010).

Functional recovery may be measured in the form of gastrointestinal function, patient mobility and health-related quality of life assessment. Early return of bowel function in enhanced recovery may be attributed to early oral nutrition, opioid-sparing analgesia with the use of regional techniques such as epidural analgesia, early mobilization and restrictive fluid management in the perioperative period. A clear benefit has not been shown yet for either laparoscopic or open surgery along with enhanced recovery in the gastrointestinal recovery or physical recovery. A definitive answer as to whether early discharge within enhanced recovery had any deleterious effect on quality of life and patient satisfaction has not been found. But from the limited evidence available, it may be suggested that enhanced recovery does not adversely influence quality of life or psychomotor functions such as sleep quality, pain and fatigue levels after surgery.

Enhanced recovery pathway consists of about 20 different component steps. Which of these have a major role in the outcome of individual patients is difficult to define. It appears that the ultimate success of the program relies on adapting as many elements of the pathway as possible and a piecemeal adoption usually results in a failure of the program (Gustafsson et al. 2011). An association between improved protocol adherence and postoperative outcomes has been demonstrated in a large observational study. It is worth noting that all preoperative elements influenced postoperative outcomes but intravenous fluid management and preoperative carbohydrate drinks appear to be the major independent predictors.

Although there appears to be high compliance with pre- and intraoperative elements, the compliance with postoperative measures is at best seen to be about 65 %. Early mobilization, feeding and discontinuation of intravenous fluids, as well as epidural analgesia, showed a compliance rate of only 40–50 %. Failure to comply with the postoperative elements appears to be influenced by the outcomes of pre- and intraoperative elements; hence, "deviation" instead of "failure of compliance" is generally used in the postoperative pathway.

In the clinical setting, it is sometimes important to consider the individual patient and modify the treatment plan according to patient status rather than following the entire protocol religiously. Some aspects of the protocol may not be suitable for some patients. This is the reason why numerous healthcare workers with different expertise need to collaborate together in the decisions made for the individual patient.

Preoperative prediction of success or failure of enhanced recovery is difficult. Observations made by the National Patient Safety Agency in the United Kingdom after reviewing the circumstances behind missed complications lead to the conclusion that in addition to standard postoperative monitoring and early warning scores, a patient safety check list during the second 12-h period should determine the presence of certain symptoms and signs (National Patient Safety Agency – NHS).

> **Symptoms and Signs During the Second 12-h Postoperative Period**
> Abdominal pain needing opioid analgesia
> Anorexia or reluctance to drink
> Reluctance to mobilize
> Nausea
> Vomiting
> Tachycardia
> Abdominal tenderness
> Abdominal distension
> Poor urine output
> Cardiac arrhythmia

Recognizing these factors is the key to identifying complications at an early stage. This does not have to lead to withdrawal of the enhanced recovery pathway but consideration may be given to tailor the pathway for individual patients. Deviation can be a warning sign providing an opportunity to detect complications or impaired functional capacity and to take remedial action at an early stage.

Conclusion

What was initially described as fast-track surgery and multimodal surgical approach has evolved into enhanced recovery pathway over the years since 1990s. Preoperative explicit information to patients encourages them to be part of their own recovery, makes them aware of the importance of the preoperative carbohydrate drinks and prepares them to mobilize and take oral nutrition early after surgery. They may be convinced that postoperative pain is taken seriously by the team looking after them and there are various ways to control pain. It is shown that these measures lead to reduced stress response and insulin resistance.

Intraoperative management concentrates on minimally invasive and less traumatic approaches depending on factors such as previous abdominal surgery, location of pathology and anticipated complications with different techniques. Anaesthetic management includes short-acting drugs and techniques avoiding

Fig. 5.5 An elderly lady on postoperative day 1 after an open anterior resection. She was given bilateral transversus abdominis plane block with continuous infusion of 0.1 % ropivacaine via elastomeric pumps. She had enhanced recovery and was discharged home on postoperative day 4

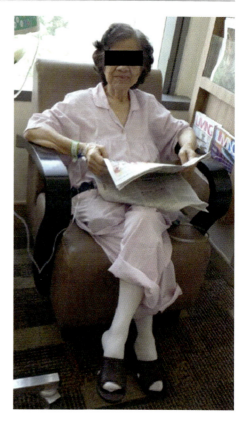

drowsiness and lethargy following surgery, hence facilitating early mobility. An important aspect of early mobility is adequate analgesia with minimal opioid usage. Mid-thoracic epidural especially in open surgery and other regional analgesic techniques such as pre-peritoneal catheters, paravertebral catheters and transversus abdominis plane catheters are preferred. A multimodal approach using oral and parenteral drugs on a regular basis is known to improve analgesia. Recent developments appear to be recommending a restrictive fluid therapy in the perioperative period replacing only the actual losses.

Satisfactory postoperative management starts in the pre- and intraoperative period. Deviations are sometimes tailored according to patient status. Reduction of incidence PONV can be achieved by intraoperative use of prophylactic medication in high-risk patients. It is suggested that antiemetics may be started when patients start early oral or enteral feeds and de-escalate once nutritional intake is well established. Patients are encouraged to mobilize very early and adequate support should be provided to prevent falls.

A team of professionals dedicated to implementing enhanced recovery pathways can range from doctors, nurses, dietitians, physiotherapists and pharmacists. This team and the patients who understand how they can contribute to a good outcome are the key stakeholders in ensuring success in the enhanced recovery program (Fig. 5.5).

References

Ahlers O et al (2008) Intraoperative thoracic epidural anaesthesia attenuates stress induced immune suppression in patients undergoing major abdominal surgery. Br J Anaesth 101:781–787

Apfel CC et al (2002) Comparison of predictive models for post operative nausea and vomiting. Br J Anaesth 88(2):234–240

Apfelbaum JL et al (1999) Practice guidelines for preoperative fasting and the use of pharmacologic agents to reduce the risk of pulmonary aspiration: application to healthy patients undergoing elective procedures: a report by the American Society of Anaesthesiologist Task Force on Preoperative Fasting. Anesthesiology 90(3):896–905

Beattie AH, Prach AT, Baxter JP, Pennigton CR (2000) A randomized controlled trial evaluating the use of enteral nutritional supplements post operatively in malnourished surgical patients. Gut 46(6):813–818

Brandstrup B, Tonnesen H, Beier-Holgersen R et al (2003) Danish Study Group on peri operative fluid therapy. Effects of intravenous fluid restriction on postoperative complications: comparison of two perioperative fluid regimens: a randomized assessor blinded multicenter trial. Ann Surg 238(5):641–648

Brandstrup B et al (2012) Which goal for fluid therapy during colorectal surgery is followed by the best outcome: near – maximal stroke volume or zero fluid balance? Br J Anaesth 109(2):191–199

Donohoe CL et al (2011) Fast-track protocols in colorectal surgery. Surgeon 9:95–103

Grantcharov TP, Rosenberg J (2001) Vertical compared with transverse incisions in abdominal surgery. Eur J Surg 167(4):260–267

Gustafsson UO et al (2011) Adherence to the enhanced recovery after surgery protocol and outcomes after colorectal cancer surgery. Arch Surg 146(5):571–577

Holte K, Nielson KG, Madsen JL, Kehlet H (2004) Physiologic effects of bowel preparation. Dis Colon Rectum 47(8):1397–1402

Jemtvedt G et al (2006) Audit and feed back: effects on professional practice and healthcare outcomes. Cochrane Database Syst Rev (2):CD000259

Karliczek A et al (2006) Drainage or non drainage in elective colorectal anastomosis: a systematic review and meta analysis. Colorectal Dis 8(4):259–265

Kehlet H (1997) Multimodal approach to control postoperative pathophysiology and rehabilitation. Br J Anaesth 87(1):62–72

Kelliher L, Jones C, Day A et al (2011) Optimising perioperative patient care 'enhanced recovery' following colorectal surgery. J Perioper Med 21(7):239–243

Khan S et al (2010) Quality of life and patient satisfaction with enhanced recovery protocols. Colorectal Dis 12(12):1175–1182

Killewich LA (2006) Strategies to minimize postoperative de conditioning in elderly surgical patients. J Am Coll Surg 203(5):735–745

Koch A et al (1997) Low molecular weight heparin and unfractionated heparin in thrombosis prophylaxis and after major surgical intervention: update of previous meta -analyses. Br J Surg 84(6):750–759

Laparoscopic surgery: failure to recognize post operative deterioration. National Patient Safety Agency – NHS (2010) National reporting and learning service. Central Alert System (CAS) reference: NPSA/2010/RRR016

Marret E et al (2007) Post operative Pain Forum Group. Meta analysis of epidural analgesia vs parenteral opioid analgesia after colorectal surgery. Br J Surg 94(6):665–667

Moiniche S et al (1998) A qualitative systematic review of incisional local anesthesia for post operative pain relief after abdominal operations. Br J Anaesth 81(3):377–383

Nelson R et al (2007) Prophylactic nasogastric decompression after abdominal surgery. Cochrane Database Syst Rev (3):CD004929

Noblett SE et al (2006) Pre operative oral carbohydrate loading in colorectal surgery: a randomized controlled trial. Colorectal Dis 8(7):563–569

Patel S et al (2012) Anaesthesia and peri operative management of colorectal surgical patients – a clinical review (part 1). J Anaesthesiol Clin Pharmacol 28(2):162–170

Rawlinson A et al (2011) A systematic review of enhanced recovery protocols in colorectal surgery. Ann R Coll Surg Engl 93:583–588

Song F, Gelnny AM (1998) Antimicrobial prophylaxis in colorectal surgery: antimicrobial prophylaxis in colorectal surgery: a systematic review of randomized controlled trials. Br J Surg 85(9):1232–1241

Tjandra JJ, Chan MK (2006) Systematic review on the short- term outcome of laparoscopic resection for colon and recto sigmoid cancer. Colorectal Dis 8(5):375–388

Zargar-Shoshtari K, Sammour T, Kahokehr A, Connolly AB, Hill AG (2009) Randomized clinical trial of the effect of glucocorticoids on peritoneal inflammation and post operative recovery after colectomy. Br J Surg 96:1253–1261

The Role of a Pharmacist in a Transdisciplinary Geriatric Surgery Team

6

Doreen Su-Yin Tan and Adeline Hsiao-Huey Wee

Take-Home Pearls
- The pharmacist plays a key role in medication reconciliation in elderly surgical patients.

6.1 Introduction: Ageing and the Use of Medication

Polypharmacy can refer to the prescribing of many medicines (five or more medicines are often quoted) or to the addition of inappropriate medicines to an existing regime. It appeared in medical literature more than 150 years ago and thus is not an unfamiliar term. Why is there a need to talk about polypharmacy in a general surgery population? The number of chronic medicine that patients receive has increased over the years. The following paragraphs will sought to explain why.

The American Food and Drug Administration approved 188 novel agents within the period of 2005–2012 (Downing et al. 2014). The explosion medications in use today, the practice of "evidence-based medicine" and the emergence of multiple guidelines have led to the use of medications in order to achieve preset goals, mostly also accepted as "key performance indicators". Unfortunately, clinical trials often "cherry-pick" subjects which enter their study, much unlike our real-world patients who often have multiple comorbid conditions. As a patient ages and "accumulates" diagnoses and/or specialty doctors whom they follow up with, it is hardly surprising that the number of medications they are taking proportionately increases with their number of comorbidities and with increasing doctors. We carried out prevalence studies of our own patients. Approximately 200 ambulatory cardiology and diabetic subjects interviewed, average age of 59 years, have an average of 6 line items. Our survey of over 400 readmission subjects to our

---

D.S.-Y. Tan, PharmD, BCPS (AQ Cardio) (✉) • A.H.-H. Wee, PharmD, BCPS
Department of Pharmacy, Khoo Teck Puat Hospital, Singapore, Singapore
e-mail: tan.doreen.sy@alexandrahealth.com.sg; wee.adeline.hh@alexandrahealth.com.sg

© Springer-Verlag Berlin Heidelberg 2015
K.-Y. Tan (ed.), *Transdisciplinary Perioperative Care in Colorectal Surgery: An Integrative Approach*, DOI 10.1007/978-3-662-44020-9_6

hospital, in the period of January to March 2013, revealed that these subjects received an average of 10 line items. Their mean age was 67 years. The average number of line items increased to 12 in our home visitation population, whose mean age is 73 years. Approximately 70 % of the 165 subjects were receiving at least 11 line items. The data seems to suggest that as people age, the number of chronic medications increase.

The probability of clinically relevant and potentially serious drug-drug interactions is strongly associated with the number of medicines dispensed (Johnell and Klarin 2007). People taking five concurrent medicines have a 50 % probability of at least one drug interaction; each additional medicine adds an additional 12 % increase in risk of drug interactions. The number of possible drug-drug interactions rises sharply when five or more medicines are concurrently administered. Small increases in number of medicines would make larger difference in the number of potential drug-drug interactions. This is of particular importance in the peri- and post-surgery period where additional medications may be administered, predisposing patients to a risk of potentially harmful drug-drug interactions.

Medication reconciliation is carried out for all patients in the Geriatric Surgical Service (GSS) by the pharmacist. Medication reconciliation (MR) is the practice of reviewing and comparing a patient's medication regimen throughout care transitions to prevent unintentional discrepancies. It has become an area of focus for patient safety organizations, such as the World Health Organization, The Joint Commission, and the Institute for Healthcare Improvement. The main goal of medication reconciliation is to develop systematic processes that will prevent omissions and duplications of medications, additionally, to reduce inappropriate therapy. For patients who may be on antihypertensives or anticoagulants and/or antiplatelets, there should be clear instructions on their management during the preoperative period as well as when these medications need to be discontinued and then when to be resumed afterward. Without such comprehensive history taking and clear instructions, adverse events can commonly occur post discharge, including incorrect resumption of medications discontinued in the hospital, failure to restart critical medications like antiplatelets for the prevention of stent thrombosis, or failure to start taking new medications. Medication reconciliation has been shown to reduce the rate of medication errors from 213 per 100 admissions to 62 per 100 admissions. The most common error made in the postoperative period was failure to order home medications (Orser et al. 2013). As such, it can be seen that careful medication reconciliation at admission and then again at discharge not only reduces preventable adverse drug events, it also reduces healthcare costs.

6.2 The Approach to the Elderly Surgical Patient

1. Work up patient's background: A list of medical problems and relevant social history (smoking, alcohol consumption, etc.) should be obtained and documented clearly.
2. Medication reconciliation: A proper and holistic medication list and doses of medications which the patient is actually taking should be solicited and matched against the patient's active problem list. Any medications without indication or indication without treatment should be investigated.

3. Determine renal function: Whenever assessing an aged surgical patient, one must always estimate renal function using the Crockroft-Gault (CG) equation. Due consideration must be paid to ensure that the patient is not too positive in his/her urine output or drains. There are quirks of medications used in poor renal function that pharmacists must be mindful of when suggesting or initiating medications which are commonly used for a younger patient with greater reserve. It is noteworthy that the CG is not accurate when renal function is rapidly fluctuating.

4. Note relevant laboratory and vital parameters: Full blood count, liver panel, lipid panel, glucose monitoring panel and glycated haemoglobin, prothrombin time/international normalised ratio (PT/INR), activated partial thromboplastin time (aPTT), and thyroid function test where applicable.

5. Note old medications and consider important drug-drug interactions which can possibly occur; examples include but are not limited to:

    (a) Antihypertensives, e.g. angiotensin-converting enzyme inhibitors (ACEi), angiotensin receptor blockers (ARBs), hydrochlorothiazide, loop diuretics, and Non-steroidal anti-inflammatory drugs/cyclooxygenase II inhibitor NSAID/COXII use or electrolyte replacement and monitoring

    (b) Sulphonylureas and/or insulins and fluoroquinolones, erythromycin, and clarithromycin

    (c) Metformin and volume contraction postoperatively

    (d) Antidiabetic medications and poor oral intake or friable blood glucose

    (e) Anticoagulant warfarin and antibiotics, NSAIDs, fever, poor oral intake, and protracted diarrhoea; how many days has warfarin been stopped? Is international normalised ratio at a level for which the surgeon is comfortable to operate on?

    (f) Baseline central nervous system suppressants (e.g. benzodiazepines, antidepressants) and opiates

The above form the basic fodder for considerations of drug dosing and adjustments and any drug-drug and drug-disease interactions which may arise in the acute course of the perioperative and postoperative periods.

6.3 Preoperative Considerations

Preoperatively, there are perhaps two key areas to pay rapt attention to. Firstly, for patients on antihypertensives, antidiabetic agents, and anticoagulants and/or antiplatelets, extra care should be taken to monitor for drug interactions and the adjustments or starting/stopping them. Secondly, patients on medications which are highly likely to interact with medications used in the postoperative setting should be highlighted and alternatives should be used.

Patients who have been on previous antihypertensives that are commonly used for patients with congestive heart failure, diabetic nephropathy, and hypertension, including angiotensin-converting enzyme inhibitors (ACEi) and angiotensin receptor blockers (ARBs), increase the risk of severe and refractory hypotension under general anaesthesia (Coriat et al. 1994; Orser et al. 2013). It has been suggested that stopping these drugs the day before surgery may reduce the risk of serious intraoperative hypotension (Orser et al. 2013). However, care should be taken to ensure that these medications may be safely withheld.

Diabetics are particularly tricky to take care of, particularly the older ones who are likely to be frail. The additional consideration of these patients who may be kept nil by mouth before and during the postoperative period makes restarting regular medications trickier. In particular, if diabetes was well-controlled with recent glycated haemoglobin levels of low 6 % or in the region of 5 %, more care needs to be taken to balance the oral intake, carefully considering nutritional supplementation postoperatively and the restarting of regular medications, particularly sulphonylureas and insulins.

The next group of patients would be those who are on anticoagulants warfarin and antiplatelets like aspirin. Special attention should be given for atrial fibrillation subjects who have been on long-term warfarin as it should be discontinued only for a minimal number of days. There are newer oral anticoagulants like apixaban, edoxaban, rivaroxaban, and dabigatran which would warrant a proper bridging plan because of the shorter half-life, more rapid onset/offset, and irreversibility of anticoagulation effects. To add on to the complexity of the situation, in order to determine how long before offset safe for surgery, the patients' renal function would have to be taken into deliberation. Some anticoagulation services should be available to advise on how to bridge anticoagulants. The avenues of bridging should be explored at least 2 weeks in advance so that there is time to arrange for coverage and counselling with the use of parenterals such as low-molecular-weight heparins. Subjects on warfarin are at risk for unintended medication discontinuation after elective ambulatory procedures and even after overnight hospital stays (Bell et al. 2006). Thus, we recommend that a clear set of instructions on when to resume therapy should be passed to the inpatient team taking care of the patient post operation, the patient, and the patient's caregivers.

Subjects with recent cardiac events, especially with a coronary stent inserted in within the last year, should be receiving two antiplatelets, usually aspirin and clopidogrel. However, new antiplatelets prasugrel and ticagrelor may be used as well.

6.4   Postoperative Care

The pharmacist continues to be an important figure in the patient's therapy even after the operation. Post-op medication management is as important to the success of the program as preoperative medication management. Postoperative complications such as blood loss resulting in hypotension may necessitate withholding antihypertensive therapy. Possible drug interactions between new post-op orders and existing therapy which require therapeutic substitution, recommending appropriate antibiotic use, reducing adverse effects from the use of opioids for analgesia, and drug dose adjustments in renal impairment, are all important roles the GSS pharmacist plays as he/she reviews the patient's medications.

Postoperative hypertension should be evaluated carefully and reversible causes like pain, volume contraction, hypercarbia, hypoxia, agitation, and bladder distension should be adequately managed prior to correction of blood pressure. This should be observed except in the setting of hypertension emergency which is

6 The Role of a Pharmacist in a Transdisciplinary Geriatric Surgery Team 97

Table 6.1 Intravenous antihypertensive medications

Drug	Dose	Time of action	Considerations and adverse effects
Labetalol	Loading dose 20 mg followed by 20–80 mg every 10 min, up to total 300 mg. May consider 1–2 mg/min infusion titrated until desired effect has been achieved (max total 300 mg)	Onset in 2–5 min, peaks at 5–15 min and lasts 2–18 h (accumulative effects) Elimination half-life:~ 5.5 h	Should not be used in patients with uncompensated heart failure, bradycardia, heart block greater than 1st degree (except if on functioning pacemaker), bronchospasm
Nitroglycerin	The starting dose is 5 μg/min; it can be titrated at 5 μg/min every 3–5 min; after dose exceeds 20 μg/min, it can be increased by 10–20 μg/min, up to max 400 μg/min	Onset almost immediate, duration of action 3–5 min	Hypotension particularly in volume depletion and right ventricular infarction and reflex tachycardia. Tachyphylaxis onset within 24–48 h. Methaemoglobinaemia with prolonged infusion
Hydralazine	IV bolus: 3–20 mg repeated every 1–4 h as needed	Onset in 5–20 min; drop in BP can last up to 12 h. Circulating half-life is 2–8 h, 7–16 h in end-stage renal failure	Reflex tachycardia in ischaemic heart disease may result in iatrogenic MI. Avoid in patients with dissecting aneurysms. Can increase intracranial pressure further in pre-existing raised ICP Use lower doses in renally impaired
Esmolol	500–1,000 μg/kg loading dose over 30 s, followed by infusion starting at 50 μg/kg/min and increasing by 50 μg/kg/min every 4 min, up to 300 μg/kg/min PRN	Onset ~2 min, lasts 10–30 min	Associated with hyperkalaemia; monitor potassium Should not be used in patients with uncompensated heart failure, bradycardia, heart block greater than first degree (except if on functioning pacemaker), bronchospasm
Sodium nitroprusside	0.25–0.3 μg/kg/min titrated by 0.5 μg/kg/min every 1–2 min, max 10 μg/kg/min	Onset <2 min, lasts 1–10 min Half-life nitroprusside ~2 min, thiocyanate ~3 days, doubled or tripled in renal failure	May increase intracranial pressure due to profound vasodilation Coronary steal and post-load reduction, caution in acute myocardial infarction Prolonged infusion iu doses >3 μg/kg/min over prolonged periods (>2 days) may result in cyanide toxicity, especially in renal and hepatic dysfunction

associated with end-organ damage. The choice of an intravenous antihypertensive to be given to the patient in this setting will depend very much on the baseline comorbidities and intercurrent issues which may be evolving in the patient at hand. Locally available options include labetalol, esmolol, nitroglycerin, sodium nitroprusside, and hydralazine. Careful considerations of concurrent issues like bradycardia, anaemia, and past medical history of ischaemic heart disease are important drug-disease interactions which can determine the decision of which agent to choose (Table 6.1) (Soto-Ruiz et al. 2011).

The postoperative patient is also at risk for venous thromboembolic (VTE) complications that can increase the patient's length of stay. This is also an area where the pharmacist plays an active role in recommending prophylaxis in consultation with the team. Depending on the type of procedure, the presence of an ileostomy may result in increased fluid and electrolyte losses and the pharmacist may recommend necessary electrolyte replacements. The pharmacist may also suggest supplementation to achieve the necessary vitamin and mineral balance for patients who are at risk for malabsorption postoperatively (Bell et al. 2006). Additionally, postoperation pain control and the maintenance of bowel movement become the prime parameters which the primary team will pay absolute attention to. The use of multimodal analgesia can assist with pain control and may at times be opioid-sparing. However, other aspects of care are crucial, for example, there are many considerations in using Non-steroidal anti-inflammatory drugs (NSAIDs) in an elderly patient and especially if volume contracted. This is where the pharmacist plays an active role in his/her review of the medication charts of the GSS patients.

Other complications that could arise, like a newly acquired infection, could mean commencement of antibiotics which would also require considerations of current renal and hepatic function. The pharmacist aids the team in necessary dose titrations and makes a recommendation with knowledge of prevalent antibiograms of resistance strains of bacteria, thus allowing for a prudent choice of empirical antibiotic.

Table 6.2 lists a suggested mnemonic, modified from the mnemonic "FASTHUGS" in critical care, to aid the team in monitoring and adjustments of various medications.

Lastly, counselling patients on side effects that may be experienced from the prescribed medications and answering any drug-related enquiries that our patients have provide the necessary reassurance for them and their loved ones. This is particularly so if old medications have been withheld or doses have changed. Clear instructions should be given to the patient with respect to when restarting of medications or if discussions are required with their usual doctors in charge or their chronic diseases like hypertension, diabetes, anticoagulation, and/or heart disease.

6.5 Evolving Roles of the Pharmacist over the Years

Indeed, the practice of pharmacy in hospital wards has changed significantly in recent years. In the early 1990s, pharmacists were responsible for drug distribution and had little involvement in patient care and they rarely communicated with

Table 6.2 Medication considerations in critical care

	Parameter	What to monitor	Medication(s) of particular interest	Action and rationale
F	Feeding	Calories in/out, tailored according to premorbid state, presence of infection or catabolic states post operation	Oral hypoglycaemic agents (e.g. glipizide, gliclazide) Insulins, in particular, long acting ones (e.g. glargine, detemir)	When oral intake is nil or poor and if BG is often below 8 mmol/L, review to take off all regular oral or injectable medications (see under "G" for more details)
A	Analgesia	Pain score, cognition, state of alertness, renal function and fluid "ins and outs", bowel movement	Opioid use NSAIDS, COXIIs Previous antihypertensives, e.g. ACE inhibitors, diuretics Previous central nervous system active agents, e.g. benzodiazepines	Caution with the use of NSAIDs and COXIIs (e.g. etoricoxib, naproxen, ibuprofen) particularly if baseline renal impairment or raised serum creatinine Elderly's response to opiates and congeners may be exaggerated; watch for constipation and nausea
T	Venous thromboembolism	Mobilization, signs and symptoms of bleeding, use of pharmacologic VTE prophylaxis (e.g. subcutaneous (SQ) enoxaparin), or intermittent pneumatic calf compressors (IPCs) if high risk of bleeding	Previous use of warfarin or other oral anticoagulants like rivaroxaban	VTE is a preventable adverse outcome. All patients should be risk-assessed daily and VTE prophylaxis considered in high-risk patients (e.g. history of previous VTE) until patient achieves full mobility

(continued)

Table 6.2 (continued)

	Parameter	What to monitor	Medication(s) of particular interest	Action and rationale
G	Glucose	Serum blood glucose, keep between 8 and 11 mmol/L (Sheehy and Gabbay 2009)	As above, under "F"	History of (H/o): oral intake resumed, may consider restarting old meds. Otherwise, sliding scale insulin may be considered. Old meds may be restarted at preadmission doses at day of discharge if was well-controlled prior to admission
				No H/O diabetes: Keep BG – blood glucose around 10 mmol/L
				Medication reconciliation, complete with a verification of most recent HbA1c, is recommended
E	Serum electrolytes and fluid balance	Sodium, potassium, renal function, and fluid "ins and outs", and if applicable, acid-base status, calcium and magnesium levels	Intravenous fluid replacements, potassium supplements, glucose supplements	Renal adjustment of certain antibiotics (e.g. vancomycin, aminoglycosides) when used, oral antidiabetic agents, anticoagulants
			Previous or current diuretic use	BP may be raised post operation due to volume contraction. Hydrate adequately before treating BP unless end-organ damage is evident
			Presence of renal dysfunction and/or acute kidney injury may influence dosing of antibiotics	Patients at risk of arrhythmias: Replace potassium, magnesium, and calcium adequately
				Patients with poor baseline nutritional status: may be at risk of refeeding syndrome. Monitor and replace phosphate, potassium, magnesium, glucose
V	Vitals	Heart rate, blood pressure (BP), postural changes in blood pressure (BP), body temperature, presence/acquisition of infections	Antihypertensives, e.g. ACE inhibitors, diuretics	Caution with restarting antihypertensives particularly if volume contracted
			Vasopressors	Elderly more prone to postural hypotension and falls
S	Stool	Bowel movement	Opioid use for post-op pain	The lack of bowel movement could be a side effect or complication of the surgery. Daily monitoring is recommended

ACE angiotensin-converting enzyme, *BG* blood glucose, *COXII* cyclo-oxygenase II inhibitors, *IPC* intermittent pneumatic calf compressors, *NSAID* nonsteroidal anti-inflammatory drugs, *SQ* subcutaneous, *VTEP* venous thromboembolic prophylaxis

6 The Role of a Pharmacist in a Transdisciplinary Geriatric Surgery Team 101

patients about their medications or disease processes. With the introduction of "clinical pharmacy," however, the pharmacist's attention began to shift from the medication itself to the interaction between the patient and the medication.

Today, the pharmacist's role in many practice settings has expanded to include not only dispensing functions but also direct contact with patients and other healthcare providers. The focus has also shifted to individualizing care for each patient. This is crucial especially in the care of the elderly patient since age-related changes in drug disposition and pharmacodynamic responses have significant clinical implications; increased use of a number of medications raises the risk that medicine-related problems may occur (Mansur 2012; Maher 2014; Roth et al. 2013).

As outlined here, the pharmacist has a significant role to play in the care of the elderly surgical patient whose care is often complicated with multiple comorbidities and polypharmacy. This model of transdisciplinary care that invites and recognizes the participation of pharmacists is an ideal platform for true collaborative care for a patient population who is otherwise at high risk of complications and adverse outcomes that extend far beyond just the acute admission for the index surgery.

References

Bell C et al (2006) Potentially unintended discontinuation of long-term medication use after elective surgical procedures. Arch Intern Med 166:2525–2531

Coriat P et al (1994) Influence of chronic angiotensin-converting enzyme inhibition on anesthetic induction. Anesthesiology 81(2):299–307

Downing N et al (2014) Clinical trial evidence supporting FDA approval of novel therapeutic agents, 2005-2012. JAMA 311:368–377

Johnell K, Klarin I (2007) The relationship between number of drugs and potential drug-drug interactions in the elderly: a study of over 600 000 elderly patients from the Swedish prescribed drug register. Drug Saf 30:911–918

Maher RL (2014) Clinical consequences of polypharmacy in elderly. Expert Opin Drug Saf 13(1):57–65

Mansur N (2012) Looking beyond polypharmacy: quantification of medication regimen complexity in the elderly. Am J Geriatr Pharm 10:223–229

Orser B et al (2013) Review article: improving drug safety for patients undergoing anesthesia and surgery. Can J Anesth 60(2):127–135

Roth MT et al (2013) Individualized medication assessment and planning: optimizing medication use in older adults in the primary care setting. Pharmacotherapy 33(8):787–797

Sheehy AM, Gabbay RA (2009) An overview of preoperative glucose evaluation, management, and perioperative impact. J Diabetes Sci Technol 3:1261–1269

Soto-Ruiz KM et al (2011) Perioperative hypertension: diagnosis and treatment. Neth J Crit Care 15:143–148

Prehabilitation and Rehabilitation in Colorectal Surgery

7

Sharon Cheng-Kuan Lim, Melissa Zhi-Yan Heng, and Gregory Heng

---

Take-Home Pearls

- Physiotherapy for colorectal patients can include preoperative management (prehabilitation) or postoperative management (rehabilitation).
- Patients undergoing colorectal surgery are a heterogenous group with varying needs. Therefore, there will not be a "one size fits all" physiotherapy intervention. Physiotherapy should be recommended for patients who are predisposed to higher risk of postoperative complications and prolonged recovery. Risk assessment and stratification may help in identification of higher-risk patients who can benefit from enhanced care and lower-risk patients who may not benefit.
- Physiotherapy component of prehabilitation includes aerobic and strength conditioning for a few weeks prior to surgery. Conditioning at moderate intensity, as recommended by the American College of Sports Medicine (ACSM), has shown some benefit. Low-intensity exercises also appear to produce benefits in the postoperative recovery. Outcomes of prehabilitation can be further enhanced with nutritional optimisation.
- Postoperative physiotherapy should include pulmonary and mobility management followed by a period of reconditioning to restore premorbid level of physical health and function. Considerations should be given to whether rehabilitation may need to continue even after discharge from the acute care setting to facilitate successful reintegration into the home and community.
- Use of objective outcome measurements to measure physical function can be useful to monitor functional status and progress the exercise prescription during prehabilitation and rehabilitation.

S.C.-K. Lim (✉) • M.Z.-Y. Heng
Department of Rehabilitation Services, Khoo Teck Puat Hospital, Singapore, Singapore
e-mail: lim.sharon.ck@alexandrahealth.com.sg

G. Heng
Department of Surgery, Khoo Teck Puat Hospital, Singapore, Singapore

© Springer-Verlag Berlin Heidelberg 2015
K.-Y. Tan (ed.), *Transdisciplinary Perioperative Care in Colorectal Surgery: An Integrative Approach*, DOI 10.1007/978-3-662-44020-9_7

- Exercise prescription has to be individualised as every older adult differs in lifestyle, disease symptoms, chronic diseases, emotional state, functional capacity and disability.

7.1 Preamble

Physiotherapy, in general, seeks to maintain and restore people's optimum movement and functional ability, across a wide span of conditions and settings, from health promotion and disease prevention to musculoskeletal and intensive care. Physiotherapists use largely physical and non-invasive approaches and take into account factors that may affect the quality of movement and function. These factors can include physical, psychological, emotional and social well-being.

In the management of surgical patients, the traditional roles of the physiotherapist have largely been focused on:

1. *Respiratory management*
   Typically in the initial postoperative setting for the prevention and treatment of chest complications. Sometimes, preoperative education is included to manage anxiety and increase compliance to rehabilitation postoperatively.
2. *Mobility and functional rehabilitation*
   This includes using the concept of early mobilisation and facilitating of the restoration of the individual's joint mobility, bed mobility, ambulation and other functional activities (Naylor et al. 2006).

In most settings, physiotherapists are activated in the patient care when referred by the doctor in a multidisciplinary setting. This is commonly initiated postoperatively, when postoperative rehabilitation is deemed necessary. In many areas where multidisciplinary involvements occur, there is a degree of reliance on the physiotherapist to ensure that patients achieve their respiratory and physical capacity postoperatively. Is current practice the best? Can patient care and outcomes be further improved (Reilly 2001)?

In this chapter, we will evaluate the current practice and discuss the role of combining prehabilitation and rehabilitation, using the transdisciplinary approach. This chapter will also further explore some of the factors, evidence and experience to put forth some changes in physiotherapy practices, especially in face of transdisciplinary approach.

7.2 Understanding How Much Physiotherapy Intervention Is Required for Colorectal Surgery: Evidence for Physiotherapy?

Physiotherapy for the colorectal surgical patient can include preoperative and postoperative rehabilitation. The concept of optimisation prior to surgery or prehabilitation in this population is relatively new and evidence of its effectiveness is still emerging. Chest physiotherapy post upper abdominal surgery has been shown by some authors to decrease the incidence of postoperative pneumonia when compared to the control group who did not receive any physiotherapy (Manzano et al. 2008; Westwood et al. 2007). However, the effectiveness of physiotherapy in the postoperative phase has been inconclusive largely due to poor methodological studies (Pasquina et al. 2006). It is also possible that subgroups exist in this heterogenous pool of patients such that some patients may benefit and some may not benefit as much from physiotherapy, thereby diluting the results. Better understanding of how risk stratification of the patients may assist with better patient selection, prognostication and development of management plans pre- and postoperatively is needed.

Colorectal surgery is required for a wide variety of conditions, such as traumatic injury of the colon, colorectal malignancies or pelvic floor pathologies. Consequently, a wide profile of patients would be expected, ranging from young and fit patients to elder and frail patients. Depending on their diagnosis, disease progression and prognosis, patients can also vary in the stages of acceptance and mental/emotional preparation. The average length of stay for patients post colorectal surgery has been reported to range from 2 days to 10.7 days (Dilworth and White 1992; Majeed et al. 1996). The length of stay can be further lengthened by about 3 days if patients develop postoperative chest infection (Dilworth and White 1992). Risk factors associated with longer periods of stay and poorer functional recovery, with or without complications, include individuals who are smokers, individuals with pre-existing lung conditions like chronic bronchitis, surgeries with vertical or oblique incisions rather than horizontal incisions, and individuals who are older (Dilworth and White 1992; Lassen et al. 2009; Li et al. 2013).

The heterogeneity in patient characteristics within the colorectal discipline explains the difficulty in attempting to stratify patients into subcategories that indicate the required level of physiotherapy. The literature available has attempted to stratify risk of surgery for individuals into two categories: high and low risk. Therefore, using this available knowledge, we attempt to clinically rationalise the level of physiotherapy intervention based on this available model (Table 7.1).

7.2.1 Low-Risk Patients with Less Rehabilitation Needs

Patients who are younger, have fewer medical co-morbidities and/or are not undergoing major colorectal procedures will likely have minimal risks of postoperative chest complications and are unlikely to have significant decrease in physical capacity. For this low-risk group, traditional levels of physiotherapy may more than suffice. In fact, with sufficient pain management and encouragement from the doctors and nurses to resume normal activities, physiotherapy may not be indicated.

7.2.2 High-Risk Patients with More Rehabilitation Needs

Patients who are older, have multiple medical co-morbidities, have had a prior period of deconditioning due to curtailment or reduction of physical function, have undergone neo-adjuvant chemo- or radiotherapy, or will be undergoing

Table 7.1 Common risk factors associated with increased postoperative complications and poorer surgical outcomes (Fearon et al. 2012; Fujita and Sakurai 1995)

High risk	Low risk
Surgical factors	Surgical factors
Upper abdominal surgery	Lower abdominal surgery
Open surgery	Laparoscopic surgery
Prolonged surgery (>3–4 h)	Short surgical duration (<3–4 h)
Vertical or oblique incisions	Horizontal incisions
Age >65 years old	Age <65 years old
Smoker	Non-smoker
Pre-existing respiratory diseases	No active or ongoing respiratory diseases
Chronic bronchitis	
Chronic obstructive pulmonary diseases	
Pre-existing metabolic diseases	Minimal systemic co-morbidities
Diabetes	
Renal diseases	
Liver cirrhosis and failure	
Malnutrition status	Good nutritional status and optimisation
Anaemia	
Sarcopenia	
Psycho-emotional factors	Positive mental and emotional preparation and outlook
Depression	
Anxiety	

surgical procedures that are prolonged or open (especially upper abdominal incisions) would have considerable higher risk of postoperative chest complications (Fujita and Sakurai 1995; Fearon et al. 2012) prolonged immobility, and poorer long-term functional outcomes. In essence, these factors appear to point towards patients who are frail. Mayo and colleagues (2012) found that patients who deteriorated during the prehabilitation phase were also more likely to have complications after surgery. These patients tended to be older (>75 years old) and more anxious.

Postoperative physiotherapy, which includes peri-operative education, has been part of standard care for patients undergoing abdominal surgery, especially for patients who are at higher risk of postoperative chest complications. For a selected group of higher-risk patients who are at risk of slower recovery, a period of a few weeks of prehabilitation for physical conditioning and boosting of the immune system via the reduction of surgical/illness-associated anxiety may reduce this risk. It is generally perceived that establishing rapport and improving the patient's understanding before their surgery can also promote postoperative compliance to rehabilitation.

7.3 Prehabilitation

Prehabilitation aims to improve the physical and functional capacity of an individual through increasing the individual's buffering capacity to withstand and recover from surgical stress. How does one do prehabilitation for colorectal surgery? Does it improve patient outcomes? Which patient group should have prehabilitation? Evidence in this area is limited but certainly emerging in the area of physiotherapy and surgery.

7.3.1 Is Prehabilitation Effective? Does It Improve Postsurgical Outcomes?

Prehabilitation has more commonly been performed in patients undergoing orthopaedic surgeries, such as periods of strengthening before total knee replacements (TKRs) and laminectomies. Prehabilitation for TKRs and laminectomies has consistently demonstrated the ability of patients with existing joint problems to improve in strength, pain, and function with a 4–8 week aerobic conditioning and strengthening programme prior to surgery (Mckay et al. 2012; Nielsen et al. 2010; Topp et al. 2009). Improvements in aerobic capacity and strength also had positive effects on functional outcomes in patients who have undergone a period of prehabilitation when compared to the control group (Topp et al. 2009). However, improvements in physical function did not necessarily result in improvements in postoperative complications, pain scores or quality of life.

With respect to colorectal discipline, there is a growing amount of evidence suggesting the beneficial role of prehabilitation in improving surgical outcomes. Carli et al. (2009) conducted a pilot study, which compared an exercise group who did under a cycling and strengthening programme with a control group who were asked to walk daily and do some breathing exercises. In this study, the control group performed better in the 6 min walk test preoperatively and at follow-up. Poorer compliance of the participants of the exercise group (~16 %) to the cycling and strengthening programme than the walking programme was cited as a possible reason for the observation. In a follow-up study, Mayo et al. (2012) found improvements in postoperative walking distances in 33 %, no changes in 38 % and actual deterioration in 29 % of the prehabilitation group. In the same paper, it was mentioned that improved functional exercise capacity prior to surgery improved postoperative recovery. Li et al. (2013) further supported the role of prehabilitation by establishing that prehabilitation intervention was found to be a significant predictor of a positive change in functional capacity when comparing preoperative and postoperative states. Kim et al. (2009) used prehabilitation with a 4-week duration for patients who were at high risk of poor bowel resection outcome. In this study, an exercise compliance of ~74 % was achieved and results indicate that the patients in the prehabilitation group achieved significant improvements in the 6MWT postoperatively. Apart from possible improvements in postoperative functional capacity, prehabilitation was also found to have positive impact on reducing anxiety and depression (Li et al. 2013; Mayo et al. 2012). Overall, there appears to be more research emerging which supports the effectiveness of prehabilitation in improving postoperative outcomes.

7.3.2 How Should Prehabilitation Be Designed?

Prehabilitation protocols in colorectal surgical populations are not well established and have variability in various studies, when compared to those in other specialist areas, such as orthopaedic surgeries (refer Table 7.2).

7.3.2.1 Frequency
Most studies asked their prehabilitation patients to exercise for two to three times a week. A few studies have used a frequency of five times a week.

7.3.2.2 Intensity
Studies have used a range of intensities from 50 to 70 % of MHR or RPE of 11–13 for aerobic exercises. Prescriptions were consistent with the general guidelines by the American College of Sports Medicine (ACSM). Interestingly, Carli et al.'s (2010) and Mayo et al.'s (2012) low-intensity exercise groups had also demonstrated benefits from baseline. In fact, the low-intensity exercise groups had performed better in the 6MWT during both the prehabilitation and rehabilitation phase, and the finding was attributed to increased compliance to the regime than a higher intensity one. For the strengthening component, exercise prescription for strengthening has been varied, ranging from 8 to 10 RM to volitional fatigue. No studies had evaluated the effect of their exercise prescription for strengthening with strength-specific outcome measures.

7.3.2.3 Type of Exercise
The majority of the studies included aerobic exercises in the form of cycling and/or walking into their exercise protocol. Some studies included upper limb and/or lower limb strengthening exercises.

7.3.2.4 Time or Duration of Exercise Session
Most studies have used 20–30 min of aerobic exercises, and if strengthening exercises were included, the entire session, inclusive of warm-ups and cool-downs, took about 60 min.

7.3.2.5 Duration of Prehabilitation
The majority of prehabilitation trials run for a 4–6 weeks. A few studies used time to surgery during prehabilitation which resulted in prehabilitation durations of 2–8 weeks.

7.3.2.6 Supervised Versus Non-supervised Setting
Studies have either used supervised outpatient-based or unsupervised home-based exercise programme. No direct comparisons have been made with regard to the

7 Prehabilitation and Rehabilitation in Colorectal Surgery

Table 7.2 Summary of prehabilitation protocols

Authors	Subject demographics	Intervention/control details	Outcome measures
Dimeo et al. (1998)	$n=5$ (4 females, 1 male)	Prehabilitation	Conducted pre-post intervention
	Age: 18–55 years old	Frequency: weekdays	Treadmill stress test with continuous ECG monitoring
	Surgery: cancer± chemotherapy	Intensity: corresponding to a lactate concentration of 3 ± 0.5 mmol L^{-1}	Walking distance per training session (m)
		Type: treadmill walking	
		Duration: 6 weeks	
		Monitoring: supervised, location not indicated	
Kim et al. (2009)	$n=21$	*Prehabilitation*	Conducted before and after intervention
	Exercise group: 14 (5 females, 9 males)	Frequency: daily	VO_2max test
	Control: 7 (3 females, 4 males)	Intensity: progressive from 40 to 65 % HRR, RPE 11–16	6MWT
	Age:	Duration: 20–30 min	
	Exercise group: average 55 years old	Type: cycling on ergometer	
	Control: average 65 years old	Total duration of intervention: 4 weeks	
	Surgery: bowel resection surgery	Monitoring: supervised, home based	
Li et al. (2013)	$n=108$	*Prehabilitation*	1 week (preoperation) and 4 and 8 weeks (post operation)
	Exercise group: 54 (32 females, 22 males)	Frequency: three times a week	6MWT
	Control group:	Intensity: moderate aerobic (50 % MHR), volitional fatigue for strengthening	CHAMPS questionnaire
	64 (35 females, 29 males)	Duration: 30 mins aerobic	SF-36
	Age:	Type: aerobic exercises (walking or other machines)+strengthening using callisthenics or resistance bands	Emotional health
	Exercise group: 67.4 ± 11 years old	Total duration of intervention: dependent on surgery lead time; median of 33 days	Complication rate
	Control group: 66.4 ± 12 years old	Monitoring: unsupervised, home based	
	Surgery: Elective surgery for primary colorectal cancer		

(continued)

Table 7.2 (continued)

Authors	Subject demographics	Intervention/control details		Outcome measures
Dronkers et al. (2010)	$n = 42$	*Prehabilitation*		Timed "up and go"
	Exercise group: 22 (7 females, 15 males)	Frequency: twice/week		Chair rise time
	Control group: 20 (4 females, 16 males)	Intensity:		Maximal inspiratory pressure
	Age: > 60 years old		Maximum of one set of 8–15 rm, consistent with 60–80 % of the one-repetition maximum for resistance training	Physical activity questionnaire
	Surgery: elective abdominal oncological surgery		55–75 % of maximal heart rate or perceived exertion between 11 and 13 on the Borg Scale for aerobic training	Maximal aerobic capacity
			Duration :60 min consisting of 20–30 mins of aerobic training	Quality of life
			Type: warm-up, lower limb extensor resistance training, inspiratory muscle training, aerobic training, functional activities training, cool-down	Fatigue
		Total duration of intervention: 2–4 weeks		
		Monitoring:		
		Exercise group; supervised in outpatient setting		
		Control: Unsupervised, home based		
Carli et al. (2010); Mayo et al. (2012)	Exercise group 1: $n = 58$	*Prehabilitation*		Conducted preoperative baseline measure and postoperatively between 2 weeks and 4 months
	Exercise group 2:	Group 1: bike/strengthening		VO_2max
	$n = 54$	Frequency: strength training at 3 times/week; aerobic 5 times/week		6MWT
	Age: 63 subjects <65 years old	Intensity: aerobic initially 50 % of MHR with gradual increase at 10 %/week; strengthening at 8RM		Hospital Anxiety and Depression Scale (HADS)
	Surgeries: 85 open; 17 laparoscopic; all upper abdominal	Duration:30 min aerobic; 10–15 min strengthening		
		Type: cycling and upper/lower limb strengthening		
		Group 2: walking/breathing		
		Frequency: daily		
		Duration: minimum of 30 min		
		Prehab duration: mean of 52 days (22–60 days)		
		Monitoring: unsupervised, home based, with weekly monitoring via phone calls		

efficacy of either, but in the study of Carli et al. (2010), compliance to the protocol when unsupervised was low. In another study (Kim et al. 2009) where regular visits were supplemented to the home-based programme, compliance was significantly higher and yielded higher improvements when compared to the control group.

There is at present no standard guidelines on how prehabilitation should be conducted for this population although elements of aerobic and strength training appear to be popular. Most studies appear to attempt to comply to the exercise prescription principles of frequency, intensity, type and time, consistent with those by the ACSM. However, achieving the prescribed volumes of exercise could be challenging for this population due to patient-related factors of fatigue, pain, frailty and motivation level. While papers have attempted to achieve a minimum training period of 4–6 weeks, as peak VO_2 has been shown to improve with a 4-week duration of physical intervention (Govindasamy et al. 1992), colorectal patients have improved in their functional outcomes with even shorter training durations of 2–4 weeks. From the current known available research, there appears to be insufficient studies evaluating the strength between supervised versus non-supervised exercise intervention. This may be attributed to the lack of use of compliance rate as an outcome measure or that the aim of the studies has not included the evaluation of the type of setting.

7.4 Rehabilitation

7.4.1 Physiotherapy: Acute Postoperative Phase

Much of the research on the role of postoperative physiotherapy has been focused on the effectiveness and/or efficacy of the management and prevention of respiratory and pulmonary complications in the first 1–2 days post surgery. Prolonged supine positioning may impair pulmonary mechanics and oxygenation (Kehlet 1997). Anaesthesia and surgical trauma of abdominal surgery alter the function of respiratory muscles (Pasquina et al. 2006). There is a large body of literature investigating the efficacy of use of physiotherapy techniques of deep breathing exercise complemented with supported/assisted cough, incentive spirometry, intermittent positive pressure breathing and postural drainage to reduce postoperative pulmonary complication (Pasquina et al. 2006; Chumillas et al. 1998; Fagevik Olsén et al. 1997). The use of incentive spirometry has shown limited value, especially if early mobilisation has been achieved (Guimarães et al. 2009). In a meta-analysis by Pasquina et al. (2006), some of the studies demonstrated that these techniques aid to reduce incidence of pulmonary complications, which include a wide diversity of pathologies such as atelectasis, pneumonia and bronchitis. Conversely, it was also challenged that once the limitations of these studies were accounted for, the strength of the evidence may be altered. An appropriate amount of patient education should be incorporated as well, to include salient information that may allay postoperative fears and anxiety, such as the possibility of being supported for ventilation or experiencing pain at the site of operation.

Early mobilisation is another technique or strategy that is increasingly recognised in the field of postsurgical rehabilitation. Early mobilisation has been recorded to include walking and sitting out of bed (Delaney et al. 2003). Early mobilisation is not only a functional activity, but it reduces the cardiac, respiratory, fluid shift, bone and joint changes associated with prolonged bed rest/supine positioning. The technique has been shown to have little adverse effects and lowers the incidence of postoperative chest infection, lowers the usage of analgesia, improves lung volumes and promotes earlier recovery (Lassen et al. 2009; Lee et al. 2011; Zafiropoulos et al. 2004).

During the acute postoperative phase, it is essential to collaborate with the anaesthetic team to optimise pain control to facilitate pain-tolerated mobilisation and eliminate pain as the limiting factor to early mobilisation. Optimal pain relief includes the use of epidural anaesthesia and/or oral medications. In recent years, concurrent improvements in surgical techniques such as laparoscopy, together with optimal pain relief, early mobilisation and nutrition, allowed for a shortening of hospital stay between 2 and 5 days (Bardram et al. 2000). The postoperative management techniques constitute a multimodal approach to postoperative care and are designed to reverse changes in endocrine, metabolic, neural and pulmonary function commonly observed post surgery (Basse et al. 2000). Postoperative rehabilitation of colorectal patients typically ceases once the patient is able to manage basic activities of daily living either independently or with minimal assistance from a caregiver.

7.4.2 Physiotherapy: Subacute Postoperative Phase to Full Independence or Achieving Premorbid Status

There is a limited body of evidence investigating the role of physiotherapy and exercise/exercise prescription in the subacute and chronic postoperative phase. Christensen et al. (1982) established that individuals experienced fatigue postoperatively and approximately one-third of their sample population continued to experience fatigue one month post surgery. Less than 50 % of the patients returned to their premorbid status. A single arm study exploring the outcomes of an accelerated programme found that while patients could be discharged early, median of 2 days, from the hospital post-colonic resection, 25 % still felt fatigued, insecure and socially isolated (Basse et al. 2000). In many of the studies cited in Table 7.2, patients were still seen to be improving in functional outcomes at 8 weeks post operation, indicating that there is still much potential for further recovery after the initial inpatient hospitalisation. This signifies that there is a role for rehabilitation even after the discharge of the patient from the hospital to facilitate maximal recovery. With regards to the lack of literature in this area, we propose that the main pointers discussed of prehabilitation be applied and the social and psychological factors of the individual be taken into consideration.

Table 7.3 Common outcome measures used in prehabilitation and rehabilitation

Outcome measures
Physical or functional
2 or 6 min walk test
VO_2max using cycling ergometer or treadmill protocol
Quality of life
Health-related quality of life (Short-Form 36)
Hospital Anxiety and Depression Scale
Others
Length of inpatient hospital stay

7.4.3 Measuring Progress and Success of Rehabilitation

Eligibility to be discharged from rehabilitation can be considered when the patient has reached his/her preoperative functional baseline or is capable of progressing independently to attain premorbid functional status. The need for continuation of rehabilitation post discharge should be taken into consideration if it was clinically reasoned that the patient has yet to achieve premorbid functional status and requires further facilitation to do so. Objective outcome measurements taken at either commencement of prehabilitation or just before the operation can be used as an evaluation tool. Outcome measures may also be used to evaluate the efficacy of prehabilitation for the individual. Commonly used outcome measurements are summarised in Table 7.3.

7.5 Enhancing Patient Recovery in Transdisciplinary Management: Whose Role Should it Be?

In care of the colorectal patient, most practices would adopt a multidisciplinary approach, where everyone is aware of each other's role in the care of the patient. The downside is that there is a reliance, and occasionally an over-reliance, on each respective professional to ensure continuity in their area of care, for example, waiting for the dietitian to prescribe optimal nutritional intake or for the physiotherapist to ensure that the patient mobilises. Care tends to be segmented and dependent on the availability of the professional, rather than catered to the patient's needs. For the patient who is fairly enabled, empowered, and in little need of additional support, a segmented approach may not be detrimental to his or her recovery. However, many patients undergoing colorectal surgery have needs influenced by multiple factors, and their journey before and after surgery requires greater support from the healthcare professional team.

A transdisciplinary approach has been advocated in many settings such as chronic disease management, paediatrics, home care and rehabilitation as it is thought to improve patient outcomes over a multidisciplinary approach (Reilly 2001). A transdisciplinary approach is a "team approach, in which responsibilities are shared and the normal boundaries of the various healthcare professions are blurred" (Reilly 2001). A transdisciplinary approach in the management of the colorectal patient has shown good results (Tan et al. 2011). The domain experts are expected to provide their area of expertise to ensure optimal recovery in that area, but if every member of the team is tuned in to the patients' holistic needs and empowered to provide continuous and consistent education, reminders and support, the patient's recovery would be enhanced.

These are a few examples:

1. During the prehabilitation phase, conditioning and strengthening would be enhanced if nutritional intake was optimised (Fiatarone et al. 1994). Dietitians could prescribe a dietary plan that takes into account the patient's strength and conditioning needs, on top of their nutritional restrictions as a result of their disease or condition. The physiotherapist needs to have a firm understanding of this dietary plan and ensure compliance during exercise sessions.

2. During the immediate postoperative period, the patient is likely to require the most assistance, and this is when a transdisciplinary approach can play an important role. The physiotherapist can assess the patient's respiratory parameters and recommend the best positioning and the ideal breathing exercise type, frequency and intensity. The Enhanced Recovery After Surgery (ERAS) group recommends for patients to be out of their beds for 2 h on the day of surgery to up to 6 h per day subsequently (Lassen et al. 2009) as part of their early mobilisation. However, given the manpower constraints in most institutions, it is unlikely that the physiotherapist can come by every few hours to ensure that his or her recommendations have been followed through. A well-informed nurse would be in a strategic position to remind the patient of the recommendations. Similarly, once the physiotherapist has ascertained cardiovascular stability and the capacity for ambulation, the nurse can ensure that for simple activities of daily living such as toileting, the patient is allowed to walk, with or without assistance.

3. Home therapy or community nursing can be a time-consuming and labour-intensive service to provide and to pay for, especially if only a basic level of care is needed. Transdisciplinary approach in the home or community setting makes both sense and cents. For instance, if the physiotherapist is armed with basic knowledge and skills to manage simple surgical wounds, then he or she can also provide wound checks and simple dressing changes while providing supervised home exercises. When the situation becomes complicated, the physiotherapist can then activate the nurse to come for a more detailed assessment. Likewise, the nurse can provide basic exercise education and supervision during his or her visits to manage a complicated wound.

7.6 What Are Some of the Challenges of Transdisciplinary Management?

"Too many cooks spoil the broth". The more players there are in a team, the greater the potential for breakdown in communication and synergy. This is especially if everyone is doing a bit of everything. This can end up in things being under- or over-done. Reilly (2011) has recommended role extension, role enrichment, role expansion, role release and role support to establish a successful transdisciplinary team. Our experience supports this and we recommend:

1. Role allocation, with each member of the team clear on his or her own role and that of other members. Transdisciplinary roles clarification and training to establish areas of cross coverage and escalation. Each respective profession should be expected to set goals and make recommendations within the domain of their expertise.
2. Platform for communication and coordination, e.g. transdisciplinary ward rounds/meetings.

In the process of establishing this, there are some other challenges to overcome, such as additional training on cross-coverage areas, individual profession's ability to let go of their area of expertise and control, and re-establishing team control. On the last point, it is convention that the surgeon is the lead in the management of the patient. However, with transdisciplinary approach, where the team recognises the multifaceted aspects of health and function, there are times in the patient's journey when other members of the transdisciplinary team, such as the nurse, physiotherapist or dietitian, may have a bigger role and hence take the lead in directing the patient's care.

7.7 Physiotherapy Clinical Experience

In Khoo Teck Puat Hospital, the transdisciplinary team identifies high-risk geriatric surgical patients with frailty, and stratified as having higher risk of postoperative mortality and morbidity. These patients are managed by a team of clinicians, which includes the surgeon, the anaesthetist, the nurse, the physiotherapist and the dietitian, all of whom intervene before operation for preoperative optimisation and education. A transdisciplinary approach has been adopted to enhance the patient outcomes.

These individuals are offered a period of prehabilitation prior to the surgery for a duration of approximately 2 weeks. The physiotherapist uses outcome measures of cardiovascular function, lower limb strength and balance to assess the functional capacity of the patient prior to and after the phase of prehabilitation. These baseline scores form the basis for exercise prescription during prehabilitation, as well as a target to be achieved postoperatively. The exercise programme options were home based or outpatient based (geriatric gym). While supervised setting may appear to be the rational/preferred option, there are limiting factors that may require unsupervised home exercise sessions to be chosen. For example, the lack of availability of family members to bring the individual to a gym, the distance from home to the gym or the cost of gym sessions versus that of home. The programme was designed to improve cardiovascular fitness, functional strength and confidence in these patients, taking into consideration any physical limitations and symptoms. The prehabilitation exercise programme was supported by nutritional optimisation. Just prior to surgery, the patients are reassessed on the same set of outcome measures mentioned above.

The therapists experienced anecdotal evidence of significant rapport being built between the family, patient and members of the transdisciplinary team starting from the prehabilitative phase, which could account for the greater level of compliance for early mobilisation postoperatively. Families were more trustful of the treatments carried out and this appeared to benefit the patient's emotional status as well.

The patients are followed through from the immediate postoperative period to rehabilitative facilities (if required) and/or back home until their premorbid status has been achieved. Follow-up reviews and calls are made during this process, and the team maintains contact with the rehabilitation facilities if required. For the immediate postoperative, the team practises early mobilisation and conditioning. Graduated strength and conditioning, taking both the forms of supervised and non-supervised forms, are prescribed to ensure recovery of premorbid levels of function.

While implementing the prehabilitation programme, we encountered a number of challenges and technical considerations. One example was transportation issues of patients with mobility issues who were willing to have their rehabilitation conducted in the outpatient gym setting. Caregivers had to reschedule their personal appointments for patients to be brought to gym facilities, which proved to be a complex issue. Coordination of the timing between the family, patient and the physiotherapist had to be made. Other issues limiting the patient from exercising at the ideal prescribed exercise prescription include symptom of the pathology (e.g. abdominal pain), fatigue and poor motivation. These were culpable in impeding patients' progress during prehabilitation. We also recognised the impact of cultural differences as a contributing factor to exercise compliance as well, for example, the older adult's perception of exercise, their role in society and in their families and their perspective of cancer and longevity. Secondary to the heterogeneity of the patient group, no two exercise programme were the same and hence evaluation of the rehabilitation was an existing challenge. Lastly, the task of evaluating the efficacy of the rehabilitation program posed as a major challenge as no two prescribed exercise programme were the same.

7.8 Future Directions

As of the current available literature, we would recommend allocating extra resources to prehabilitation for higher-risk patients. Clinicians should take extra effort in reconciling the patients' holistic health and function prior to onset of their diseases, current health and function, and prognostication on postsurgical health and function to establish realistic and achievable short-term and long-term goals with the patients and their families. Patients who have already experienced a significant decline, which will only be exacerbated by trauma from a surgery, should be given additional support. Continued efforts to investigate the optimal exercise prescription at different stages of prehabilitation and rehabilitation should be conducted. An expansion of the literature investigating the role of physiotherapy in the subacute phase of physiotherapy may assist therapist to further facilitate the complete recovery of the patient post surgery and reduce the impact of decline. Further evaluation of the appropriateness of the outcome measures that evaluated various components of strength, functional capacity and endurance and its sensitivity to small amount of change in the systems would be deemed useful. With regard to the rehabilitation programme that we are currently conducting, it may also be recommended that more resources be allocated to address frailty-associated domains of social and psychological health.

References

Bardram L, Funch-Jenson P, Kehlet H (2000) Rapid rehabilitation in elderly patients after laparoscopic colonic resection. Br J Surg 87:1540–1545

Basse L, Jakobsen DH, Billesbolle P, Werner M, Kehlet H (2000) A clinical pathway to accelerate recovery after colonic resection. Ann Surg 232(1):51–57

Carli F, Charlebois P, Stein B, Zavorsky G, Kim DJ, Scott S, Mayo NE (2010) Randomized clinical trial of prehabilitation in colorectal surgery. Br J Surg 97:1187–1197

Christensen T, Bendix T, Kehlet H (1982) Fatigue and cardiorespiratory function following abdominal surgery. Br J Surg 69:417–419

Chumillas S, Ponce JL, Delgado F, Viciano V, Mateu M (1998) Prevention of postoperative pulmonary complications through respiratory rehabilitation: a controlled study. Arch Phys Med Rehabil 79:5–9

Delaney CP, Zutshi M, Senagore AJ, Remzi FH, Hammel J, Fazio VW (2003) Prospective, randomized, controlled trial between a pathway of controlled rehabilitation with early ambulation and diet and traditional postoperative care after laparotomy and intestinal resection. Dis Colon Rectum 46(7):851–859

Dilworth JP, White RJ (1992) Postoperative chest infection after upper abdominal surgery: an important problem for smokers. Respir Med 86:205–210

Dimeo F, Rumberger GB, Keul J (1998) Aerobic exercise as therapy for cancer fatigue. Med Sci Sports Exerc 30(4):475–478

Dronkers JJ et al (2010) Preoperative therapeutic programme for elderly patients scheduled for elective abdominal oncological surgery: a randomized controlled pilot study. Clin Rehabil 24(7):614–622

Fagevik Olsén M et al (1997) Randomized controlled trial of prophylactic chest physiotherapy in major abdominal surgery. Br J Surg 84(11):1535–1538

Fearon KC, Jenkins JT, Carli F, Lassen K (2012) Patient optimization for gastrointestinal cancer surgery. Br J Surg 100:15–27

Fiatarone MA, O'Neill EF, Ryan ND, Clements KM, Solares GR, Nelson ME, Roberts SB, Kehaylas JJ, Lipsitz LA, Evans WJ (1994) Exercise training and nutritional supplementation for physical frailty in very elderly people. N Engl J Med 330(25):1769–1775

Fujita T, Sakurai K (1995) Multivariate analysis of risk factors for postoperative pneumonia. Am J Surg 169:305–307

Govindasamy D, Paterson DH, Poulin MJ, Cunningham DA (1992) Cardiorespiratory adaptation with short term training in older men. Eur J Appl Physiol 65:203–208

Guimarães MMF, Dib RPE, Smith AF, Matos D (2009) Incentive spirometry for prevention of postoperative pulmonary complications in upper abdominal surgery. Cochrane Database Syst Rev (3):CD006058

Kehlet H (1997) Multimodal approach to control postoperative pathophysiology and rehabilitation. Br J Anaesth 78:606–617

Kim DJ, Mayo NE, Carli F, Montgomery DL, Zavorsky GS (2009) Responsive measures to prehabilitation in patients undergoing bowel resection surgery. Tohoku J Exp Med 217(2):109–115

Lassen K, Soop M, Nygren J, Cox BW, Hendy PO, Spies C, von Meyenfeldt MF, Fearon KCH, Revhaug A, Norderval S, Ljungqvist O, Lobo DN, Dejong CHC (2009) Consensus review of optimal perioperative care in colorectal surgery. Enhanced recovery after surgery (ERAS) group recommendations. Arch Surg 144(10):961–969

Lee TG, Kang SB, Kim DW, Hong S, Heo SC, Park KJ (2011) Comparison of early mobilization and diet rehabilitation program with conventional care after laparoscopic colon surgery: a prospective randomized controlled trial. Dis Colon Rectum 54(1):21–28

Li C, Carli F, Lee L, Charlebois P, Stein B, Liberman AS, Kaneva P, Augustin B, Wongyingshinn M, Gamsa A, Kim DJ, Vassiliou MC, Feldman LS (2013) Impact of a trimodal prehabilitation program on functional recovery after colorectal cancer surgery: a pilot study. Surg Endosc 27:1071–1082

Majeed AW, Troy G, Nicholl JP, Smythe A, Reed MWR, Stoddard CJ, Peacock J, Johnson AG (1996) Randomised, prospective, single-blind comparison study of laparoscopic versus small-incision cholecystectomy. Lancet 347:989–994

Manzano RM, de Carvalho CRF, Saraiva-Romanholo BM, Vieira JE (2008) Chest physiotherapy during immediate postoperative period among patients undergoing upper abdominal surgery: randomized clinical trial. San Paulo Med J 126(5):269–273

Mayo NE, Feldman L, Scott S, Zavorsky G, Kim DJ, Charlebois P, Stein B, Carli F (2012) Impact of preoperative change in physical function on postoperative recovery: argument supporting prehabilitation for colorectal surgery. Surgery 150:505–514

McKay C, Prapavesis H, Doherty T (2012) The effect of a prehabilitation exercise program on quadriceps strength for patients undergoing total knee arthroplasty: a randomized controlled pilot study. Phys Med Rehabil 4:647–656

Naylor J, Harmer A, Fransen M, Crosbie J, Innes L (2006) Status of physiotherapy rehabilitation after total knee replacement in Australia. Physiother Res Int 11(1):35–47

Nielsen PR, Joegensen LD, Dahl B, Pedersen T, Tonnesen H (2010) Prehabilitation and early rehabilitation after spinal surgery: randomized clinical trial. Clin Rehabil 24:137–148

Pasquina P, Tramer MR, Granier J, Walder B (2006) Respiratory physiotherapy to prevent pulmonary complications after abdominal surgery. A systematic review. Chest 130:1887–1899

Reilly C (2001) Transdisciplinary approach: an atypical strategy for improving outcomes in rehabilitative and long-term acute care settings. Rehabil Nurs 26(6):216–244

Tan KY, Tan P, Tan L (2011) A collaborative transdisciplinary "geriatric surgery service" ensures consistent successful outcomes in elderly colorectal surgery patients. World J Surg 35(7):1608–1614

Topp R, Swank AM, Quesada PM, Nyland J, Malkani A (2009) The effect of prehabilitation exercise on strength and functioning after total knee arthroplasty. Phys Med Rehabil 1:729–735

Westwood K, Griffin M, Roberts K, Williams M, Yoong K, Digger T (2007) Incentive spirometry decreases respiratory complications following major abdominal surgery. Surgeon 5(6):339–342

Zafiropoulos B, Alison JA, McCarren B (2004) Physiological responses to the early mobilisation of the intubated, ventilated abdominal surgery patient. Aust J Physiother 50:95–100

Integrative Approach to Laparoscopic Surgery for Colorectal Cancer

8

Fumio Konishi, Takayoshi Yoshida, Yusuke Komekami, and Chunyong Lee

Take-Home Pearls

- A transdisciplinary approach involving the systemic participation of the various medical specialty members in the care of the patients is indispensable for achieving successful surgical treatment.
- Prehabilitation in elderly patients is particularly important to improve the physical fitness and maintain good nutritional and psychosocial condition in elderly patients.
- For those with obstruction due to colorectal cancer, decompression procedures should be considered before performing laparoscopic colorectal surgery.
- Patients who undergo minimally invasive procedures are good candidates for fast-track (FT) perioperative care.
- FT care reduces the incidence of postoperative organ dysfunction and morbidity resulting in a faster recovery after surgery.

8.1 Introduction

Since the first report by Jacobs et al. in 1991 (1991), laparoscopic colorectal surgery has been performed in an increasing number of cases each year not only in Asian countries including Japan but also in other countries worldwide (Fig. 8.1). According to nationwide statistics in Japan, in 2011 over 19,000 cases of laparoscopic colorectal cancer surgery were performed. Among the various laparoscopic surgical

---

F. Konishi (✉)
Department of Surgery, Nerima Hikarigaoka Hospital, Tokyo, Japan

Department of Surgery, Saitama Medical Center Jichi Medical University, Saitama, Japan
e-mail: DZD00740@nifty.ne.jp

T. Yoshida • Y. Komekami • C. Lee
Department of Surgery, Nerima Hikarigaoka Hospital, Tokyo, Japan

© Springer-Verlag Berlin Heidelberg 2015
K.-Y. Tan (ed.), *Transdisciplinary Perioperative Care in Colorectal Surgery: An Integrative Approach*, DOI 10.1007/978-3-662-44020-9_8

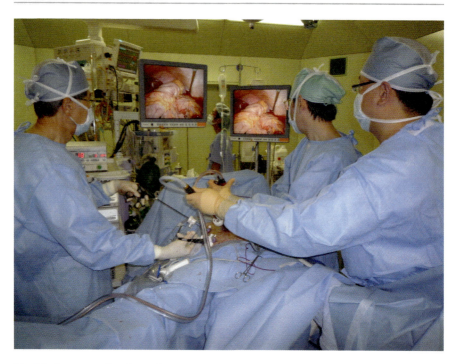

Fig. 8.1 Laparoscopic colorectal surgery

procedures, laparoscopic colorectal surgery is the second most commonly performed procedure in Japan next to laparoscopic cholecystectomy. In general most laparoscopic colorectal surgeries were performed in cancer patients. The Japan Society of Endoscopic Surgery distributed questionnaires to approximately 500 member hospitals and institutions and collected data regarding the take-up rate of laparoscopic colectomy and laparoscopic rectal resection. The results showed an increase in take-up rate of both laparoscopic colectomy and laparoscopic rectal resection. The take-up rate of laparoscopic colectomy in 2011 was 48 % and that of the rectal resection was 45 % (Fig. 8.2) (Japan Society for Endoscopic Surgery 2012). Reasons for the increasing number of patients treated with laparoscopic colorectal surgery include the minimally invasive nature of the procedure which results in reduced pain, improved cosmesis, earlier recovery, and shorter hospital stay. Another important reason for the increasing adoption of this technique is the fact that the long-term outcomes of colorectal cancer patients are comparable to those observed after open surgery (The Colon Cancer Laparoscopic or Open Resection Study Group 2009; Fleshman et al. 2007). This finding has been documented in several large-scale randomized controlled trials worldwide.

In this chapter the perioperative care of patients who undergo laparoscopic colorectal surgery is presented and discussed focusing on areas of integrative approach. The fundamental perioperative care of the patients who undergo laparoscopic colorectal surgery should be provided not only by surgeons, gastroenterologists,

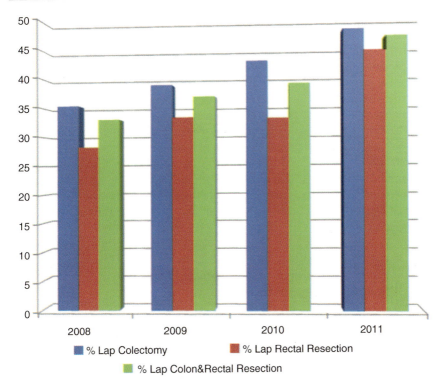

Fig. 8.2 Penetration rate of laparoscopic colon and rectal cancer surgery (Nationwide survey, Japan Society of Endoscopic Surgery (JSES) 2012)

anesthesiologists, and nurses in the wards and the theaters but also by rehabilitation trainers, dietitians, cardiologists, pulmonary physicians, and nephrologists depending on the condition of the patients. A transdisciplinary approach involving the systemic and active participation of the various specialty members in the perioperative care of the patients is truly indispensable for achieving successful surgical treatment and also obtaining a good quality of life for the patients after surgery.

8.2 Potential Advantages of Laparoscopic Colorectal Surgery

8.2.1 The Less Invasive Nature

First, the small surgical wound created in laparoscopic colorectal surgery results in less tissue damage than that observed in open surgery. The reduced tissue damage results in lower cytokine and immune responses, which leads to a faster recovery after surgery. In laparoscopic surgery CO_2 is used to insufflate the abdominal cavity. By using CO_2 insufflation, surgeons can prevent the direct exposure of intraperitoneal organs to the air. Exposure of the intraperitoneal organs to air may suppress immune response which is detrimental to the patient's postoperative recovery, and performing pneumoperitoneum using CO_2 may prevent such changes (Hanly et al. 2003). In most previous studies, the amount of blood loss was significantly less in patients undergoing laparoscopic colectomy than in those treated with open surgery. This is due to the ability to precisely observe the intraperitoneal organs and tissue using the laparoscope and meticulous operative maneuvers. Reducing the amount of blood loss is beneficial for improving the patient's recovery from the surgical intervention. Open colectomy involves the manual manipulation of the intestines by the surgeons which induces a significant inflammatory response, possibly leading to paralytic ileus and postoperative adhesions of the intestine (Schwarz et al. 2004). Because the amount of bowel manipulation in laparoscopic surgery is much less than that observed in open surgery, the invasiveness of laparoscopic surgery is considered to be minimized.

8.2.2 Immune, Cytokine, and Hormone Response Following Laparoscopic Colectomy

Surgical intervention is generally considered to result in the suppression of cell-mediated immunity, an increased level of cytokines, and an enhanced inflammatory response. It has been reported that in patients undergoing laparoscopic colectomy, the postoperative rise in levels of IL-6, IL-8, IL-10, and CRP is less than observed in open colectomy (Wichmann et al. 2005). This finding is considered to be due to the reduced invasiveness of laparoscopic surgery comparing to open surgery.

In our previous study comparing laparoscopic vs. open surgery with respect to the cytokine response and inflammatory changes, the rise in the IL-6 levels was significantly lower in the lap colectomy than in the open colectomy group. Similar data have been reported in a number of previous papers. As for the hormonal response, the rise in the ADH and ACTH levels did not differ between the laparoscopic group and the open surgery group (Fig. 8.3) (Ozawa et al. 2000).

8.3 Areas of Integrative Approach

8.3.1 Evaluation of Surgical Risks

The evaluation of surgical risks in patients undergoing laparoscopic colectomy is usually performed in a similar manner to that of open surgery. There is a tendency toward longer operation time in cases of laparoscopic colorectal surgery. Performing pneumoperitoneum using CO_2 may cause hypercapnia and decrease the cardiac output. Therefore, in patients with severe cardiovascular and pulmonary dysfunction, the indication for laparoscopic colorectal surgery should be carefully evaluated.

There are several assessment tools commonly used to evaluate surgical risks. Some of these tools require specific assessment and interventions using an

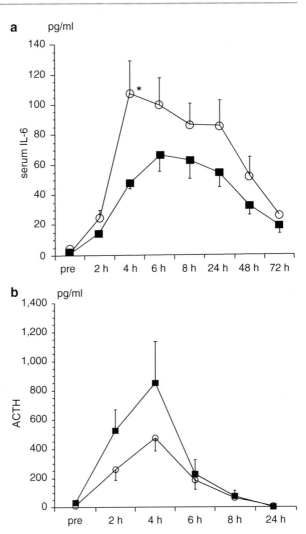

Fig. 8.3 The postoperative changes of serum IL-6 (**a**) and ACTH. *$P<0.05$ (**b**) (Ozawa et al. 2000)

integrative and team-based approach. Various factors including symptoms, comorbidities, and laboratory data have been identified to be important surgical risk factors. The patient's age itself may not be a risk factor; however, comorbidities and frailty associated with old age are considered to be risk factors in surgical patients. The followings are representative operative risk assessment tools.

8.3.1.1 American Society of Anesthesiologists (ASA) Scores

This is the most widely used scoring system (Bowles et al. 2008). This scoring system classifies patients into five categories and determines the surgical risk based on a simple assessment of the patients' condition; therefore, it is easy to use. The mortality rates for and ASA status of I, II, III, and IV have been reported to be 0.08, 1.8,

7.8, and 9.8 %, respectively. In general, conducting preoperative assessments of patients with a Class II or III status is important. Although widely used, this scoring system is a crude method of assessment and offers little opportunities of developing specific preoperative interventions for higher-risk patients.

8.3.1.2 Physiological and Operative Severity Score for the Enumeration of Mortality and Morbidity (POSSUM, CR-POSSUM)

The efficacy of the POSSUM score in predicting the postoperative outcome has been proven. This scoring system is widely used due to its relative simplicity and proven efficacy. There are 12 preoperative and six intraoperative variables including age, respiratory and cardiac comorbidities, ECG, blood pressure, BUN, Hb, WBC, grade of operative intervention, amount of blood loss, and the presence of malignant tumors and intraperitoneal bacterial contamination (Copeland et al. 1991). In the scoring system, the postoperative morbidity and mortality rates are automatically calculated. The CR-POSSUM was subsequently developed using multivariate models of colorectal surgery based on the same principles (Tekkis et al. 2004).

8.3.1.3 Charlson Weighted Comorbidity Index

This index is more commonly used by geriatricians. It gives each comorbidity a different weight according to the long-term outcome of patients with that particular comorbidity, which is helpful for quantifying comorbidities in elderly patients (Charlson et al. 1987). Our recent study of colorectal surgery patients showed that the risk of postoperative comorbidities was almost four times higher if the weighted comorbidity index score is 5 or greater (Tan et al. 2009).

8.3.1.4 Frailty

"Frailty" is a new concept for assessing the surgical risks of elderly patients. It is interesting to note that some elderly patients without comorbidities may exhibit higher frailty index. The presence of frailty is determined based on the activity level, grip strength, and walking speed and others as suggested by Fried et al. (2001).

The assessment of comorbidity index and frailty do not fall within the usual competence of a standard surgical team. Individuals trained in the assessment of geriatric patients may be more appropriate. Nonetheless, they may well offer more sensitive measures of increased perioperative vulnerability. It is becoming clearer that these assessments may become indispensible in the assessment of the elderly surgical patient. Integrating individuals well versed in geriatric assessment into the surgical team may well be advantageous.

8.3.2 Decompression of the Colon Proximal to the Tumor Causing Stenosis

Stenosis or obstruction due to colorectal cancer should be dealt with somewhat differently than using open surgery. This is because the ability to expose the operating

Fig. 8.4 Stenting in a case of rectosigmoid carcinoma

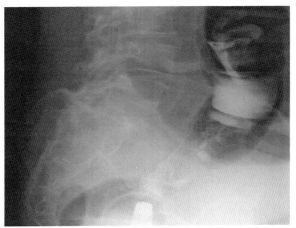

field during laparoscopic procedures is difficult in the presence of distension of the large or small bowel or both. Therefore, in cases of laparoscopic colorectal surgery, stenosis or obstruction should be managed to resolve distension in the bowel proximal to the tumor. When there is stenosis without symptoms of bowel obstruction, the patient is advised to stop taking solid food and to consume only liquids. This allows the feces accumulated in the bowel proximal to the tumor to be eventually passed through the stenotic segment. It usually takes approximately a week for the accumulated feces to pass through the stenosis.

On the other hand, when there is obstruction due to a tumor, decompression of the distended bowel proximal to the tumor should be attempted before resection. The most effective way to decompress the bowel is to either construct a stoma or place a self-expandable colonic stent via a colonoscopic procedure. Stenting is effective for achieving decompression and is useful as a bridge to surgical resection. The procedure requires a high level of technique and is usually performed by a well-trained colonoscopist to avoid complications during stent insertion (Fig. 8.4) (Sarkar et al. 2013). Therefore, collaboration between surgeons and endoscopists is essential. There are certain limitations associated with this procedure. When the tumor is situated around the acute bend of the colon, inserting the stent is technically difficult. In addition, if the obstruction is severe and it is not possible to pass a guidewire through the tumor, it is technically impossible to place a stent. As for the site of the tumor, the patients with mid to lower rectal tumors are usually not indicated for stenting. This is because the distal portion of the stent may project into the lower rectum causing difficulty performing rectal resection. Although not always unsuccessful, performing stent insertion of the transverse or the right colon can be difficult due to the instability in colonoscopic manipulation. Although there are technical problems and the long-term outcomes of colon cancer patients who undergo stenting as a bridge to surgery are still controversial (Sabbagh et al. 2013), colonic stenting is an effective modality for decompressing the obstructed colon before laparoscopic surgery.

Fig. 8.5 Transanal decompression tube

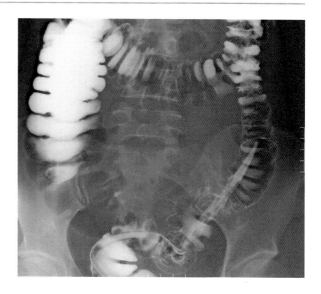

When stent insertion is technically difficult, a transanal decompression tube can be used to treat obstructing tumors in the left side or in the rectum, although the effectiveness of decompression is not always sufficient and the time required for a decompression will be longer (Fig. 8.5). The usage of transanal decompression tube before laparoscopic colectomy was reported by Shingu et al. (2013). The insertion of the decompression tube is performed during a colonoscopic procedure and by a well-trained colonoscopist.

All the above described techniques may carry a significant risk of tumor perforation and failed decompression mandating more emergent surgical intervention, and thus constant communication between the endoscopist and the surgeon needs to be established.

8.3.3 Laparoscopic Colorectal Cancer Surgery in the Elderly

As the age of patients with colorectal cancer is becoming higher, the perioperative care of elderly patients is a particularly important issue (Tan and Tan 2013). In Japan the Ministry of Health defines "elderly" as an age of 65 or higher. Elderly individuals are further divided into two groups. Patients between 65 and 74 years of age are defined as "young old," and those 75 or over are defined as "old old." Therefore, in Japan an age of 75 or older is an appropriate definition of "elderly." In the UK, a colorectal cancer collaborative group reported that patients between 65 and 70 years of age should not be considered old from physiological and functional point of view. Due to the less invasive nature of laparoscopic colorectal cancer surgery, elderly patients are considered to be good candidates for laparoscopic colectomy. Previous studies have evaluated octogenarians who underwent laparoscopic colectomy. The authors reported that although the operative time of laparoscopic

8 Integrative Approach to Laparoscopic Surgery for Colorectal Cancer

surgery is longer, the length of hospital stay is significantly shorter and the rate of postoperative complications tends to be lower than that observe in open colectomy (Tan et al. 2009; Issa et al. 2011). However, there is a higher incidence of comorbidities in elderly patients; therefore, the transdisciplinary perioperative care of elderly patients who undergo laparoscopic colectomy is of significant importance. The potential systemic effects of prolonged laparoscopy may potentially lead to medical complications including complications in the cardiovascular and respiratory system, and these require interventions from physicians best delivered through a transdisciplinary approach.

8.3.4 Prehabilitation in Elderly Patients

Strengthening of the functional capacity before surgery can be achieved with the process of "prehabilitation." Such preoperative care is particularly required when operating on elderly patients (Carli and Zavorsky 2005). A poor level of preoperative fitness is associated with an increased rate of morbidity and delayed recovery after surgery. Prehabilitation aims to improve the patient's physical fitness and obtain a good nutritional and psychosocial condition (Tan 2013). Although laparoscopic colectomy is considered to be less invasive than open surgery, the use of "prehabilitation" should be considered in order to minimize surgical complications and to achieve a good quality of life after surgery particularly in elderly patients. There are two reports on the use of prehabilitation before colorectal surgery. Li et al. reported the results of their trial of "trimodal prehabilitation program" in laparoscopic colectomy patients. In their study exercise, anxiety reduction and nutritional therapy were adopted as methods of prehabilitation, and the outcomes were compared with those observed in the control patients treated without prehabilitation. The results showed that exercise was significantly effective in improving the preoperative 6MWT (6 min walking test) values (Li et al. 2013). Although only a few randomized trials have evaluated the effects of prehabilitation in patients undergoing colorectal surgery, it is expected that such treatment will reduce the number of postoperative complications, shorten the length of hospital stay, reduce disability, and improve the quality of life. Carli et al. compared simple walking and breathing with biking and strengthening exercises and found no differences in postoperative walking capacity between the two groups (Polle et al. 2007). The implementation of prehabilitation demands integration of nursing and physiotherapy support into the preoperative care of patients. To obtain best results, care delivery has to be holistic. Sharing of goals and reviews of achievement of targets between the providers delivering prehabilitation and the surgeons is indispensible.

8.3.5 Anesthesia

Although anesthesia is performed in a similar manner as that used in open surgery, there should be specific considerations of anesthesia techniques to facilitate laparoscopic colorectal surgery. During the induction of anesthesia, ventilation of the patients is performed by pressing the anesthesia bag. During this procedure, oxygen gas is pushed into the stomach, and it can eventually reach the small intestine. This may cause distension of the small bowel, resulting in serious difficulties in exposing the operative field during laparoscopic colorectal surgery. The role of the anesthesiologists is important in preventing such situations. If a nasogastric tube is placed before anesthesia is induced, the oxygen gas insufflated into the stomach will automatically be evacuated through the nasogastric tube, resulting in a minimal distension of the stomach and small intestine. Alternatively, the surgeons may ask the anesthetists to perform "crash induction" in which the patient is intubated immediately following muscle relaxation without ventilation using the anesthesia bag.

As previously stated, performing pneumoperitoneum using CO_2 may cause hypercapnia during the surgical procedure. Therefore, depending on the patient's condition during anesthesia, the frequency of ventilation should be increased if there is a risk of hypercapnia.

It is important that the anesthetist understands the difficulties of laparoscopic colorectal surgery and takes steps to facilitate easier laparoscopy, and thus the anesthetist needs to be constantly engaged into the laparoscopic surgical team.

8.3.6 Enhanced Recovery After Surgery (ERAS)

The use of fast-track perioperative care was initially reported in the mid-1990s. The fast-track perioperative care programs consist of multidisciplinary approaches, including the participation of dieticians, nurses, surgeons, and anesthesiologists. Its aim is to reduce the surgical stress response and incidence of organ dysfunction and morbidities, thereby promoting a faster recovery after surgery (Vlug et al. 2011). Due to the less invasive nature of laparoscopic procedures including laparoscopic colorectal surgery, patients treated with such procedures are good candidates of the fast-track perioperative care. The Enhanced Recovery After Surgery (ERAS) system was created during the development of fast-track perioperative care by Kehlet and Wilmore (2002). Fast-track perioperative care consists of the following items: preoperative counseling of the patients, no usage of mechanical bowel preparation, no usage of sedatives, administration of liquid containing carbohydrate solution until 2 h before surgery in place of preoperative fasting, the use of epidural anesthesia during and after surgery in place of opioid pain control, restrictions on the perioperative administration of intravenous fluid, restriction on the routine use of drains and nasogastric tubes, and the early removal of Foley catheter (Wind et al. 2006a).

There are a number of reports on the use of fast-track perioperative care in patients undergoing laparoscopic colorectal surgery. The LAFA (laparoscopic fast track) randomized controlled trial reported in 2011 is the highest level study to prospectively compare four groups, i.e., Lap (Laparoscopic)/FT (Fast Track), Open/FT, Lap/Standard, and Open/Standard (Wind et al. 2006a; Vlug et al. 2011). A total of 472 patients from nine Dutch hospitals were randomized among the four groups. This trial is special because the four groups were blinded as much as possible. The abdomen was covered with a large dressing to hide the type of surgical procedure to blind the surgeons, patients, and nurses. The fast-track patients were treated in a ward specialized in fast-track perioperative care. The criteria for discharge were predetermined in the protocol. As a result, the combination of laparoscopic surgery with fast-track care resulted in a significantly faster recovery after surgery than that observed in the other three combinations, resulting in the shortest length of hospitalization. Therefore, it is considered that both laparoscopic surgery and the fast-track care contributed to achieving a faster recovery after surgery. Similar results were found in the meta-analysis reported by Li et al. (2012). Regarding the incidence of postoperative morbidities in LAFA trial, there were no differences among the four groups. However, in one meta-analysis and one systematic review of colorectal surgery, reduced incidence of morbidity and mortality was observed in the patients treated with fast-track care than in those treated with standard care (Gouvas et al. 2009; Wind et al. 2006b). Discussions on a team-based integrative approach to enhanced recovery have been presented in a previous chapter.

Conclusions

Laparoscopic colorectal surgery is technically well established and is beneficial for the patients due to the reduced invasiveness compared to that observed in open surgery. Patients who undergo minimally invasive procedures are good candidates for fast-track (FT) perioperative care, and FT care reduces the incidence of postoperative organ dysfunction and morbidity resulting in a faster recovery after surgery. The use of transdisciplinary perioperative care involving the systemic and holistic participation of various specialty members is indispensable for achieving successful surgical treatment and obtaining good quality of life for the patients after laparoscopic colorectal surgery.

References

Bowles TA, Sanders KM et al (2008) Simplified risk stratification in elective colorectal surgery. ANZ J Surg 78(1–2):24–27

Carli F, Zavorsky GS (2005) Optimizing functional exercise capacity in the elderly surgical population. Curr Opin Clin Nutr Metab Care 8(1):23–32

Charlson ME, Pompei P et al (1987) A new method of classifying prognostic comorbidity in longitudinal studies: development and validation. J Chronic Dis 40(5):373–383

Copeland GP, Jones D et al (1991) POSSUM: a scoring system for surgical audit. Br J Surg 78(3):355–360

Fleshman J, Sargent DJ et al (2007) Laparoscopic colectomy for cancer is not inferior to open surgery based on 5-year data from the COST Study Group trial. Ann Surg 246(4):655–662; discussion 662–654

Fried LP, Tangen CM et al (2001) Frailty in older adults: evidence for a phenotype. J Gerontol A Biol Sci Med Sci 56(3):M146–M156

Gouvas N, Tan E et al (2009) Fast-track vs standard care in colorectal surgery: a meta-analysis update. Int J Colorectal Dis 24(10):1119–1131

Hanly EJ, Mendoza-Sagaon M et al (2003) CO2 Pneumoperitoneum modifies the inflammatory response to sepsis. Ann Surg 237(3):343–350

Issa N, Grassi C et al (2011) Laparoscopic colectomy for carcinoma of the colon in octogenarians. J Gastrointest Surg 15(11):2011–2015

Jacobs M, Verdeja JC et al (1991) Minimally invasive colon resection (laparoscopic colectomy). Surg Laparosc Endosc 1(3):144–150

Japan Society for Endoscopic Surgery (2012) 11th Nationwide survey of endoscopic surgery in Japan. J Jpn Soc Endosc Surg 17(5):571–687

Kehlet H, Wilmore DW (2002) Multimodal strategies to improve surgical outcome. Am J Surg 183(6):630–641

Li MZ, Xiao LB et al (2012) Meta-analysis of laparoscopic versus open colorectal surgery within fast-track perioperative care. Dis Colon Rectum 55(7):821–827

Li C, Carli F et al (2013) Impact of a trimodal prehabilitation program on functional recovery after colorectal cancer surgery: a pilot study. Surg Endosc 27(4):1072–1082

Ozawa A, Konishi F et al (2000) Cytokine and hormonal responses in laparoscopic-assisted colectomy and conventional open colectomy. Surg Today 30(2):107–111

Polle SW, Wind J et al (2007) Implementation of a fast-track perioperative care program: what are the difficulties? Dig Surg 24(6):441–449

Sabbagh C, Browet F et al (2013) Is stenting as "a bridge to surgery" an oncologically safe strategy for the management of acute, left-sided, malignant, colonic obstruction? A comparative study with a propensity score analysis. Ann Surg 258(1):107–115

Sarkar S, Geraghty J, Rooney P (2013) Colonic stenting: a practical update. Frontline Gastroenterology 4(3):219–226

Schwarz NT, Kalff JC et al (2004) Selective jejunal manipulation causes postoperative pan-enteric inflammation and dysmotility. Gastroenterology 126(1):159–169

Shingu Y, Hasegawa H et al (2013) Clinical and oncologic safety of laparoscopic surgery for obstructive left colorectal cancer following transanal endoscopic tube decompression. Surg Endosc 27(9):3359–3363

Tan L (2013) Prehabilitation. In: Tan K-Y (ed) Colorectal cancer in the elderly. Springer, Heidelberg/New York/Dordrecht/London, pp 73–81

Tan KY, Tan P (2013) Transdisciplinary care for elderly surgical patients. In: Tan K-Y (ed) Colorectal cancer in the elderly. Springer, Heidelberg/New York/Dordrecht/London, pp 83–92

Tan KY, Kawamura Y et al (2009) Colorectal surgery in octogenarian patients–outcomes and predictors of morbidity. Int J Colorectal Dis 24(2):185–189

Tekkis PP, Prytherch DR et al (2004) Development of a dedicated risk-adjustment scoring system for colorectal surgery (colorectal POSSUM). Br J Surg 91(9):1174–1182

The Colon Cancer Laparoscopic or Open Resection Study Group, Buunen M, Veldkamp R et al (2009) Survival after laparoscopic surgery versus open surgery for colon cancer: long-term outcome of a randomised clinical trial. Lancet Oncol 10(1):44–52

Vlug MS, Wind J et al (2011) Laparoscopy in combination with fast track multimodal management is the best perioperative strategy in patients undergoing colonic surgery: a randomized clinical trial (LAFA-study). Ann Surg 254(6):868–875

Wichmann MW, Huttl TP et al (2005) Immunological effects of laparoscopic vs open colorectal surgery: a prospective clinical study. Arch Surg 140(7):692–697

Wind J, Hofland J et al (2006a) Perioperative strategy in colonic surgery; LAparoscopy and/or FAst track multimodal management versus standard care (LAFA trial). BMC Surg 6:16

Wind J, Polle SW et al (2006b) Systematic review of enhanced recovery programmes in colonic surgery. Br J Surg 93(7):800–809

Team-Based Integrative Care for Recurrent and Locally Advanced Rectal Cancer Surgery

9

Min-Hoe Chew

Take-Home Pearls

- Locally advanced primary rectal cancers and recurrent rectal cancers require multifaceted preoperative planning to achieve R0 resections.
- Intraoperative considerations are based on a compartment-based approach.
- Subspecialties required include orthopedics, vascular surgery, urology, plastic surgery, and gyne-oncology.
- Recovery and rehabilitation require appropriate preoperative psychological assessment and preparation and stoma and wound care with the aim to improve quality of life, which is as important an outcome as disease-free survival.

9.1 Background

Surgical management for rectal cancer remains challenging despite significant technical advances in the past few decades. The narrow confines of the bony pelvis with other pelvic organs in close proximity pose significant technical challenges, leading to increased local recurrence rates compared to colon cancers. With the routine adoption of meticulous mesorectal dissection in rectal cancer surgery, local recurrence rates have improved significantly, and there is an increased rate of anal sphincter preservation whenever technically and oncologically feasible. However, despite the use of pre- or postoperative adjuvant chemoradiotherapy, there remains a relatively high local and distant tumor recurrence rate, and up to 32 % of patients with rectal cancers may eventually develop tumor recurrence after curative resection (Mirnezami et al. 2010). Furthermore, newly diagnosed primary locally advanced

---

M.-H. Chew
Department of Colorectal Surgery, Singapore General Hospital,
Singapore, Singapore
e-mail: chew.min.hoe@sgh.com.sg

© Springer-Verlag Berlin Heidelberg 2015
K.-Y. Tan (ed.), *Transdisciplinary Perioperative Care in Colorectal Surgery:
An Integrative Approach*, DOI 10.1007/978-3-662-44020-9_9

rectal cancers that invade contiguous organs are not uncommon, and incidence can range from 25 to 64 % (AIHW 2009; Mercury Study Group 2006).

Surgery has been the only potentially curative option offering a chance for long-term survival, and pelvic exenteration is a procedure usually offered for advanced primary (APC) and locally recurrent rectal cancers (LRC). Pelvic exenteration (PE) surgery was first introduced by Brunswick in 1948 for advanced cervical cancer (Brunschwig 1948) but was associated with high morbidity, perioperative mortality of 23 %, as well as poor postoperative quality of life. In the last two decades, there has been improvement in outcomes and survival rates. This has largely been due to meticulous planning with an interdisciplinary pelvic oncology team comprising a colorectal surgeon, urologist, gyne-oncology surgeon, plastic surgeon, and vascular and orthopedic surgeons. Preoperative workup using appropriate imaging with CT, MRI and PET scans provides important information to aid in decision making algorithms as well as surgical expertise required. In addition, anesthetic evaluation to determine whether the patient is a suitable operative candidate as well as good intraoperative communication with the surgical team are vital in this physiologically and physically demanding procedure. The postoperative recovery team, including stoma nurses to manage both colostomies and urinary conduits, wound nurses for flap reconstructions, physiotherapists for physical rehabilitation, as well as dieticians for nutritional enhancement and guidance, provides confidence to the patient in the recovery process, which often may take a considerable period of time.

9.2 Planning Preoperatively

In an evaluation of a patient for PE surgery, tumor location is largely classified according to the four main compartments of the pelvis – anterior (involving gynecological or urological organs), axial/central, posterior (involving sacrum and coccyx), and lateral (involving pelvic sidewall structures) (Moore et al. 2004) (Fig. 9.1).

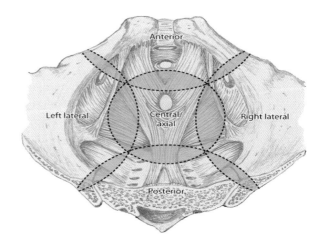

Fig. 9.1 Compartment approach for pelvic exenteration surgery

While this classification was designed for recurrent cancers, it can intuitively be utilized for planning in locally advanced primary cancers. There are a multitude of considerations while evaluating whether a patient is suitable for PE surgery, and decision-making for such a procedure requires several facets. To date, uniform consensus regarding the optimal surgical management of APC and LRC patients has yet to be developed. While there are several guidelines and recommendations published, these are constantly evolving and may lag behind current standards in therapy. Furthermore, differences in practices within the same country and across international borders lead to different strategies and a wide variety of opinions on selection criteria and surgical approaches. Nonetheless, it is widely accepted that superior results are achieved with R0 resections during complete or partial removal of pelvic viscera. The surgeon is required to evaluate and decide whether en bloc resection of pelvic bones as well as ligaments and muscles, nerves, and vessels would achieve good surgical clearance. On the other hand, the narrow confines of the bony pelvis as well as adhesions from radiotherapy and previous surgery may lead to loss of the usual surgical planes and create technical difficulties during resection that may result in considerable morbidity and mortality (Lopez et al. 1994; Nielsen et al. 2012). Much of the decision-making process requires a thorough clinical evaluation and, together with a good radiologist, is guided by information provided by pelvic magnetic resonance imaging (MRI) and positron emission tomography (PET) scans. The surgeon is thus required to balance the pros and cons of various parameters during evaluation and also determine whether the procedure performed would lead to better quality-of-life outcomes.

There have been several predictive factors described that may determine R0 resections. These include for LRC, original margin status, site of pelvic recurrence, number of points of fixity, lymph node status at primary surgery, intraoperative radiotherapy, preoperative and postoperative adjuvant therapy, increased serum CEA levels, extent of resection, and operation type at primary resection (Heriot et al. 2008; Ike et al. 2003; Moore et al. 2004; Pacelli et al. 2010). Besides clinical parameters, pelvic MRIs are crucial in the decision-making process for PE surgery. This is largely because the use of MRI allows clear appreciation of surgical planes and has advantages of good delineation of bony and soft tissue structures. These features allow the surgeon to determine resectability as well as the need for extrafascial dissection to achieve clear circumferential margins. Interestingly, while MRI is the first-choice staging modality for primary rectal cancer (Beets-Tan et al. 2000, 2001), there is little literature about its performance for predicting extent of tumor invasion in local recurrences. Dresen et al. (2010) has demonstrated that preoperative MRI for recurrent lesions is accurate, with a negative predictive value of 93–100 % for invasion into critical structures. However, there was a trend towards over-staging of recurrent tumors and this was mainly attributed to misinterpretation of diffuse fibrosis, especially at the lateral pelvic sidewall.

PET scans provide useful information with regard to presence of metastatic disease and is also an accurate modality for detecting pelvic recurrence with advantages over CT or MRI in differentiating scar/fibrosis from viable tumor (Schaefer and Langer 2007; Huebner et al. 2000). Nonetheless false-positive interpretations of physiologic FDG uptake in displaced pelvic organs like bladder, seminal vesicles, uterus, and small bowel loops as well as radiation-induced inflammation reduce specificity. Both the PET and pelvic MRI thus require expert assessment together with a dedicated radiologist and often, the decision to proceed requires a period of evaluation.

To aid in summarizing what factors are useful in PE surgery, a survey involving an international panel of 36 colorectal surgeons that perform PE surgery was conducted. Ninety-nine clinical and radiological criteria were evaluated based on a Likert scale. Clinical factors suggestive of systemic disease, symptoms of advanced local recurrence, surgical fitness, and cognitive impairment were considered important by the panel when considering suitability for surgery. For radiological features, strong agreement was achieved for factors associated with tumor involvement in the axial and anterior compartments. Agreement, however, was not obtained for resectable metastatic disease as well as lateral and posterior compartment tumor involvement. These features will require further evaluation before consensus may be obtained (Chew et al. 2013).

9.3 Surgical Approach Unique for Pelvic Exenteration Surgery

9.3.1 Sacrectomy

A sacrectomy may be considered if the tumor is adherent or has invaded the presacral fascia especially if previous rectal resection has been performed. Oncological benefits (Wells et al. 2007; Melton et al. 2006; Feresnchild et al. 2009) have been purported with improved overall survival and disease-free survival. Traditionally, sacropelvic resection at or below the level of S3 was considered the limit of resection, but there have been increasing number of reports for high sacrum (at or above level of S2) (Dozois et al. 2011; Colibaseanu et al. 2014). Outcomes in these series have shown that for higher sacrum resection, 5-year survival rates (17–31 %) are as good as those for lower sacrum resections (20–26 %).

The orthopedic surgeon has frequently been called for assistance at this portion of the procedure, which requires the patient to be turned prone following completion of the abdominal and perineal phases of the procedure. In total sacrectomies, pelvic stability reconstruction of the lumbar spine and the iliac bone is required with titanium rods supplemented by bone grafts. Recently, abdominal approaches have been suggested for S3 and below (Solomon et al. 2014). The multiple logistic advantages described include reducing general anesthetic time as turning a patient prone on an already prolonged operation (on average >9 h per case), with multiple invasive monitoring lines, is often arduous, complex, and challenging. The ability to better dissect off lateral compartment structures transabdominally and vascular control and hemostasis argue in favor of an abdominal approach for lower sacrectomies.

Complication rate remains high, however, and major complications such as pelvic sepsis range from 15 to 39 % and increase if the patient has had radiotherapy.

Fig. 9.2 Anatomy displayed required for lateral exenteration

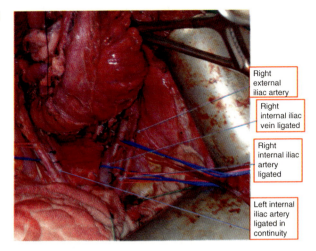

Wound dehiscence rates also range from 31 to 58 %. For postoperative neurological deficits, higher sacrectomies have been found to cause higher incidences of urinary and bowel dysfunction, but there was no observed functional difference in postoperative ambulation between high or low sacrectomies (Harji et al. 2013). Postoperative rehabilitation and physiotherapy are evidently vital in all patients who undergo sacrectomies.

9.3.2 Vascular Resection and Reconstruction

Various studies suggest that lateral pelvic sidewall recurrence is a very poor prognostic variable, with the inability to achieve R0 resection as one of the main deterring reasons (Mirnezami et al. 2010). These inferior results have been described largely due to anatomical restrictions from the bone or major pelvic sidewall vessels that limit extent of resection. Certainly, improved techniques and imaging permit en bloc resection with some encouraging results for lateral pelvic recurrences. Recent results have suggested that R0 resection rates can approach as high as 53 % with overall survival of 69 % at 19 months follow-up (Austin and Solomon 2009) and can be achieved with extended radical resections including en bloc iliac vessels as well as lateral pelvic bone and ligament resection.

In this technique, "preparation" of the pelvis often requires the mobilizing the iliac vessels free. Typically, the external iliac artery and vein are slung and mobilized off the lateral wall (Fig. 9.2). This allows access to the obturator canal and structures such as the sciatic nerve, femoral nerve, psoas, obturator internus, sacrospinous ligaments, and lateral bony structures such as the ischial spine. The internal iliac ligation usually begins with the artery followed by the vein (Fig. 9.2). If tumor is noted to have extended to the common or external iliac vessels, a vascular surgeon usually performs reconstruction with patch grafts or bypass surgery (Austin and Solomon 2009). This approach has been described in sarcoma surgery and graft patency rates are high at 58–93 % (McKay et al. 2007).

9.3.3 Reconstruction

Reconstruction after PE surgery is necessary on several fronts. Urogenital tract and perineal defects often require decisions based on the quality of the tissue, which is often impaired after chemoradiotherapy, and the functional status of the remnant organ.

Ureteric reconstruction can be performed using either ileal or colonic conduits. Complication rate may be high during conduit formation (16 %), and factors identified include R2 resection margins, magnitude of exenteration, and presence of cardiovascular history (Teixeira et al. 2012). Comparisons between ileal and colonic conduits, however, have noted no difference in glomerular filtration rates or stenotic complications at the ureterointestinal anastomosis. To avoid a permanent urinary ostomy bag, some options of urinary diversion to form a continent reservoir include a Miami pouch, which is reported 93 % continence rate. Other procedures include Kock pouch, Florida pouch, and Mainz pouch but this may be challenging in an irradiated pelvis. A detailed discussion with the urologist is paramount.

The perineal wound can be large after PE surgery. This is especially if the tumor originally is fungating through the perineum, after sacrectomies, or presence of unhealthy tissue after radiotherapy requiring larger-than-planned excisions. Suggested methods may be the use of omentum flaps, biological meshes, or using a pedicled flap with the aid of a plastic surgeon. Common flaps used include, transpelvic rectus abdominis myocutaneous flaps, gracilis myocutaneous flaps, and gluteal myocutaneous advancement or rotational flaps (Mirnezami et al. 2010). Other novel methods include the use of mammary implants in the pelvic cavity (Valle et al. 2011), or the use of a colonic flap with the mucosa removed has been described with good outcome in nine patients (Sahakitrungruang and Atittharnsakul 2012).

9.4 Postoperative Care and Quality of Life

The radical nature of the surgery often creates a toll on the patient and their caregivers. While clear surgical margins are important facets in planning, once confirmation of safety is established in the preoperative phase, assessment of the quality of life of the survivor has been suggested to be equally an important indicator compared with survival (Fraser 1993). The long hospital stay, high complication rates, and the creation of both colostomy and conduits in the patient are important considerations when counseling the patient preoperatively. Psychological preparation of the patient is required and aided often by a dedicated nurse clinician or coordinator and what to expect in the recovery phase should be clearly defined. The rehabilitation team incorporates the physiotherapists, stoma nurses, wound

9 Team-Based Integrative Care for Recurrent and Locally Advanced Rectal Cancer

care nurses, and dieticians as well as potentially psychologists to help the patient cope are key determinants in the successful outcome. It is important in this recovery team to understand too that while the immediate recovery phase can be difficult, long-term QOL is good. This is corroborated by Austin and Solomon (2009) who, in a study of 37 patients, noted that longer-term survivors of PE surgery for advanced primary and recurrent rectal cancers have comparable QOL to those undergoing routine rectal cancer surgery and the population at large. In particular, while physical well-being was slightly poorer compared with the general populace, mental well-being was noted to be good or comparable. This once again demonstrates the importance of preparation preoperatively as well as the postoperative recovery team.

Conclusion

The feasibility of such radical surgery options has been clearly proven and provides potential survival benefits for patients whom have been defined to be "incurable." The associated risks of the surgery discussed with the patient need to be balanced against the benefits of symptoms control, survival outcomes as well as quality-of-life issues. Successful surgery in APC and LRC requires skill sets and expertise beyond that of a single colorectal surgeon. The numerous specialties involved, and discussions with meticulous planning using detailed MRI and PET scans, are best done in tumor board settings. Trained nurse clinicians may best coordinate psychological preparation of the patient as well as coordinate rehabilitation and care of wounds, flaps, and stomas. It is likely in this integrative team-based care for such patients that success is raised in these surgeries.

References

Austin KK, Solomon MJ (2009) Pelvic exenteration with en bloc iliac vessel resection for lateral pelvic wall involvement. Dis Colon Rectum 52(7):1223–1233

Austin KK, Young JM, Solomon MJ (2010) Quality of life survivors after pelvic exenteration for rectal cancer. Dis Colon Rectum 53:1121–1126

Australian Institute of Health and Welfare (AIHW) (2009) Rectosigmoid junction and rectum for Australia. AIHW, Canberra

Beets-Tan RG, Beets GL, Borstlap AC et al (2000) Preoperative assessment of local tumour extent in local advanced rectal cancer: CT or high resolution MRI? Abdom Imaging 25(5):533–541

Beets-Tan RG, Beets GL, Vliegen RF et al (2001) Accuracy of magnetic resonance imaging in prediction of tumour-free resection margin in rectal cancer surgery. Lancet 357(9255):497–504

Brunschwig A (1948) Complete excision of pelvic viscera for advanced carcinoma. Cancer 1:77

Chew MH, Brown WE, Masya L et al (2013) Clinical, MRI, and PET-CT criteria used by surgeons to determine suitability for pelvic exenteration surgery for recurrent rectal cancers: a Delphi study. Dis Colon Rectum 56(6):717–725

Colibaseanu DT, Dozois EJ, Mathis KL et al (2014) Extended sacropelvic resection for locally recurrent rectal cancer: can it be done safely and with good oncologic outcomes? Dis Colon Rectum 57(1):47–55

Dozois EJ, Privitera A, Holubar SD et al (2011) High sacrectomy for locally recurrent rectal cancer: can long-term survival be achieved? J Surg Oncol 103:105–109

Dresen RC, Kusters M, Daniels-Gooszen AW et al (2010) Absence of tumor invasion into pelvic structures in locally recurrent rectal cancer: prediction with preoperative MR imaging. Radiology 256(1):143–150

Feresnchild FT, Vermaas M, Verhoeft C et al (2009) Abdominosacral resection for locally advanced and recurrent rectal cancer. Br J Surg 96:1341–1347

Fraser SCA (1993) Quality-of-life measurement in surgical practice. Br J Surg 80:163–169

Harji DP, Griffiths B, McArthur DR, Sagar PM (2013) Surgery for recurrent rectal cancer: higher and wider? Colorectal Dis 15(2):139–145

Heriot AG, Byrne CM, Lee P et al (2008) Extended radical resection: the choice for locally recurrent rectal cancer. Dis Colon Rectum 51(3):284–291

Huebner RH, Park KC, Shepherd JE et al (2000) A meta-analysis of the literature for whole-body FDG PET detection of recurrent colorectal cancer. J Nucl Med 41(7):1177–1189

Ike H, Shimada H, Yamaguchi S et al (2003) Outcome of total pelvic exenteration for primary rectal cancer. Dis Colon Rectum 46:474–480

Lopez MJ, Standiford SB, Skibba JL (1994) Total pelvic exenteration. A 50-year experience at the Ellis Fischel Cancer Centre. Arch Surg 129(4):395–396

McKay A, Motamedi M, Temple W et al (2007) Vascular reconstruction with the superficial femoral vein following major oncologic resection. J Surg Oncol 96:151–159

Melton GB, Paty PB, Boland PJ et al (2006) Sacral resection for recurrent rectal cancer: analysis of morbidity and treatment results. Dis Colon Rectum 49:1099–1107

Mercury Study Group (2006) Diagnostic accuracy of preoperative magnetic resonance imaging in predicting curative resection of rectal cancer: prospective observational study. BMJ 333:779

Mirnezami AH, Sagar PM, Kavanagh D et al (2010) Clinical algorithms for the surgical management of locally recurrent rectal cancer. Dis Colon Rectum 53(9):1248–1257

Moore HG, Shoup M, Riedel E et al (2004) Colorectal cancer pelvic recurrences: determinants of resectability. Dis Colon Rectum 47(10):1599–1606

Nielsen M, Rasmussen P, Lindegaard J, Laurberg S (2012) A 10-year experience of total pelvic exenteration for primary advanced and locally recurrent rectal cancer based on a prospective database. Colorectal Dis 14(9):1076–1083

Pacelli F, Tortorelli AP, Rosa F et al (2010) Locally recurrent rectal cancer: prognostic factors and long-term outcomes of multimodal therapy. Ann Surg Oncol 17(1):152–162

Sahakitrungruang C, Atittharnsakul P (2012) Colonic flap with mucosa removed: a novel technique for pelvic reconstruction after exenteration of advanced pelvic malignancy. Tech Coloproctol 16:373–378

Schaefer O, Langer M (2007) Detection of recurrent rectal cancer with CT, MRI and PET/CT. Eur Radiol 17(8):2044–2054

Solomon MJ, Tan KK, Bromilow RG et al (2014) Sacrectomy via the abdominal approach during pelvic exenteration. Dis Colon Rectum 57(2):272–277

Teixeira SC, Ferenschild FT, Solomon MJ et al (2012) Urological leaks after pelvic exenterations comparing formation of colonic and ileal conduits. Eur J Surg Oncol 38(4):361–366

Valle M, Federici O, Ialongo P et al (2011) Prevention of complications following pelvic exenteration with the use of mammary implants in the pelvic cavity: technique and results of 28 cases. J Surg Oncol 103:34–38

Wells BJ, Stotland P, Ko MA et al (2007) Results of an aggressive approach to resection of locally recurrent rectal cancer. Ann Surg Oncol 14:390–395

Multimodal Approach to Familial Colorectal Cancer

10

Sarah Jane Walton and Sue Clark

Take-Home Pearls

- Early referral to specialist centres improves patient outcome in familial CRC.
- Geneticists and counsellors have a key role in diagnosis.
- Management of polyposis syndromes can begin in childhood, involving paediatric and adolescent transition expertise.
- High-quality endoscopy and advanced endoscopic therapies are key in managing those with Lynch and polyposis syndromes.
- Most individuals with FAP, MAP and some with Lynch syndrome and hamartomatous polyposis syndromes require surgery, with well-informed and nuanced decision-making central.
- Lynch syndrome and all of the polyposis syndromes are associated with extraintestinal manifestations, necessitating involvement of a wide network of experienced clinicians.

10.1 Introduction

Colorectal cancer (CRC) development depends upon complex interaction between genetic predisposition and environment. Most tumours occur by chance, and environmental factors are thought largely responsible. Familial CRC arises in individuals where genetics plays a more influential role. This group may be categorised into low, moderate or high risk for CRC. This risk is higher in families with more relatives affected by cancer, and when tumours arise at a young age. About 5 % of CRC falls

---

S. Clark (✉)
The Polyposis Registry, St Mark's Hospital,
Harrow, Middlesex, UK
e-mail: s.clark8@nhs.net

S.J. Walton
Department of Surgery, St Mark's Hospital, Harrow, Middlesex, UK

© Springer-Verlag Berlin Heidelberg 2015
K.-Y. Tan (ed.), *Transdisciplinary Perioperative Care in Colorectal Surgery: An Integrative Approach*, DOI 10.1007/978-3-662-44020-9_10

into the high-risk group, where genotype plays a fundamental role in the inheritance of bowel cancer. Lynch syndrome and polyposis syndromes fall into this group.

10.2 Evaluating Risk

Individuals should be risk stratified for CRC development to enable clinicians to determine appropriate surveillance and management (Fig. 10.1). It is imperative that an accurate family history is obtained detailing affected family members, sites of all tumours and the age at which they occurred (Houlston et al. 1990). A detailed personal history must be sought, including previous polyps, cancers or risk factors for CRC development (e.g. inflammatory bowel disease). This is best done in a specialist family cancer clinic where sufficient time can be given to gather accurate information and counsel patients (Lips 1998).

Evaluating cancer risk within a family is a dynamic process. Individuals may move to a higher-risk group as more cancers develop within the same family over time or as more information is gathered for existing relatives.

In the high-risk group of Lynch and polyposis syndromes, there is a one in two chances of inheriting a lifetime risk of bowel cancer of more than 50 %. The polyposis syndromes can usually be diagnosed without too much difficulty through a

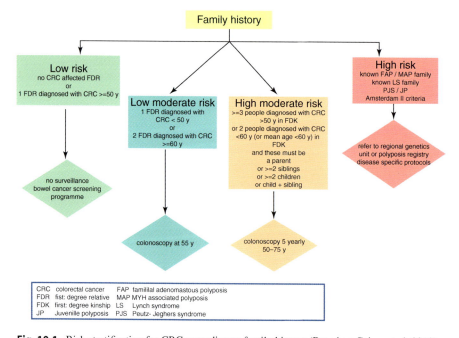

Fig. 10.1 Risk stratification for CRC according to family history (Based on Cairns et al. 2010)

recognisable phenotype, but Lynch syndrome can be more difficult because there is no distinguishing feature, only the presence of cancer.

10.3 Lynch Syndrome

This autosomal dominantly inherited condition accounts for approximately 2–4 % of all CRCs and the majority of inherited colonic tumours. Lynch syndrome was previously termed hereditary non-polyposis colorectal cancer (HNPCC), but as some adenomatous polyps can arise in this condition, this term has been largely discarded (Jass 2006).

Lynch syndrome typically presents with CRC in the fourth decade of life with a tendency towards right-sided, poorly differentiated, mucinous colonic tumours with lymphocytic infiltrates. There are often multiple cancers within the colon and elsewhere including the endometrium, stomach, ovaries, renal tract, pancreas, small bowel and brain (Aarnio et al. 1999).

10.3.1 Genetics

Lynch syndrome results from germline mutations in tumour suppressing mismatch repair (MMR) genes coding for proteins that either correct base pair mistakes during DNA replication or stimulate apoptosis when it is irreparable (Jass 2006). Affected individuals inherit a defective copy. MMR function is lost in a cell when the remaining normal gene becomes mutated. A lack of MMR proteins stimulates tumourigenesis by allowing rapid accumulation of mutations in other genes. Microsatellites, regions of short DNA sequence repeats, characteristically become mutated as a result of deficiency in MMR proteins, resulting in microsatellite instability (MSI). MSI is a key feature of tumours that lack MMR and is seen in approximately 15 % of sporadic CRCs as well as those arising in Lynch syndrome.

10.3.2 Diagnosis

A diagnosis of Lynch syndrome can be made using a combination of family history, tumour analysis (to detect MSI) and/or genetic testing. Whilst families fulfilling the Amsterdam II criteria (Box 10.1) may have Lynch syndrome, these will only identify half of those with the syndrome, as 50 % of those affected will fail to meet the criteria. Of those meeting the criteria, half will not have Lynch syndrome (Simmang et al. 1999). Nearly all Lynch syndrome tumours will be MSI high due to MMR mutation and show lack of MMR protein expression on immunohistochemistry (MMR-IHC). The Bethesda criteria (Box 10.2) help in deciding when to test tumours for MSI or MMR-IHC. This will usually identify up to 90 % of people with CRC due to Lynch syndrome (Umar et al. 2004).

Box 10.1. Amsterdam Criteria II (Vasen et al. 1999)

At least *three relatives* with a Lynch syndrome-associated cancer (colorectal, endometrial, small bowel, ureteral, renal pelvis). One should be a first-degree relative of the other two

At least *two successive generations* should be affected

At least 1 CRC should be diagnosed <*50 years*

FAP should be excluded

Tumours should be verified by pathological examination

Box 10.2. Bethesda Criteria

CRC diagnosed in a patient <*50 years old*

The presence of *multiple* colorectal or other Lynch syndrome-associated tumours, either synchronous or metachronous at *any age*

CRC with *high MSI* histology in a patient <*60 years* old

CRC diagnosed in *one or more* first-degree relatives with a Lynch syndrome-associated tumour, with one of the cancers diagnosed <*50 years* of age

CRC diagnosed in *two or more* first-degree or second-degree relatives with Lynch syndrome-associated tumours, at *any age*

MMR gene mutation detection is expensive, and the decision to test will depend upon individual circumstances. This requires a multidisciplinary team approach with specialist nurses and doctors working within the field of inherited bowel cancer and genetics (Scholefield et al. 1998; Burke et al. 1997). A histopathologist, specialising in inherited CRC, is important when determining which tumours require further testing to achieve an accurate diagnosis. Patients require appropriate counselling, informing them of the possible outcomes from genetic testing, from insurance to family and work life issues. If a mutation is found, appropriate surveillance can be arranged, and other family members can be offered predictive testing to establish whether they carry the abnormal gene. If they do not, they can be discharged from follow-up. In high-risk families where no mutation can be identified, individuals should continue with colonoscopic surveillance.

The complex nature of inherited CRC requires a multidisciplinary approach, particularly in cases of diagnostic difficulty. Regular meetings to discuss complicated cases will require contributions from specialist nurses/counsellors, gastroenterologists/endoscopists, paediatric services, geneticists, radiologists, histopathologists and surgeons. This creates a forum where team members can discuss cases amongst other specialists and consensus can be reached regarding diagnosis, appropriate investigations and management, supported where possible with evidence-based practice. A chairperson directs the team. Where further endoscopies may be required for tissue diagnosis/genetic testing, they can be arranged efficiently and results discussed within the same forum when available. Recommendations can then be communicated to the patient through specialist nurses, gastroenterologists or surgeons as appropriate. This ensures the delivery of a high-quality service where accurate diagnoses can be reached, appropriate surveillance can be arranged and optimal management instituted.

10.3.3 Surveillance

Where screening has been undertaken, significant benefits to life expectancy have been demonstrated in MMR mutation carriers. This is estimated to be an additional 13.5 years, and after prophylactic proctocolectomy, 15.6 years, when compared with no intervention (Syngal et al. 1998).

Colonoscopy is recommended for at-risk individuals every 1–2 years from 25 years of age or 5 years younger than the youngest affected family member, whichever is earlier. This continues until 75 years of age, or where a causative mutation found in a family is excluded from the individual (Vasen et al. 2007). There is no evidence to support surveillance for extracolonic cancers.

10.3.4 Medical Intervention

The Colorectal Adenoma/Carcinoma Prevention Programme 2 (CAPP2) study evaluated aspirin as a chemopreventative agent in Lynch syndrome and found a reduction in CRC rate. However, more data are required to determine optimal dose and treatment duration (Burn et al. 2011).

Some cytotoxic chemotherapy agents are of questionable benefit in Lynch syndrome-associated cancer. It is imperative that oncologists are aware of the underlying diagnosis (Vasen et al. 2007).

10.3.5 Surgical Intervention

Prophylactic surgery should be discussed with high-risk individuals. This may include prophylactic colectomy, hysterectomy and/or bilateral salpingo-oophorectomy. The options for addressing CRC risk include subtotal colectomy or total colectomy with restorative proctocolectomy (RPC).

There is a 16 % risk of metachronous bowel tumours after 10 years follow-up (Ruschoff et al. 1998). For those with a colonic tumour, the surgical options are segmental colonic resection or colectomy with ileorectal anastomosis (IRA). A segmental resection may result in a better function, but full colonoscopic surveillance is still required due to a risk of further CRC development. Colectomy with IRA reduces this risk. Because the rectum is retained, the morbidity associated with proctectomy is avoided and surveillance made easier. A proctocolectomy, in the form of an end ileostomy or RPC, is recommended for rectal cancers.

10.4 Familial Colorectal Cancer Type X

Lindor et al. introduced this term to describe individuals meeting the Amsterdam criteria with MSI negative colorectal cancers (Lindor et al. 2005). Family members meeting these criteria are at lower risk of developing CRC than in Lynch syndrome but will still require 3–5-yearly colonoscopic surveillance (Dove-Edwin et al. 2006).

10.5 Familial Adenomatous Polyposis (FAP)

FAP is a rare, autosomal, dominantly inherited condition characterised by the development of hundreds to thousands of colorectal adenomas. The population prevalence of FAP is between 1/7,500 and 1/13,000 with almost 100 % disease penetrance by 40 years of age (Bisgaard et al. 1994).

Without prophylactic colectomy, almost all individuals affected will develop CRC by the fourth decade of life (Petersen et al. 1991). Polyps also occur in the stomach and duodenum. Fundic gland polyps in the stomach pose no malignant risk (Wu et al. 1998b). Ninety per cent of those with FAP develop duodenal adenomas, and in 10 % of cases these can become malignant (Wallace and Phillips 1998). They are mostly peri-ampullary and associated with poor prognosis if they progress to cancer (Clark 2009).

Extra-intestinal manifestations of FAP include osteomas, dental abnormalities (e.g. supernumerary teeth), congenital hypertrophy of the retinal pigment epithelium (CHRPE), epidermoid cysts, adrenal adenomas, cancers (including thyroid, central nervous system tumours and hepatoblastoma) and desmoid tumours (Half et al. 2009).

10.5.1 Genetics

FAP is due to germline mutation in one of the copies of the tumour suppressing adenomatous polyposis coli (*APC*) gene.

10.5.2 Diagnosis

Traditionally, FAP was diagnosed by the presence of more than 100 colorectal adenomas, but this definition fails to incorporate all cases: i.e., in attenuated FAP only 10–100 polyps may occur, and CRC presents at a later age (Hernegger et al. 2002). In up to 80 % of cases, FAP can be confirmed genetically by identifying the *APC* mutation responsible. Most will originate from previously known FAP families but 20 % arise as a new mutation (Bisgaard et al. 1994).

An expert endoscopist is important in the accurate assessment and diagnosis of FAP. The use of chromoendoscopy (dye spray) can avoid under reporting of polyp burden and misdiagnosis (Wallace et al. 1999). An upper gastrointestinal (GI) endoscopy can be helpful in confirming the diagnosis of FAP as the majority will have duodenal adenomas and fundic gland polyps.

Registries play a fundamental role in ensuring the welfare of people with polyposis syndromes, from identifying at-risk family members through detailed family pedigrees to arranging regular follow-up and offering genetic testing and counselling where appropriate. When genetic testing is not appropriately delivered, there may be adverse consequences to patient care including inaccurate information giving and inadequate counselling (Giardiello et al. 1997). The affected individual should be genetically tested, and where the mutation is identified, other family members can be offered predictive testing; if negative, they can be discharged from follow-up (Berk et al. 1999). Predictive testing is typically offered to children around the age of 12 years as it is rare for advanced colorectal adenomas to develop before this time. If no mutation is identified, then clinical surveillance is required for at-risk individuals.

10.5.3 Surveillance

Annual flexible sigmoidoscopy is recommended from 13 to 15 years but should be undertaken earlier should symptoms develop (e.g. change in bowel function, anaemia or bleeding per rectum). Screening for FAP at a younger age is not recommended due to ethical considerations and because intervention is rarely necessary in the asymptomatic (Tudyka and Clark 2012). Children should be followed up by a specialist paediatric gastroenterologist who will ensure they receive appropriate endoscopic assessment and management. Those developing more or larger polyps than expected for their age may require earlier referral for surgical intervention.

Provided no polyps are seen at flexible sigmoidoscopy, colonoscopy should commence from 20 years of age and continue at 5-yearly intervals with annual flexible sigmoidoscopy in the intervening periods. This algorithm also applies for at-risk individuals where no mutation can be identified.

10.5.4 Surgical Intervention

It is important to appreciate the genotype-phenotype correlation in FAP when planning surgery. The *APC* gene mutation site can affect phenotypic expression (Wu et al. 1998a). Mutations located between codons 1251 and 1309 predispose to a higher colorectal polyp burden, particularly in the rectum, and cancer often develops earlier. In contrast, mutations at the 3′ and 5′ ends of the gene tend to result in a milder 'attenuated' phenotype (Soravia et al. 1998; Nieuwenhuis and Vasen 2007). Some individuals with identical mutations exhibit different phenotypic expression which suggests that environmental factors or other genes are important in disease manifestation. Mutations 3′ of 1399 are associated with a higher risk of desmoid development, which can lead to significant morbidity (Sinha et al. 2010). This knowledge may impact upon surgical decision-making, influencing the timing and type of surgery offered.

Once a diagnosis is confirmed, prophylactic colectomy or proctocolectomy is usually offered. A thorough colonoscopy is required to determine polyp burden prior to surgery. Unless this is high or polyps cause symptoms, surgery can be planned for a convenient time, e.g. during school holidays, to minimise impact on education and other activities. For the majority, surgery will be undertaken around mid to late teens.

Until the late 1970s, the only surgical options were a total proctocolectomy (TPC) with end ileostomy or a colectomy with IRA. 1978 saw the advent of RPC with ileo-anal anastomosis (Parks and Nicholls 1978). More recently, a laparoscopic approach has become a surgical option, with the advantage of improved cosmesis.

10.5.5 Surgical Options

For the majority of people facing surgery, a permanent ileostomy will not be a real consideration, and so the decision regarding the type of surgery will come down to either RPC or colectomy and IRA. The advantages and disadvantages of these procedures are listed in Box 10.3.

10.5.5.1 TPC

The whole of the large bowel is excised and a permanent end ileostomy formed, completely removing the risk of CRC. This will rarely be performed prophylactically but is appropriate for very low rectal cancers.

Box 10.3. Comparing Advantages and Drawbacks of Colectomy and IRA and RPC

	Colectomy and IRA	RPC
Advantages	One-stage procedure, no ileostomy	Less frequent endoscopic surveillance
	Acceptable bowel frequency (×3/day). Incontinence rare	Lowered cancer risk
	Technically easier to perform laparoscopically/open	
	Lower perioperative morbidity	
	No effect on fertility/erectile function	
Disadvantages	Intensive endoscopic follow-up	Bowel frequency typically ×5/day. Impaired continence common
	Completion proctectomy sometimes needed	Usually two-stage procedure with temporary ileostomy. Complex surgery
	Rectal cancer risk (Nugent and Phillips 1992)	Higher perioperative morbidity (Björk et al. 2001)
		50 % reduction in female fertility (Olsen et al. 2003)
		2 % risk of erectile/ejaculatory dysfunction
		10 % risk pouch failure resulting in permanent ileostomy (Von Roon et al. 2007)
		Can develop cancer in the pouch/anastomosis (Van Duijvendijk et al. 1999a)

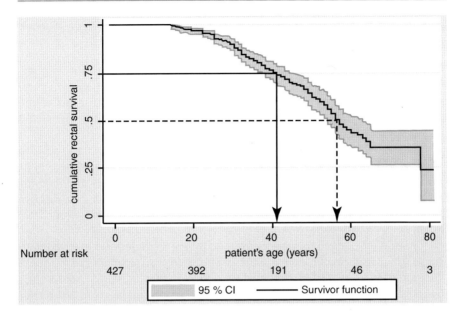

Fig. 10.2 Kaplan-Meier plot showing survival of a healthy rectum (i.e., not requiring removal because of cancer or high adenoma burden) plotted against patient age following IRA. St Mark's Hospital data 1948–2007. Tudyka and Clark (2012) (Reproduced with permission from Hellenic Society of Gastroenterology)

10.5.5.2 Colectomy and IRA

This can be a laparoscopic or open procedure. Defaecatory frequency and leakage are less when compared to RPC (Aziz et al. 2006). The major disadvantage is the carcinoma risk in the retained rectum, which rises sharply after 50 years of age (Fig. 10.2) (Tudyka and Clark 2012; Nugent and Phillips 1992; Nugent et al. 1993). For those requiring subsequent rectal excision, an ileo-anal pouch may be suitable or otherwise a completion proctectomy with end ileostomy will be necessary.

10.5.5.3 RPC

This operation is an attractive option as nearly the entire large bowel is removed. However, RPC can significantly reduce female fecundity and in 1–2 % of men lead to erectile or ejaculatory dysfunction (Aziz et al. 2006; Cornish et al. 2007). Controversy remains regarding the best technique for anastomosing the pouch and anus. Stapling leaves a small cuff of rectal mucosa where tumours can develop (Van Duijvendijk et al. 1999a). Performing a mucosectomy and a handsewn anastomosis instead is technically challenging, may affect functional outcome and does not abolish cancer risk. Adenomas and carcinomas can also occur in the pouch itself (Church 2005).

10.5.6 Other Considerations and Multidisciplinary Surgical Decision-Making

Historical data found a cumulative rectal cancer risk in the retained rectum after IRA of up to 30 % by 60 years of age. Before RPC, there was no alternative to permanent ileostomy following colectomy other than IRA, so many chose this, regardless of polyp burden. Managing the rectum post-surgery was difficult before flexible endoscopy became available.

It is known that some groups with FAP carry a higher risk of CRC development, e.g. those with codon 1309 mutation. RPC is recommended here rather than IRA, as the risk of developing significant rectal polyposis and requiring proctectomy is high. RPC is also recommended in severe phenotypes, e.g. over 500 colonic adenomas or more than 20 rectal adenomas (Church et al. 2003; Sinha et al. 2010).

It is vital that a multidisciplinary team (MDT) of specialists are involved in the surgical management of patients. In the first instance, it is important that the geneticist can identify the *APC* mutation where possible. Then, a skilled endoscopist is essential in determining the true extent of polyp burden in the colon and rectum. A pathologist must assess all histology accurately as this may influence the timing of surgery. Specialist nurses and paediatric gastroenterologists often build bonds with patients over years of clinic attendance and may act as patient advocates during MDT discussions. Finally, all available information is presented and discussed within the MDT meeting and surgical recommendations offered to the patient. In cases of attenuated polyposis, surgery may be deferred to a later stage if polyp burden remains small. Some can remain endoscopically manageable with annual surveillance. This may be particularly relevant for those with a desmoid prone mutation in whom trauma from surgery may stimulate desmoid development. Complex cases such as these highlight the importance of MDT discussion and the provision of patient-tailored care.

Patients are counselled about the advantages and disadvantages of each procedure in a specialist clinic setting so they can make an informed decision regarding their surgery. No significant difference has been demonstrated in bowel function and quality of life when comparing RPC and IRA (Aziz et al. 2006; Van Duijvendijk et al. 1999b; Ko et al. 2000; Günther et al. 2003; Hassan et al. 2005). A selective patient-tailored approach results in a better outcome following IRA (Church et al. 2003).

Lifelong follow-up is necessary for individuals with FAP, with endoscopic and clinical examination of the rectum or pouch. After colectomy, the major causes of morbidity and mortality are duodenal cancer and desmoid tumours (Nugent et al. 1993; Bertario et al. 1994), and it is important that these are monitored in a specialist, multidisciplinary setting too.

10.5.7 Managing Extra-colonic Manifestations of FAP

10.5.7.1 Duodenal Disease

Duodenal adenomas develop in nearly all people with FAP and become invasive in 10 % (Groves et al. 2002). Surveillance is recommended with endoscopy after 30 years of age in asymptomatic individuals (Cairns et al. 2010). Intervals between endoscopies will vary between 6 months and 5 years, determined by the Spigelman stage (Box 10.4) (Burke et al. 1999; Spigelman et al. 1989). Expert endoscopists using a side-viewing scope are essential in the assessment of the ampulla, and its surrounding area, that is at particular risk of tumour development. Thorough histological analysis by expert pathologists is necessary to determine the stage of disease. The cancer risk in stages I–II disease is minimal, but approaches one third with Spigelman stage IV disease over a 10-year period (Groves et al. 2002). Where cancer arises, prognosis is poor (Latchford et al. 2009). Expert endoscopic management using advanced techniques to control peri-ampullary polyps can be employed in severe diseases to delay definitive surgery, such as prophylactic pancreatico-duodenectomy or pancreas-sparing duodenectomy, that is associated with significant morbidity and mortality (Gallagher et al. 2004; Mackey et al. 2005). However, there are no data currently that show endoscopic therapies alter long-term cancer risk and the management of duodenal adenomatous polyps remains a challenge for clinicians.

Box 10.4. Spigelman Staging and Recommended Endoscopy Intervals

	Points allocated		
	1	**2**	**3**
Number of polyps	1–4	5–20	>20
Polyp size (mm)	1–4	5–10	>10
Histological type	Tubular	Tubulovillous	Villous
Degree of dysplasia	Mild	Moderate	Severe
Total points	**Spigelman stage**	**Recommended follow-up interval**	
0	0	5 years	
1–4	I	5 years	
5–6	II	3 years	
7–8	III	1 year and consider endoscopic therapy	
9–12	IV	6 monthly. Consider prophylactic duodenectomy	

10.5.7.2 Desmoid Disease

Desmoid tumours are benign, locally infiltrating, fibromatous tumours arising in connective tissue. They occur in approximately 15 % of patients with FAP, and although the majority are not associated with significant morbidity, there is an associated mortality rate of 10 % (Clark et al. 1999; Church et al. 1999). Most occur in the abdominal wall or mesentery, and associated complications include ureteric obstruction, bowel obstruction, perforation, fistulation, ischaemia and even death. Risk factors for desmoid development include trauma (e.g. surgery), female gender, particular germline mutations as well as other genetic factors (Sinha et al. 2010). Some desmoids grow and regress, whilst many remain in a stable state, and for these it is preferable to minimise surgical intervention that may otherwise stimulate further growth. Some grow relentlessly and remain a challenge to treat. The management of desmoid disease, particularly in severe cases, may require input from other disciplines. Expert radiologists are important in the identification and occasional radiological intervention of desmoids and their associated complications (e.g. intra-abdominal collections). Ureteric obstruction is not uncommon, and so regular radiological renal tract assessment with an ultrasound scan is recommended. Where obstruction occurs, ureteric stenting is required. For imaging assessment of abdominal desmoids, MRI is at least equivalent to CT and avoids radiation (Sinha et al. 2012).

Management options include nonsteroidal anti-inflammatory drugs, anti-oestrogens, cytotoxic chemotherapy and surgical excision. Good evidence for these is lacking due to desmoid rarity and variable course, but some specialist oncologists do provide chemotherapy for aggressively growing desmoids. Surgery may be considered as first-line treatment for actively growing extra-abdominal and abdominal wall desmoids, but recurrence is frequent. Desmoids growing on limbs may require specialist orthopaedic input if removal is necessary. Breast desmoids usually require referral to an expert breast unit so that lesions can be assessed and unnecessary removal avoided or significant lesions excised. For progressive mesenteric disease, referral to a specialist centre, where expert surgeons, gastroenterologists, urologists and intestinal failure specialists are available, should be sought. Surgery should only be considered in carefully selected cases due to high rates of obstructive complications, fistulation and short gut syndrome (Latchford et al. 2006). Referral to a small bowel transplant centre may be necessary when considering appropriate intervention in complicated cases.

10.6 MUTYH-Associated Polyposis (MAP)

This autosomal recessive adenomatous polyposis was described in 2002 after studying a family with FAP phenotype and no identifiable mutation (Al-Tassan et al. 2002). Similar to FAP, the development of colonic adenomas and carcinomas is the main feature of MAP. Approximately half of cases are phenotypically similar to attenuated FAP, presenting with fewer colonic polyps, whilst the remainder resemble classic FAP. Interestingly, some develop cancer, with a tendency towards right-sided colonic lesions by middle age, despite having fewer than ten polyps (Cheadle and Sampson 2007). Fewer upper duodenal adenomas occur in association with MAP compared with FAP (30 and 90 %, respectively) (Kanter-Smoler et al. 2006).

10.6.1 Genetics

MAP is due to biallelic mutation of the mutY human homologue gene (*MUTYH*). As it is a recessive condition, there may be no significant family history.

10.6.2 Surveillance and Surgery

Both colonic and upper GI surveillance are the same as for FAP currently, although there may be a more attenuated phenotype in many with MAP. This can allow for some to be monitored and managed endoscopically for longer before considering a prophylactic colectomy. The risk of developing CRC in heterozygotes is not thought to be significantly higher than the general population, and surveillance is not currently recommended.

10.7 Peutz-Jeghers Syndrome (PJS)

This autosomal dominant condition classically features mucocutaneous pigmentation (95 % of affected individuals) and GI hamartomatous polyps, predominantly in the small bowel. In up to 94 % of cases, a mutation is found in *STK11* (Beggs et al. 2010). A diagnosis of PJS can be made when one of the features in Box 10.5 is seen.

Box 10.5. Diagnosing PJS

Diagnostic criteria for PJS

Two or more PJS polyps confirmed on histology

Any number of PJS polyps found and a family history of PJS in a close relative

Mucocutaneous pigmentation found and a family history of PJS in a close relative

Any number of PJS polyps and mucocutaneous pigmentation

Bowel obstruction is a common feature of PJS due to intussusception or adhesions from multiple laparotomies. This can be reduced by intra-operative enteroscopy to clear all polyps present at the time of surgery.

The cancer risk from PJS is significant, particularly for GI, pancreatic and breast tumours. The risk for CRC with advancing age is in the order of 40 % by the age of 70 years (Hearle et al. 2006). Surveillance is recommended from an early age both to identify and remove intestinal polyps before obstruction or cancer develops. A specialist paediatric gastroenterologist is imperative in the follow-up of children with PJS to identify and manage bowel polyps and PJS-associated cancers. Most centres undertake annual clinical examination (including breast and testicular examinations) with routine blood tests. A thorough baseline OGD and colonoscopy at the age of 8 should be considered. If polyps are present, upper and lower GI endoscopic surveillance continues 3 yearly. If no polyps are seen, 3-yearly surveillance should resume at 18 years. Capsule endoscopy or MR enterography should be performed 3 yearly from 8 years of age. Annual breast imaging is recommended from 25 years with mammography and/or MRI (Beggs et al. 2010).

10.8 Juvenile Polyposis

Juvenile polyposis is characterised by multiple hamartomatous juvenile polyps in the colon and upper GI tract and, for some, haemorrhagic telangiectasia. It is an autosomal dominant condition with germline mutations in *SMAD4*, *BMPR1A* or *ENG*. Regular upper and lower GI endoscopic surveillance is necessary, with polypectomy for larger polyps. Surgery is required when polyps are unmanageable endoscopically (Patel and Ahnen 2012).

10.9 Serrated Polyposis

In serrated polyposis (previously known as hyperplastic polyposis), multiple serrated colonic polyps are seen. The genetic basis is unclear and the CRC risk difficult to ascertain due to limited data but is so far thought to be between 37 and 69 % (Jass 2007). No consensus has been reached regarding surveillance intervals, but colonoscopic screening with polyp removal every 1–2 years is reasonable.

Conclusion

Familial CRC requires a multimodal approach in its management. A specialist service improves patient outcome through the provision of patient-tailored care, delivered by a team of dedicated experts able to identify, counsel and manage inherited bowel cancer syndromes. It requires skilled endoscopists, not only for diagnosis but for on-going surveillance and intervention. Specialist histopathology and genetic services are necessary for accurate diagnosis in this complicated patient cohort. Meticulous analysis of tissue for dysplasia and cancer is vital for successful surveillance and management. Finally, a decision

10 Multimodal Approach to Familial Colorectal Cancer

must be made regarding the need for surgery and, when it is required, the type and timing of it. It is through these measures that the outcomes from familial CRC have seen significant improvement in recent years and should continue to do so.

References

Aarnio M, Sankila R, Pukkala E et al (1999) Cancer risk in mutation carriers of DNA-mismatch repair genes. Int J Cancer 81:214–218

Al-Tassan N, Chmiel NH, Maynard J et al (2002) Inherited variants of MYH associated with somatic G:C–T:A mutations in colorectal tumours. Nat Genet 30:227–232

Aziz O, Athanasiou T, Fazio VW et al (2006) Meta-analysis of observational studies of ileorectal versus ileal pouch-anal anastomosis for familial adenomatous polyposis. Br J Surg 93:407–417

Beggs A, Latchford A, Vasen H (2010) Peutz-Jeghers syndrome: a systematic review and recommendations for management. Gut 59:975–986

Berk T, Cohen Z, Bapat B et al (1999) Negative genetic test results in familial adenomatous polyposis: clinical screening implications. Dis Colon Rectum 42:307–310

Bertario L, Presciuttini S, Sala P et al (1994) Causes of death and postsurgical survival in familial adenomatous polyposis: results from the Italian Registry. Italian Registry of Familial Polyposis Writing Committee. Semin Surg Oncol 10:225–234

Bisgaard ML, Fenger K, Bulow S et al (1994) Familial adenomatous polyposis (FAP): frequency, penetrance and mutation rate. Hum Mutat 3:121–125

Björk J, Akerbrant H, Iselius L et al (2001) Outcome of primary and secondary ileal pouch-anal anastomosis and ileorectal anastomosis in patients with familial adenomatous polyposis. Dis Colon Rectum 44:984–992

Burke W, Petersen G, Lynch P et al (1997) Recommendations for follow-up care of individuals with an inherited predisposition to cancer: I. Hereditary nonpolyposis colon cancer. JAMA 277:915–919

Burke CA, Beck GJ, Church JM et al (1999) The natural history of untreated duodenal and ampullary adenomas in patients with familial adenomatous polyposis followed in an endoscopic surveillance program. Gastrointest Endosc 49:358–364

Burn J, Gerdes AM, Macrae F et al (2011) Long-term effect of aspirin on cancer risk in carriers of hereditary colorectal cancer: an analysis from the CAPP2 randomised controlled trial. Lancet 378(9809):2081–2087

Cairns S, Scholefield J, Steele R et al (2010) Guidelines for colorectal cancer screening and surveillance in moderate and high risk groups (update from 2002). Gut 59:666–690

Cheadle J, Sampson J (2007) MUTYH-associated polyposis—from defect in base excision repair to clinical genetic testing. DNA Repair (Amst) 6:274–279

Church J (2005) Ileoanal pouch neoplasia in familial adenomatous polyposis: an underestimated threat. Dis Colon Rectum 48:1708–1713

Church JM, McGannon E, Ozuner G (1999) The clinical course of intra-abdominal desmoid tumours in patients with familial adenomatous polyposis. Colorectal Dis 1:168–173

Church J, Burke C, McGannon E, Pastean O, Clark B (2003) Risk of rectal cancer in patients after colectomy and ileorectal anastomosis for familial adenomatous polyposis: a function of available surgical options. Dis Colon Rectum 46:1175–1181

Clark SK (2009) A guide to cancer genetics in clinical practice. TFM Publishing Limited, Harley, UK. ISBN 978-1903378540

Clark SK, Neale KF, Landgrebe JC et al (1999) Desmoid tumours complicating familial adenomatous polyposis. Br J Surg 86:1185–1189

Cornish JA, Tan E, Teare J et al (2007) The effect of restorative proctocolectomy on sexual function, urinary function, fertility, pregnancy and delivery – a systematic review. Dis Colon Rectum 50:1128–1138

Dove-Edwin I, de Jong AE, Adams J et al (2006) Prospective results of surveillance colonoscopy in dominant familial colorectal cancer with and without Lynch syndrome. Gastroenterology 130:1995–2000

Gallagher M, Shankar A, Groves C et al (2004) Pylorus-preserving pancreatico-duodenectomy for advanced duodenal disease in familial adenomatous polyposis. Br J Surg 91:1157–1164

Giardiello FM, Brensinger JD, Petersen GM et al (1997) The use and interpretation of commercial APC gene testing for familial adenomatous polyposis. N Engl J Med 336:823–827

Groves CJ, Saunders BP, Spigelman AD et al (2002) Duodenal cancer in patients with familial adenomatous polyposis (FAP): results of a 10 year prospective study. Gut 50:636–641

Günther K, Braunrieder G, Bittorf BR, Hohenberger W, Matzel KE (2003) Patients with familial adenomatous polyposis experience better bowel function and quality of life after ileorectal anastomosis than after ileoanal pouch. Colorectal Dis 5:38–44

Half E, Bercovich D, Rozen P (2009) Familial adenomatous polyposis. Orphanet J Rare Dis 4:22

Hassan I, Chua HK, Wolff BG et al (2005) Quality of life after ileal pouchanal anastomosis and ileorectal anastomosis in patients with familial adenomatous polyposis. Dis Colon Rectum 48:2032–2037

Hearle N, Schumacher V, Menko FH et al (2006) Frequency and spectrum of cancers in the Peutz Jeghers syndrome. Clin Cancer Res 12:3209–3215

Hernegger GS, Moore HG, Guillem JG (2002) Attenuated familial adenomatous polyposis: an evolving and poorly understood entity. Dis Colon Rectum 45:127–134

Houlston RS, Murday V, Harocopos C et al (1990) Screening and genetic counselling for relatives of patients with colorectal cancer in a family cancer clinic. Br Med J 301:366–368

Jass JR (2006) Hereditary non-polyposis colorectal cancer: the rise and fall of a confusing term. World J Gastroenterol 12:4943–4950

Jass JR (2007) Classification of colorectal cancer based on correlation of clinical, morphological and molecular features. Histopathology 50(1):113–130

Kanter-Smoler G, Bjork J, Fritzell K et al (2006) Novel findings in Swedish patients with MYH-associated polyposis: mutation detection and clinical characterization. Clin Gastroenterol Hepatol 4:499–506

Ko CY, Rusin LC, Schoetz DJ Jr et al (2000) Does better functional result equate with better quality of life? Implications for surgical treatment in familial adenomatous polyposis. Dis Colon Rectum 43:829–835

Latchford A, Sturt N, Neale K et al (2006) A 10-year review of surgery for desmoid with familial adenomatous polyposis. Br J Surg 93:1258–1264

Latchford A, Neale K, Spigelman A, Phillips R, Clark S (2009) Features of duodenal cancer in patients with familial adenomatous polyposis. Clin Gastroenterol Hepatol 7:659–663

Lindor NM, Rabe K, Petersen GM et al (2005) Lower cancer incidence in Amsterdam-I criteria families without mismatch repair deficiency: familial colorectal cancer type X. JAMA 293(16):1979–1985

Lips CJM (1998) Registers for patients with familial tumours: from controversial areas to common guidelines. Br J Surg 85:1316–1318

Mackey R, Walsh M, Chung R et al (2005) Pancreas-sparing duodenectomy is effective management for familial adenomatous polyposis. J Gastrointest Surg 9:1088–1093

Nieuwenhuis MH, Vasen HF (2007) Correlations between mutation site in APC and phenotype of familial adenomatous polyposis (FAP): a review of the literature. Crit Rev Oncol Hematol 61:153–161

Nugent KP, Phillips RK (1992) Rectal cancer risk in older patients with familial adenomatous polyposis and an ileorectal anastomosis: a cause for concern. Br J Surg 79:1204–1206

Nugent KP, Spigelman AD, Phillips RKS (1993) Life expectancy after colectomy and ileorectal anastomosis for familial adenomatous polyposis. Dis Colon Rectum 36:1059–1062

Olsen KO, Juul S, Bulow S et al (2003) Female fecundity before and after operation for familial adenomatous polyposis. Br J Surg 90:227–231

10 Multimodal Approach to Familial Colorectal Cancer

Parks AG, Nicholls RJ (1978) Proctocolectomy without ileostomy for ulcerative colitis. BMJ 2:85–88

Patel S, Ahnen D (2012) Familial colon cancer syndromes: an update of a rapidly evolving field. Curr Gastroenterol Rep 14:428–438

Petersen GM, Slack J, Nakamura Y (1991) Screening guidelines and premorbid diagnosis of familial adenomatous polyposis using linkage. Gastroenterology 100:1658–1664

Ruschoff J, Wallinger S, Dietmaier W et al (1998) Aspirin suppresses the mutator phenotype associated with hereditary nonpolyposis colorectal cancer by genetic selection. Proc Natl Acad Sci U S A 95:11301–11306

Scholefield JH, Johnson AG, Shorthouse AJ (1998) Current surgical practice in screening for colorectal cancer based on family history criteria. Br J Surg 85:1543–1546

Simmang CL et al; Standards Committee of the American Society of Colon and Rectal Surgeons (1999) Practice parameters for detection of colorectal neoplasms. Dis Colon Rectum 42:1123–1129.

Sinha A, Tekkis PP, Gibbons DC, Phillips RK, Clark SK (2010) Risk factors predicting desmoid occurrence in patients with familial adenomatous polyposis: a meta-analysis. Colorectal Dis 13(11):1222–1229

Sinha A, Hansmann A, Bhandari S et al (2012) Imaging assessment of desmoid tumours in familial adenomatous polyposis: is state-of-the-art 1.5 T MRI better than 64-MDCT? Br J Radiol 85:e254–e261

Soravia C, Berk T, Madlensky L et al (1998) Genotype–phenotype correlations in attenuated adenomatous polyposis coli. Am J Hum Genet 62:1290–1301

Spigelman AD, Williams CB, Talbot IC et al (1989) Upper gastrointestinal cancer in patients with familial adenomatous polyposis. Lancet 2:783–785

Syngal S, Weeks JC, Schrag D et al (1998) Benefits of colonoscopic surveillance and prophylactic colectomy in patients with hereditary nonpolyposis colorectal cancer mutations. Ann Intern Med 129:787–796

Tudyka V, Clark S (2012) Surgical treatment in familial adenomatous polyposis. Ann Gastroenterol 25:1–6

Umar A, Boland CR, Terdiman JP et al (2004) Revised Bethesda Guidelines for hereditary nonpolyposis colorectal cancer (Lynch syndrome) and microsatellite instability. J Natl Cancer Inst 96(4):261–268

Van Duijvendijk P, Vasen HA, Bertario L et al (1999a) Cumulative risk of developing polyps or malignancy at the ileal pouch–anal anastomosis in patients with familial adenomatous polyposis. J Gastrointest Surg 3:325–330

Van Duijvendijk P, Slors JF, Taat CW, Oosterveld P, Vasen HF (1999b) Functional outcome after colectomy and ileorectal anastomosis compared with proctocolectomy and ileal pouch-anal anastomosis in familial adenomatous polyposis. Ann Surg 230:648–654

Vasen HFA, Watson P, Mecklin J-P et al (1999) New clinical criteria for hereditary nonpolyposis colorectal cancer (HNPCC, Lynch syndrome) proposed by the International Collaborative Group on HNPCC. Gastroenterology 116:1453–1456

Vasen HFA, Moslein G, Alonso A et al (2007) Guidelines for the clinical management of Lynch syndrome (hereditary non-polyposis colorectal cancer). J Med Genet 44:353–362

Von Roon AC, Tekkis PP, Clark SK (2007) The impact of technical factors on outcome of restorative proctocolectomy for familial adenomatous polyposis. Dis Colon Rectum 50:952–961

Wallace MH, Phillips RKS (1998) Upper gastrointestinal disease in patients with familial adenomatous polyposis. Br J Surg 85:742–750

Wallace MH, Frayling IM, Clark SK et al (1999) Attenuated adenomatous polyposis coli: the role of ascertainment bias through failure to dye-spray at colonoscopy. Dis Colon Rectum 42:1078–1080

Wu JS, Paul P, McGannon EA et al (1998a) APC genotype, polyp number, and surgical options in familial adenomatous polyposis. Ann Surg 227:57–62

Wu TT, Rashid A, Luce MC, Sani N, Mishra L, Moskaluk CA, Yardley JH, Hamilton SR (1998b) Dysplasia and dysregulation of proliferation in foveolar and surface epithelia of fundic gland polyps from patients with familial adenomatous polyposis. Am J Surg Pathol 22:293–298

Transdisciplinary Fecal Incontinence Management

11

Surendra Kumar Mantoo and Paul Antoine Lehur

Take-Home Pearls

- Fecal incontinence (FI) is an embarrassing condition resulting in a detrimental effect on psychological, social, and physical functioning with significant reduction in quality of life.
- Healthcare professionals working with people with FI should be aware of the physical and emotional impact of this condition.
- General physicians and nurses play a frontline role in identifying the patients with FI or at risk of FI.
- Transdisciplinary approach is aptly suited for FI, where multiple expert opinions are required, to come up with the most effective plan of management for an individual patient.
- The aim of assessment is to determine the type of FI, its impact on function and quality of life, and the likely etiology.
- The goal of treatment should be to restore fecal continence in order to improve quality of life.
- Initial basic management includes patient and family education, dietary advice, regular bowel habit training, and medical treatment.
- Specialist management allows identification of patients who can benefit from behavioral retraining and, in case of insufficient results, from more invasive options, i.e., surgical approaches.

S.K. Mantoo (✉)
Department of Surgery, Khoo Teck Puat Hospital, Singapore, Singapore
e-mail: kumar.mantoo@alexandrahealth.com.sg

P.A. Lehur
Department of Digestive Surgery, University Hospital of Nantes, Nantes, France
e-mail: paulantoine.lehur@chu-nantes.fr

© Springer-Verlag Berlin Heidelberg 2015
K.-Y. Tan (ed.), *Transdisciplinary Perioperative Care in Colorectal Surgery: An Integrative Approach*, DOI 10.1007/978-3-662-44020-9_11

- FI is more common in the elderly and is often dismissed as a normal part of aging.
- Creation of a "dedicated pelvic floor clinic" allows key members of the transdisciplinary team to come together from the beginning to jointly communicate, exchange opinions, and work together to come up with the most effective solutions.
- Patients with severe and or double (urinary and fecal) incontinence are best managed in such a setting.
- This also creates an environment for teaching and training in a specialty which has been ignored for long.

11.1 Introduction

Transdisciplinary approach is attractive and necessary for optimal and successful management of fecal incontinence (FI). Incontinence usually results from diverse pathophysiological processes and is multifactorial in etiology. Structural abnormalities like anal sphincter muscle injury and prolapse disorders of the anorectum, functional abnormalities like impaired rectal sensation, change in stool characteristics, dietary influences, and medications, or even aging with impairment of cognitive function can all result in deranged bowel function. This multifactorial etiology results in different types of FI and thereby the need for multiple management options.

Management of disorders like FI is becoming more challenging, owing to developments in surgical options, information available, and patient and social factors. The last two decades have been very exciting for pelvic floor disorders especially FI in terms of diagnosis, investigations, and management. This mandates the need for a well-coordinated multi-subspecialty and allied healthcare team. Multidisciplinary and recently transdisciplinary approach for management of FI addresses complex patient problems and management issues in a way that each member can use his/her expertise and work together as a team to come up with a "tailor-made" management plan in the long run for each individual patient.

Healthcare professionals involved in the treatment of incontinence whether bowel, bladder, or both should include colorectal surgeons, urologists, gynecologists, incontinence nurses, social workers, dietitians, pharmacists, stoma therapists, and eventually psychologists and/or psychiatrists in some patients for optimal results.

All members of this team work together to determine the most effective plan of care, and each provides a unique role in the transdisciplinary care. The uniqueness of transdisciplinary approach allows team members to come together from the beginning to jointly communicate, exchange ideas, and come up with adaptable solutions and support for the patient and family members.

11.2 Prevalence, Risk Factors, and Economics

Fecal incontinence (FI) is an embarrassing condition resulting in a detrimental effect on psychological, social, and physical functioning with significant reduction in quality of life. Prevalence of FI varies considerably as many patients either do not report it or relate it to aging. Conservative estimates based on a systematic review suggested a prevalence rate of 11–15 % among community-dwelling adults (Macmillan et al. 2004). FI is predominantly reported in female patients with a significant increase in prevalence with increasing age (Whitehead et al. 2009).

Old age is one of the most important risk factors for FI (Bharucha et al. 2006). Other independent risk factors based on multivariate analysis in different studies include poor general health, rectal urgency, and sequelae from obstetrical injuries such as prolonged labor, difficult vaginal delivery, use of forceps, and episiotomy. Frequent association of FI with irritable bowel syndrome, urinary incontinence, colectomy and/or rectal resection, and chronic diarrhea has also been reported (Markland et al. 2010). This multifactorial etiology reinforces the importance of transdisciplinary approach including behavioral, dietary, pharmacological, and other measures to manage FI.

Most developed countries around the world are facing a problem of aging population resulting in substantial economic costs in managing health-related problems such as FI. Millions of dollars are spent annually on diapers, medications, and on a limited number of patients on surgical treatment of FI. Loss of work hours, admission to healthcare facilities like nursing homes, and salary of staff to look after these patients considerably add to this economic burden. Xu et al. reported an estimated expenditure of USD 4110 per patient annually as the economic cost associated with management of FI. Breakup of expenditure into direct medical and nonmedical costs averaged USD 2562, whereas the indirect cost due to loss of productivity averaged $1549 per patient annually. Multivariate regression analyses suggested that severe FI was significantly associated with higher annual direct costs (Xu et al. 2012). Studies have reported FI as one of the leading causes for admission to nursing homes, putting a strain on the healthcare spending (Nelson et al. 1998). Thus, a pressing and clear need exists to pay attention to the prevention and effective management of this condition.

11.3 Awareness and Role of Education

There is a general lack of information and awareness about FI among the patients, family, and community and to a great extent among the physicians as well. This may be due to the fact that few patients and even physicians are comfortable in discussing the issue of incontinence whether fecal or urinary. Even though majority of articles published on incontinence discuss the physical, mental, and social impact of this disorder, more than 50 % of incontinent patients do not seek help for their condition (Bharucha et al. 2005; Crowell et al. 2007). Multiple factors have been held responsible for this like embarrassment at reporting symptoms, lack of awareness of treatment options, and fear of surgical interventions, and many a time patients consider FI as a normal part of aging. Few studies have evaluated this in FI but a study involving patients with urinary incontinence reported that nearly 70 % of patients do not voluntarily report their problem, but when asked by the physician, nearly 75 % are willing to discuss the problem (Johanson and Lafferty 1996; Hajjar 2004). This is compounded by a lack of current knowledge on continence management among majority of physicians.

Transdisciplinary approach involving multiple partners is suited to break these barriers. Patients and their family members can unmask the real magnitude of incontinence by speaking about it without shame or prejudice. Healthcare workers need to understand that sympathetic interaction and communication is required to help incontinent patients. Care of these patients should not be reflected as a professional burden. Over the past 15–20 years, numerous professional societies/bodies have contributed in breaking these barriers by improving awareness and educating the public and healthcare workers and professionals about incontinence. The International Continence Society has even propagated the concept of primary prevention in FI (Newman et al. 2005). As an example, traumatic vaginal delivery is an important risk factor in the development of FI. FI can potentially be prevented if obstetric, gynecological, and colorectal surgeons are educated about interventions that may lead to the development of FI (Collings and Norton 2004). Similarly, prevention of fecal impaction in the elderly by ensuring regular clearing of bowels can prevent one of the commonest causes for spurious FI. Also, prevention of excessive straining by treating chronic constipation and instructing people on the benefit of regular nontraumatic bowel evacuation with the help of adequate intake of fiber and fluids is worthwhile.

All preventive measures require public education, community awareness, and health professional education with allocation of adequate resources.

11.4 Pathophysiology and Types of Bowel Incontinence

Maintenance of FI is a complex process involving not only the colonic, rectal, and anal functions like colonic transit, rectal distensibility, anal sphincter function, anorectal sensation, and anorectal reflexes but other factors like stool volume, stool consistency, and the higher control by brain centers and reflexes. Derangement in any one or more of the above can lead to FI, and based on the predominant dysfunction, FI has been subdivided into three major groups: functional, sphincter weakness, and sensory dysfunction. There is no consensus clinical definition of FI due to varied presentation and interpretation by both patients and healthcare professionals. One of the proposed definitions is continuous or recurrent uncontrolled passage of fecal material (>10 mL) for at least 1 month in an individual older than 3 years of age. Taking into account the multiple definitions by various authors, it is important to assess the severity of FI and differentiate minor FI from more severe levels of FI in which there is a serious disruption of daily life. Minor to moderate FI is defined as occasional fecal leakage or soiling, flatus incontinence, liquid stool incontinence, or rectal urgency. Major incontinence on the other extreme is defined as frequent and involuntary leakage of solid stools. Bowel diaries provide additional insights like bowel habits and daily routine in FI (Bharucha et al. 2008).

Several incontinence severity scales have been proposed for a better clinical distinction and comparison of treatment options. Park's system is a simple scale grading incontinent patients from Grade I (fully continent) to Grade IV (incontinent to solid stools) but has the disadvantages of not taking into consideration the frequency of leakage episodes (Parks 1975). Cleveland Clinic Florida Fecal Incontinence Score (CCF-FIS) is a more commonly used scale as it not only considers the nature of FI (gas, liquid, solid) but also the frequency of leakage and questions on use of pads and lifestyle alteration (Jorge and Wexner 1993). Assessing severity of FI may not be the real indicator of the impact on quality of life. More recently, multiple comprehensive quality-of-life scores have been proposed in addition to severity scales to assess the impact of FI (Thompson 1999).

At present, there is a general agreement that patient-based outcome measures are most appropriate for research studies on FI. However, standardization of the optimal instrument or combination of instruments (severity and quality of life) remains a central challenge in clinical incontinence research.

A transdisciplinary approach can help in better understanding of the pathophysiology and categorization required for an effective management of FI.

11.5 Assessment, Initial Management, and Referral

FI is a condition that presents unusual challenges in evaluation and detection largely due to underreporting by patients and underestimation by healthcare professionals. Challenges like taboo and stigmatization associated with FI need to be overcome to realize the real problem (Brown et al. 2012). Patients are often reluctant to discuss the topic of FI, mandating physicians, nurses, and other healthcare workers to take the lead. They need to explore their patients especially high-risk groups like postmenopausal women, elderly patients, and nursing home residents about bowel and bladder function, about the patient's ability to control it, and whether it is affecting their lifestyle. This is to ensure that effective therapies are available not only to patients with FI who seek treatment.

General physicians and nurses play a frontline role in identifying the patients with FI or at risk of FI. Simple questionnaires directed at FI should be offered to patients attending a clinic or any healthcare facility to identify the real burden of this problem. Studies have shown that a self-administered anonymous questionnaire yields results of greater validity when compared with face-to-face interviews for conditions deemed embarrassing by the patients (Tourangeau and Yan 2007).

The aim of assessment is to determine the type of FI, its impact on function and quality of life, and the likely etiology. Once established, management of FI begins with a careful medical and bowel history followed by a thorough physical examination. It is especially important to check patient's medication list for drugs that cause constipation or diarrhea and review their diet (fiber and fluid) and use of laxatives.

Table 11.1 Key points of assessment

Key point	What to look for?
Medical and surgical history	General health
	Comorbidities like diabetes, immunosuppressive disorders, inflammatory bowel disorders
	Previous abdominal and anorectal surgery
	Neurological disease (e.g., MS, cauda equina lesions)
Neurological status	Dementia
	Depression
	Ambulatory status
Presenting complaints related to FI	Duration
	Type of leak – gas/liquid/solid
	Number of leaks per day/week
	Quantity – minor/major FI
	Aggravating factors – laxatives, stress
	Awareness of leak
	Impact on lifestyle
Medications	Laxatives, over the counter, fiber
Social support	Presence of caregiver
	Access to toilet
	Access to healthcare facility
	Family support
Expectation and goals of treatment	Motivation of patient and family
	Fitness for any intervention

Patient's level of psychological stress and loss of self-esteem should be discussed. Key points of assessment are suggested in Table 11.1. Most patients initially are managed conservatively and referred to an appropriate specialist if the initial management fails or FI is severe.

Based on the carefully taken history (obstetrical, gynecological, any anal or colorectal surgery, urological complaints), FI can be divided into two main groups: those with an anatomical damage to the anal sphincter complex and those without. The common etiological factors are listed in Table 11.2. Physical examination should be guided by the likely etiology. General physical examination is warranted in all patients, and a complete neurological examination should be performed if neurological disease or diabetes is suspected. Careful per rectal examination is mandatory in all patients to look for surgical scars, fistulae, patulous anus, and the degree of descent on straining. Fecal impaction should also be excluded. An assessment of the resting anal tone and squeeze pressure should be made by digital rectal examination. Anal sensation should be tested along with the anocutaneous reflex. Vaginal examination should be performed to evaluate for presence of any pelvic floor disorder such rectocele/enterocele, cystocele, or vaginal prolapse.

Initial basic management includes patient and family education, dietary and fluid advice, regular bowel habit training, and medical treatment including antidiarrheals and stool-bulking agents like fiber (Omar and Alexander 2013). Simple exercises (pelvic floor muscle training or PFMT) to enhance awareness and strengthening of

11 Transdisciplinary Fecal Incontinence Management

Table 11.2 Etiology of fecal incontinence

I. Anatomical	Obstetric injury
	Post-anorectal surgery injury (lateral internal sphincterotomy, hemorrhoidectomy, fistulotomy, low anterior resection)
	Congenital anorectal malformations (imperforate anus, Hirschsprung's disease)
	Pelvic radiation
	Rectal prolapse, large hemorrhoids
	Anorectal cancer
II. Non-anatomical	Neurogenic (multiple sclerosis, diabetes mellitus)
	Spinal cord (spina bifida, meningomyelocele, lumbar sacral spinal defects)
	Aging, dementia, laxative abuse, constipation/fecal impaction
	Inflammatory bowel disease

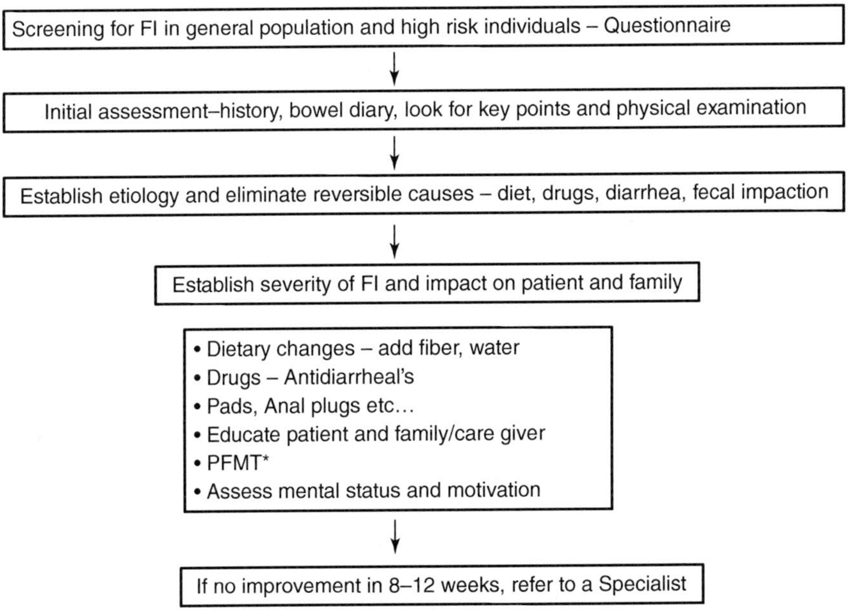

Screening for FI in general population and high risk individuals – Questionnaire

↓

Initial assessment–history, bowel diary, look for key points and physical examination

↓

Establish etiology and eliminate reversible causes – diet, drugs, diarrhea, fecal impaction

↓

Establish severity of FI and impact on patient and family

- Dietary changes – add fiber, water
- Drugs – Antidiarrheal's
- Pads, Anal plugs etc…
- Educate patient and family/care giver
- PFMT*
- Assess mental status and motivation

↓

If no improvement in 8–12 weeks, refer to a Specialist

Fig. 11.1 Basic management of fecal incontinence. *PFMT* pelvic floor muscle training

the external anal sphincter and levator ani muscles can be initiated in the primary care setting. PFMT is a simple and low-cost management option but with a weak evidence to support its efficacy (Christensen et al. 2006). Small retrograde enemas and suppositories are used in some patients for improved bowel emptying and reduced rectal soiling. Regular enemas using a special apparatus have been reported to be very effective in patients with spinal cord injury with severe constipation resulting in overflow FI (Heymen et al. 2009).

Figure 11.1 summarizes the initial management of FI.

When symptoms persist or worsen despite 8–12 weeks of conservative treatment, the patient should be referred to a specialist with interest in management of

FI. Aim is to assess and identify the patients who can benefit from surgical or more invasive options. Earlier referrals should be made when patients present with severe symptoms or when patients present with multiple problems like combined fecal and urinary incontinence and/or pelvic organ prolapse.

11.6 Further Evaluation and Specialist Management

A transdisciplinary approach is preferable to diagnose the cause and assess the severity and impact of FI before any treatment is initiated. All members of the team could work together to determine the most effective plan of care, and each provides a unique role in the team. Specialist assessment of FI is based on investigations in selected patients to quantify the severity, impact on quality of life, and likely available management options. General fitness for surgery and mental well-being should be ascertained in all patients before any invasive treatment. Most patients will need inspection of the colon and anorectum with flexible sigmoidoscopy or full colonoscopy preceding specific tests for FI.

Anorectal manometry and neurophysiologic studies like pudendal nerve terminal motor latency (PNTML) are the first-line tests to study the physiology of defecation and continence (Jones et al. 2007; Simpson et al. 2006). Anorectal manometry provides information on resting pressure, squeeze pressure, and rectoanal inhibitory reflex but does not reliably demonstrate the integrity of anal sphincter complex. Endoanal ultrasound (EAUS) using sophisticated 3D software programs and transperineal ultrasound (TPUS) reliably assess the integrity and structure of anorectal sphincter complex (Christensen et al. 2005). EAUS has better diagnostic specificity and sensitivity when compared with digital examination. Magnetic resonance imaging (MRI) with endoanal coil is used as an alternative but is more expensive and in our opinion should be used in more complex cases to demonstrate additional information like pelvic organ prolapse, etc. Defecography is used to measure the anorectal angle, evaluate pelvic floor descent, and detect occult or overt rectal prolapse that could cause FI. MRI defecography (also known as dynamic MR imaging) is an alternative which provides additional information on full static and dynamic imaging of the pelvic organs and pelvic floor components (Hetzer et al. 2006).

Biofeedback involves specific retraining of pelvic floor and abdominal wall muscles and is initiated as a first-line specialist management in most patients with FI (Byrne et al. 2007). Patients are trained to improve the control of these muscles by electromyographic stimulation under the supervision of a trained pelvic floor physiologist or a physiotherapist. Biofeedback may improve FI by enhanced contraction of the striated pelvic floor muscles and improvement in the ability to perceive rectal distension and improved coordination of the sensory and motor components required for continence. However, the role of biofeedback in FI is unsettled as the rates of success show a considerable variation in published literature (Norton et al. 2000; Madoff et al. 2004). Despite lack of unequivocal evidence, many guidelines still recommend biofeedback as "safe and effective" and its use in patients with weak sphincters and/or impaired rectal sensation (Rao 2004; Landefeld et al. 2008).

Failure of biofeedback to relieve symptoms and improve quality of life paves way for discussion of surgical or invasive options with the patient. Multiple surgical options including anal sphincteroplasty, levatorplasty, anal encirclement, implantation of an artificial anal sphincter, and muscle transfer procedures with or without electrical stimulation have been described (Christiansen 1998; Madoff et al. 1999; Grey et al. 2007). Most have become redundant with the introduction of sacral nerve stimulation (SNS). For instance with sphincteroplasty, the initial reported success rates of more than 90 % have been shown to drop significantly in studies with longer follow-up (Zorcolo et al. 2005). The role of anal sphincteroplasty is currently debated due to poor long-term efficacy and recent evidence reporting success of sacral nerve stimulation even in patients with larger sphincter defects (Matzel et al. 1995).

SNS involves low-grade electrical stimulation of sacral nerve roots via an electrode inserted in close vicinity through the third or fourth sacral foramen and connected to an implanted stimulator (Chan and Tjandra 2008). It has the unique advantage of a test phase before implanting a definitive stimulator. However, it is recognized as a high-cost, high-maintenance therapy. The mechanism of action remains unclear, but there is enough evidence to support the use of SNS as a first-line option of surgical management of FI. Two randomized controlled trials and multiple prospective trials have shown that the use of SNS in FI was associated with a significantly greater improvement in incontinence episodes and quality of life (Tjandra et al. 2008). SNS has been in use in Europe since 1995 and was approved by FDA in 2011 for the treatment of FI in patients who have failed or are not candidates for more conservative treatments. Posterior tibial nerve stimulation (PTNS), an outpatient treatment, has also been proposed as a low-cost and less-invasive alternative to SNS and has been reported to improve FI at least in short term (Hotouras et al. 2012).

Several injectable or bulking agents have been used to augment the sphincters including autologous fat, polytetrafluoroethylene (PTFE), silicone, carbon beads, etc., with moderate success (Maeda et al. 2013). Recently, a novel bulking agent anal Gatekeeper(™) (polyacrylonitrile cylinders) inserted around the anal canal has been shown to be safe and reliable with clinical improvement in FI (Ratto et al. 2011). Magnetic anal sphincter is a new option for augmenting the anal sphincters, and recent evidence supports its use in selected patients (Mantoo et al. 2012; Barussaud et al. 2013).

With the possible exception of SNS, recommendations for use of other options in FI are mostly based on case series or reports, and there is very little evidence based on randomized controlled trials. Well-designed randomized trials are desired to evaluate each of these surgical options as well as compare surgical and conservative options of management. Re-routing of fecal stream by creating a stoma is the last resort in some patients. Based on the current available evidence, Fig. 11.2 summarizes the specialist management in patients with FI.

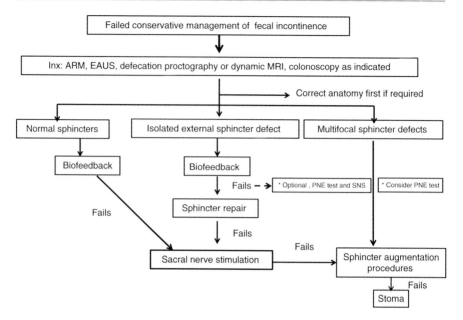

Fig. 11.2 Specialist management of fecal incontinence. *PNE* Percutaneous Nerve Evaluation; *SNS* Sacral Nerve Stimulation

11.7 Bowel Incontinence in the Elderly

FI in the elderly is often dismissed as a normal part of aging. Elderly patients may be reluctant to admit FI, so clinicians and other healthcare providers need to ask about it. Large population surveys reveal a prevalence of 3–16.9 % among people age 65 and over (Black 2007). The prevalence is as high as 50 % in elderly patients in nursing homes (Talley et al. 1992).

In contrast to the younger patients, the pathophysiology of FI in the elderly is difficult to assess and quantify due to mental, social, and physical limitations. Modern physiologic and functional assessment tools have been successfully used to overcome some of these limitations. An accurate and objective pretreatment assessment with consideration of multiple factors in a transdisciplinary environment can successfully manage the expectations of an elderly patient. As an example, medical social workers and psychologists are important in determining the family dynamics and support available to elders. They can determine the impact of incontinence on patient's social activities and relationships and also provide counseling to assist them in expressing feelings about their incontinence problems.

Speech and language therapists can help the elderly in overcoming communication problems either verbal or nonverbal to make their needs known in a timely and effective manner. Training of elderly patients to use gestures and communication aids and training of caregiver to understand can break the communication barrier.

Physiotherapists are required to provide a comprehensive musculoskeletal and functional mobility assessment. This is important to assess whether the elderly can benefit from the use of an assistive device such as a walking frame, stick, etc., to improve the patient's ability to ambulate to the bathroom. PFMT and biofeedback to strengthen the muscles involved in maintaining continence are also part of the physical therapy intervention.

Fecal impaction in nursing home patients and anal sphincter dysfunction due to muscle laxity or diabetic neuropathy are the two prime causes of FI in the elderly. Both conditions can be treated effectively with a transdisciplinary approach. Higher prevalence of comorbidities like diabetes, cardiac, renal, and respiratory problems makes it necessary to involve other specialists to optimize these conditions before any invasive procedures can be offered. Less invasive procedures with limited care required by the patient are favored in elderly patients with significant comorbidities.

11.8 Role of the Transdisciplinary Team

Traditionally, multidisciplinary model of team practice has been used to manage most of the health-related conditions. A potential drawback in multidisciplinary approach is that individual team members approach a situation or a problem from their own perspective and then share their findings. Transdisciplinary team approach seeks to build upon and improve on the existing model of multidisciplinary care. Reilly et al. have described the fundamentals of transdisciplinary care, emphasizing the importance of role extension, role enrichment, role expansion, role release, and role support of individual team members in a transdisciplinary team. The underlying principles include blurring of disciplinary lines with members coming together from the beginning to jointly communicate, exchange ideas, and work together to come up with solutions to problems (Reilly 2001). Tan et al. have successfully used the transdisciplinary model of care for geriatric surgical patients (Wang et al. 2013).

This approach is aptly suited for a health-related problem like FI, where multiple expert opinions are required and can be discussed face to face even in the presence of the patient and family, to come up with the most effective plan of management for an individual.

Multiple healthcare providers involved in the treatment of FI include nurses, social workers, and general or family physicians in the primary care setting. At a specialist center, colorectal surgeons, urologists, gynecologists, radiologists, and pelvic floor physiologists and physiotherapists work as a team in the best interest of patients with FI. Psychiatrists, specially trained continence nurses, psychologists, dietitians, pharmacists, and stoma therapists complement this team to provide a comprehensive care of FI. Transdisciplinary model of care in FI is illustrated in Fig. 11.3, and the role of individual team members is described in Table 11.3. It needs to be stressed here that in transdisciplinary care, all members can readily expand and extend their role in the best interest of patient care.

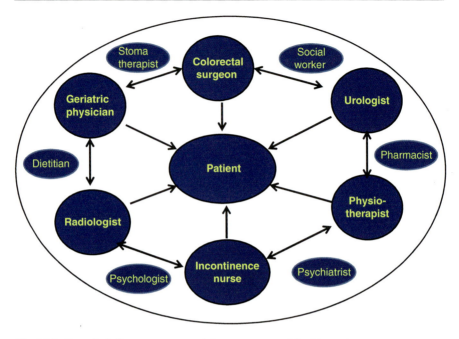

Fig. 11.3 Transdisciplinary team approach in management of fecal incontinence

Table 11.3 Transdisciplinary team members and their role in management of FI

Team member	Main role
Incontinence nurse	Frontline to identify the patients
	Counseling
	Care planning
	Follow-up
Colorectal surgeon	Assessment
	Investigations
	Treatment – nonsurgical and surgical
Urologist	Assessment
	Investigations
	Treatment – nonsurgical and surgical
Radiologist	Special investigations like dynamic MRI, DP
	Interpretation of results
Geriatric physician	Identification of patients and at risk patients
	Optimization of medical conditions
Physiotherapist	Biofeedback
	Follow-up
	Referral
Dietitian	Optimization of diet to avoid constipation and loose stools
Pharmacist	Omit offending drugs
	Long-term medication plan

11 Transdisciplinary Fecal Incontinence Management

Creation of a "dedicated pelvic floor clinic" allows key members of the transdisciplinary team to be present in the clinic at the same time and create an environment where complex patients can be discussed in detail and more efficient manner. The patients can feel reassured and develop the much required trust to allow a thorough discussion of their problems and clinical assessment. More generous time slots offered to these patients allow a detailed review and discussion of the clinical findings, imaging, and input from all members of the team. This creates an environment for teaching and training in a specialty which has been ignored for long. Lastly, development of a transdisciplinary team gives the clinic an identity to which other healthcare workers can readily refer their patients.

References

Barussaud ML, Mantoo S et al (2013) The magnetic anal sphincter in faecal incontinence: is initial success sustained over time? Colorectal Dis 15(12):1499–1503

Bharucha AE, Seide BM et al (2008) Melton LJ 3rd. Insights into normal and disordered bowel habits from bowel diaries. Am J Gastroenterol. Mar;103(3):692–8

Bharucha AE, Zinsmeister AR et al (2005) Prevalence and burden of fecal incontinence: a population-based study in women. Gastroenterology 129(1):42–49

Bharucha AE, Zinsmeister AR et al (2006) Risk factors for fecal incontinence: a population-based study in women. Am J Gastroenterol 101(6):1305–1312

Black D (2007) Faecal incontinence. Age Ageing 36(3):239–240

Brown HW, Wexner SD et al (2012) Quality of life impact in women with accidental bowel leakage. Int J Clin Pract 66(11):1109–1116

Byrne CM, Solomon MJ et al (2007) Biofeedback for fecal incontinence: short-term outcomes of 513 consecutive patients and predictors of successful treatment. Dis Colon Rectum 50(4):417–427

Chan MK, Tjandra JJ. (2008) Sacral nerve stimulation for fecal incontinence. Dis Colon Rectum 51:1015–1025.

Christensen AF, Nyhuus B et al (2005) Three-dimensional anal endosonography may improve diagnostic confidence of detecting damage to the anal sphincter complex. Br J Radiol 78(928): 308–311

Christensen P, Bazzocchi G et al (2006) A randomized, controlled trial of transanal irrigation versus conservative bowel management in spinal cord-injured patients. Gastroenterology 131(3):738–747

Christiansen J (1998) Modern surgical treatment of anal incontinence. Ann Med 30(3): 273–277

Collings S, Norton C (2004) Women's experiences of faecal incontinence: a study. Br J Community Nurs 9(12):520–523

Crowell MD, Schettler VA et al (2007) Impact of anal incontinence on psychosocial function and health-related quality of life. Dig Dis Sci 52(7):1627–1631

Grey BR, Sheldon RR et al (2007) Anterior anal sphincter repair can be of long term benefit: a 12-year case cohort from a single surgeon. BMC Surg 7:1

Hajjar RR (2004) Psychosocial impact of urinary incontinence in the elderly population. Clin Geriatr Med 20(3):553–564, viii

Hetzer FH, Andreisek G et al (2006) MR defecography in patients with fecal incontinence: imaging findings and their effect on surgical management. Radiology 240(2):449–457

Heymen S, Scarlett Y et al (2009) Randomized controlled trial shows biofeedback to be superior to pelvic floor exercises for fecal incontinence. Dis Colon Rectum 52(10):1730–1737

Hotouras A, Allison M et al (2012) Percutaneous tibial nerve stimulation for fecal incontinence: a video demonstration. Dis Colon Rectum 55(6):711–713

Johanson JF, Lafferty J (1996) Epidemiology of fecal incontinence: the silent affliction. Am J Gastroenterol 91(1):33–36

Jones MP, Post J et al (2007) High-resolution manometry in the evaluation of anorectal disorders: a simultaneous comparison with water-perfused manometry. Am J Gastroenterol 102(4): 850–855

Jorge JM, Wexner SD (1993) Etiology and management of fecal incontinence. Dis Colon Rectum 36(1):77–97

Landefeld CS, Bowers BJ et al (2008) National Institutes of Health state-of-the-science conference statement: prevention of fecal and urinary incontinence in adults. Ann Intern Med 148(6): 449–458

Macmillan AK, Merrie AE et al (2004) The prevalence of fecal incontinence in community-dwelling adults: a systematic review of the literature. Dis Colon Rectum 47(8):1341–1349

Madoff RD, Rosen HR et al (1999) Safety and efficacy of dynamic muscle plasty for anal incontinence: lessons from a prospective, multicenter trial. Gastroenterology 116(3):549–556

Madoff RD, Parker SC et al (2004) Faecal incontinence in adults. Lancet 364(9434):621–632

Maeda Y, Laurberg S et al (2013) Perianal injectable bulking agents as treatment for faecal incontinence in adults. Cochrane Database Syst Rev (2):CD007959

Mantoo S, Meurette G et al (2012) The magnetic anal sphincter: a new device in the management of severe fecal incontinence. Expert Rev Med Devices 9(5):483–490

Markland AD, Goode PS et al (2010) Incidence and risk factors for fecal incontinence in black and white older adults: a population-based study. J Am Geriatr Soc 58(7):1341–1346

Matzel KE, Stadelmaier U et al (1995) Electrical stimulation of sacral spinal nerves for treatment of faecal incontinence. Lancet 346(8983):1124–1127

Nelson R, Furner S et al (1998) Fecal incontinence in Wisconsin nursing homes: prevalence and associations. Dis Colon Rectum 41(10):1226–1229

Newman DK, Gaines T et al (2005) Innovation in bladder assessment: use of technology in extended care. J Gerontol Nurs 31(12):33–41; quiz 42–43

Norton C, Hosker G et al (2000) Biofeedback and/or sphincter exercises for the treatment of faecal incontinence in adults. Cochrane Database Syst Rev (2):CD002111

Omar MI, Alexander CE (2013) Drug treatment for faecal incontinence in adults. Cochrane Database Syst Rev (6):CD002116

Parks AG. (1975) Anorectal incontinence. J R Soc Med;68:21–30

Rao SS (2004) Diagnosis and management of fecal incontinence. American College of Gastroenterology Practice Parameters Committee. Am J Gastroenterol 99(8):1585–1604

Ratto C, Parello A et al (2011) Novel bulking agent for faecal incontinence. Br J Surg 98(11): 1644–1652

Reilly C (2001) Transdisciplinary approach: an atypical strategy for improving outcomes in rehabilitative and long-term acute care settings. Rehabil Nurs 26(6):216–220, 244

Simpson RR, Kennedy ML et al (2006) Anal manometry: a comparison of techniques. Dis Colon Rectum 49(7):1033–1038

Talley NJ, O'Keefe EA et al (1992) Prevalence of gastrointestinal symptoms in the elderly: a population-based study. Gastroenterology 102(3):895–901

Thompson WG (1999) Irritable bowel syndrome: a management strategy. Baillieres Best Pract Res Clin Gastroenterol 13(3):453–460

Tjandra JJ, Chan MK et al (2008) Sacral nerve stimulation is more effective than optimal medical therapy for severe fecal incontinence: a randomized, controlled study. Dis Colon Rectum 51(5):494–502

Tourangeau R, Yan T (2007) Sensitive questions in surveys. Psychol Bull 133(5):859–883

Wang Z, Tan KY et al (2013) Functional outcomes in elderly adults who have undergone major colorectal surgery. J Am Geriatr Soc 61(12):2249–2250

Whitehead WE, Borrud L et al (2009) Fecal incontinence in US adults: epidemiology and risk factors. Gastroenterology 137(2):512–517, 517.e511–512

Xu X, Menees SB et al (2012) Economic cost of fecal incontinence. Dis Colon Rectum 55(5):586–598

Zorcolo L, Covotta L et al (2005) Outcome of anterior sphincter repair for obstetric injury: comparison of early and late results. Dis Colon Rectum 48(3):524–531

Integrating Science and Technology to Proctology

12

Frederick H. Koh and Ker-Kan Tan

> **Take-Home Pearls**
> - Fistulotomy remained the standard of care in low fistula.
> - Technological innovation has improved our understanding of the anatomy of anal fistula.
> - Many new treatment modalities have been proposed for the management of anal fistula. But none has yet become standard of care.
> - Technological advancement has given us more options of treatment for haemorrhoids.

12.1 Anal Fistula

Historical records of the surgical treatment of anal fistula date back to the time of Hippocrates in 430 BC, when the use of seton was first described. Since then, the management of this complex condition has intrigued many physicians, including Eisenhammer, Goodsall and Parks, all of whom made observations which have helped shaped the understanding and management of this condition.

Successful management of any condition requires the understanding of its pathogenesis. In anal fistula, the cryptoglandular theory remains the most quoted hypothesis that accounts for the majority of anal fistulas. Some of the other predisposing factors leading to formation of anal fistula include Crohn's disease, tuberculosis and malignancy. In the cryptoglandular theory, the spread of sepsis from the infected crypt gland in the intersphincteric space can occur in three planes – vertical, horizontal and circumferential. The direction of the spread often denotes the type of abscesses seen. A caudal spread of the sepsis will result in a perianal abscess, while

---

F.H. Koh • K.-K. Tan (✉)
Division of Colorectal Surgery, Department of Surgery, University Surgical Cluster,
National University Health System, Singapore, Singapore
e-mail: ker_kan_tan@nuhs.edu.sg

© Springer-Verlag Berlin Heidelberg 2015
K.-Y. Tan (ed.), *Transdisciplinary Perioperative Care in Colorectal Surgery:
An Integrative Approach*, DOI 10.1007/978-3-662-44020-9_12

a cephalad spread will result into either a high intermuscular or supralevator pararectal abscess. Horizontal or lateral spread through the external sphincter will result in an ischiorectal abscess. Circumferential spread can occur in any of the above-mentioned planes.

The presence of an external opening near the anus often denotes the presence of an underlying anal fistula. Patients typically present with a persistent discharging lump or occasionally following previous surgery that was performed to drain an associated abscess. Apart from the location of the external opening, it is important to exclude any underlying abscess that will require a drainage procedure. At the same time, one should palpate for the presence of an indurated tract medial to the external opening as it veers towards the anus. This would indicate the presence of an underlying fistula tract. It is also vital to perform a digital rectal examination to evaluate and document the passive and active anal tone.

The importance of the location of the external opening is highlighted by David Henry Goodsall back in the 1900s. The Goodsall rule states that, with a patient lying in a lithotomy position, an external opening anterior to the line passing through the middle of the anus would have a straight radial course to the dentate line, while an external opening posterior to the same line would have a curved tract towards the posterior midline (Goodsall and Miles 1990).

Another classification that has withstood the test of time and technology is the Parks classification described by Sir Alan Parks in the 1970s. On the basis of the cryptoglandular theory, the Parks classification divides anal fistula into intersphincteric, transsphincteric, suprasphincteric and extrasphincteric (Parks et al. 1976). This classification guides subsequent surgical management. In intersphincteric and low transsphincteric fistulas where there is no or minimal involvement of the external sphincter muscles, respectively, a lay-open fistulotomy can be safely performed with excellent success rates. However, in situations where the amount of external sphincter muscle involvement is deemed considerable, as in high transsphincteric and suprasphincteric fistulas, a lay-open fistulotomy will result in considerable sphincter damage and could increase the risk of developing anal incontinence subsequently. Hence, numerous sphincter-saving procedures have been proposed to prevent this morbidity.

12.2 Technological Advancement in the Preoperative Assessment of Anal Fistula

As we continue to advocate surgical interventions based on the Goodsall rule and Parks classification, there remain instances whereby the fistulas may actually deviate from the norm. This could have detrimental effects when the severity of the fistulas was only ascertained intraoperatively. With the continual advancement in diagnostic radiology, it is now possible to garner imaging for depicting the anatomy of the anal fistula preoperatively. This would definitely aid in understanding the anatomy of the fistula, the planning of the surgery and preoperative counselling for the patients. Endoanal ultrasonography (EAUS) and magnetic resonance imaging (MRI) are two such modalities used in the assessment of anal fistula.

Fig. 12.1 Endoanal ultrasonographic picture showing the course of the fistula with respect to the sphincter musculature

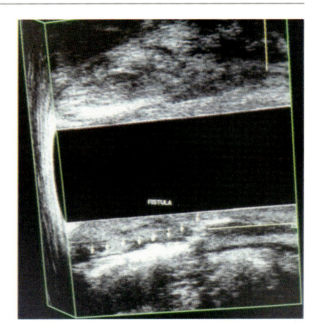

12.2.1 Endoanal Ultrasound (Fig. 12.1)

Endoanal ultrasound (EAUS), also known as anal endosonography, has been shown to be a cheap and accurate diagnostic modality that enables preoperative visualisation of the fistula tract (Nevler et al. 2013). One of its main advantages is the ability to delineate the anatomy of the fistula tract distinctly and to correlate its path with respect to the integrity and relation of the internal and external sphincters. The use of hydrogen peroxide coupled with the advent of 3-dimensional images also increase the accuracy of the test and help to better identify the location of the internal opening and determine the presence of any secondary fistula tracts (Kim and Park 2009). When used properly, the radiological findings correspond closely with the surgical findings, and the images provide a blueprint to plan the optimal surgical intervention.

As in all sonographic modalities, the main disadvantage lies in its heavy dependence on the competency of the operator. In addition, EAUS has a limited focal range whereby pathology beyond the anal sphincters complex may not be as clearly visualised.

12.2.2 Magnetic Resonance Imaging

The superior ability to discern soft tissue planes has resulted in magnetic resonance imaging (MRI) being used in various specialties. With a reported concordance rate of over 90 % with operative findings, MRI has slowly become a recognised modality in the preoperative assessment of recurrent and complex anal fistulas (Holzer et al. 2000). It is also able to evaluate the deeper surgical planes, underlying

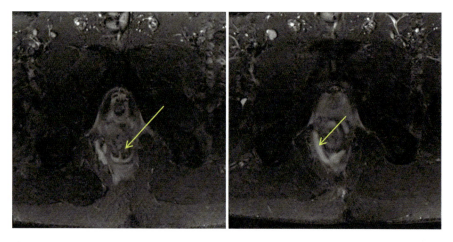

Fig. 12.2 MRI images of the pelvis. Image on the *left* shows an intersphincteric fistula tract at the 6 o'clock position (*arrowed*), and image on the *right* shows a right ischiorectal abscess (*arrowed*), which is communicating with the fistula tract

pathologies and complex characteristics of the anal fistulas more accurately than EAUS (Fig. 12.2). The availability of the MRI, or the lack of it, and its significant cost are its main limitations.

12.3 Surgical Management for Anal Fistula: A Journey Through Time and Innovation

The principles of surgical management in anal fistulas are the eradication of sepsis, prevention of recurrence and preservation of continence. While numerous evolving techniques have sprung up over the years in the hope of replacing lay-open fistulotomy as the standard of care in the management of all anal fistulas, none has succeeded thus far. We hereby evaluate the various techniques that have been advocated for anal fistula over the past years.

12.3.1 Fistulotomy

Lay-open fistulotomy was first described by John Arderne, an English surgeon, in the fourteenth century. As the name implies, this technique essentially involves laying open the fistula tract after establishing the path of the fistula from the external opening to the internal opening. This would facilitate drainage of the perianal sepsis and enables the wound to heal by secondary intention. A recent study demonstrated a 3-year recurrence rate of as low as 7 % with this technique (Benjelloun et al. 2013). The key component of this technique involves curetting the fistula tract to eradicate any infected and unhealthy tissue. A variation of the technique involves marsupialisation of the edges to prevent the skin from closing over the wound before healing from the wound bed, thereby reducing recurrence rates. This approach has been shown to be associated with faster wound healing and shorter duration of wound discharge (Ho et al. 1998).

Despite its high success rates, the risk of subsequent faecal incontinence increases if this technique is performed in fistulas with considerable involvement of the external anal sphincter or in patients with predisposing impaired anal continence. It has been reported that mild incontinence occurred in 9 % while severe incontinence is documented in up to 4 % of the patients (Stremitzer et al. 2011). This has a detrimental impact on the patients' quality of life. Thus, lay-open fistulotomy has gradually fallen out of favour in patients with high anal fistula if considerable amount of anal sphincter muscles would be divided (Mylonakis et al. 2001; Cavanaugh et al. 2002).

12.3.2 Seton

First described by Hippocrates, seton placement within the fistula tract, either loosely or tightly, has been around for a long time. It is often used either as a bridging procedure to fistulotomy or a single modality in high complex anal fistula to avoid upfront division of excessive amount of sphincter muscle (McCourtney and Finlay 1995; Memon et al. 2011). There are two ways to insert a seton – draining (loose) and cutting (tight). The primary aim of inserting a seton within the fistula tract is to enable drainage of the sepsis.

Although a draining seton effectively relieves the perianal sepsis, it is often not definitive. A subsequent procedure such as fistulotomy is typically performed when the seton has migrated more superficially. A recent meta-analysis actually highlighted a fistula recurrence rate of 3–5 %, depending on whether the anal sphincters were divided with placement of seton. The group that had their anal sphincters divided had slightly better outcomes. But the faecal incontinence rate was also significantly higher in the group that had their anal sphincter divided compared with those who only had seton without division of sphincters (25.2 % vs. 5.2 %) (Vial et al. 2010).

Conversely, when a cutting seton is used, one of the aims is to exteriorise a deep tract by inducing fibrosis superficial to the seton. This would gradually make the tract more superficial as the seton is tightened sequentially in intervals after its insertion. Apart from significant pain and discomfort arising from the rigidity of the seton coupled with the frequent tightening procedures, the reported incontinence rates are actually considerable in spite of its purported sphincter-sparing properties. The faecal incontinence rate of as high as 12 %, with almost 60 % of patients complaining of minor persistent loss of continence to flatus and fluid, has been reported (Ritchie et al. 2009). This complication is likely secondary to the disruption of the anal sphincters as the tightening process of the seton actually cuts through the sphincters gradually, and the ensuing fibrosis and scarring of the muscle fibres resulted in suboptimal function of the sphincters.

12.3.3 Mucosal Advancement Flap

This technique was first described for the repair of rectovaginal fistulas in 1902 which later extended to the treatment of complex anal fistulas. The two primary aims of this technique are to disrupt any communication of the tract with the anal canal and to completely remove the diseased and inflamed tissue from the anal mucosal surface (Elting 1912). A meta-analysis review of the success rate for anal fistula following mucosal advancement flap procedures revealed a recurrence rate from 7.0 to 51.7 %, while the wound healing time was reported to be 24.5 (±5.5) days. The incontinence rate was documented to be from 3.7 to 13.4 %. But as this technique is typically reserved for mainly the recurrent and/or complex high anal fistulas, one would expect their success rates to be less than first-line options such as fistulotomy.

One of the limitations precluding its widespread adoption is the technical difficulties in mastering this procedure. A thorough understanding of the anal anatomy and the underlying pathology is critical to maximise the success and minimise its complication rates (Golub et al. 1997; Leng and Jin 2012). To pursue a higher success rate for this technique, some surgeons have combined the mucosal advancement flap with the administration of platelet-rich plasma which is an autologous form of tissue glue. A 16.0 % recurrence rate after a median follow-up period of 27 months was reported which did not appear to improve the procedural outcome significantly (Göttgens et al. 2014).

12.3.4 Utilising Technology for Anal Fistula Treatment

The problems of the aforementioned techniques are apparent. Anal fistulas involving minimal sphincter muscles can be easily dealt with by the fistulotomy procedure. But none of the "traditional" methods have been deemed safe and effective in the treatment of high, complex and recurrent anal fistulas. With the continual advancement in science and technology, newer and innovative techniques have been introduced with the aim to improve the success rates following the treatment of this difficult condition while preserving the anal sphincter function.

12.3.4.1 Fibrin Glue

The rationale of fibrin glue in anal fistula is the application of an adhesive substance into the fistula tract with the aim to facilitate its closure by laying down a fibrin network. If proven to be successful, this is an attractive, fast and non-invasive method for treating anal fistulas. In the initial years following its introduction in the 1990s, the overall closure rate reported could be as high as 85–100 % after single or multiple treatments (Sentovich 2001). However, longer-term follow-up studies revealed suboptimal results with one study reporting a healing rate of 39.1 % at 12 weeks post-operatively. Another randomised study highlighted a 27-month post-operative healing rate of only 21 % (Singer et al. 2005; Chung et al. 2009).

It is postulated that the high failure rates could be attributed to its inability to eradicate the infected and inflamed tissue and its failure to tackle complex fistulas with secondary extensions. Coupled with the high failure and recurrence rates and the cost of the fibrin glue, this technique has largely fallen out of favour (Swinscoe et al. 2005).

12.3.4.2 Fistula Plug

As we enter the new millennium, a bioprosthetic plug (Fig. 12.3) was introduced to address the liquid nature of the fibrin glue which was one of the postulated reasons for its poor outcome. These plugs are placed within the fistula tract, typically after perianal sepsis has subsided with the aid of a draining seton. The fistula plug is then sutured in place at the internal opening with the excess plug material being removed if it extrudes from the external opening (Fig. 12.4).

Initial interest was overwhelming following a prospectively conducted study which involved a cohort of 25 patients, where 15 patients were treated with plug and 10 with glue. A 6-month fistula closure success rate of 87 % was reported with plug

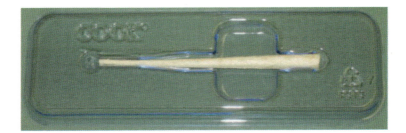

Fig. 12.3 Anal fistula plug

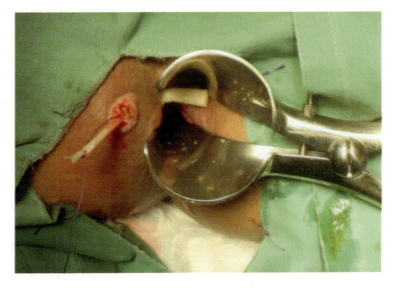

Fig. 12.4 Placement of the fistula plug within the fistula tract

treatment, compared to 40 % in those who had glue application (Johnson et al. 2006). Just like the fibrin glue, varying institutions and longer-term follow-up failed to replicate the success shared by the initial group. A retrospective review in an Australian centre reported a failure rate of 86.7 % at 59 weeks (Tan et al. 2013). A meta-analysis including three retrospective and two randomised studies also demonstrated that the incidence of recurrence for the anal fistula plug was 62.1 % compared to 47 % for conventional surgical approach (Pu et al. 2012).

A multicentre study of 126 patients over 5 years attempted to evaluate the risk factors that could predispose to failure of the fistula plug. While they concurred with the very low success rates, they found that anteriorly located fistula tends to have a lower chance of closure (12 %, hazard ratio = 2.98, confidence interval [CI] 1.01–8.78) (Blom et al. 2014). Other factors that have been reported as risk factors for failures included the extrusion of the fistula plug and its inability to deal with fistulas with secondary extensions.

12.3.4.3 Video-Assisted Anal Fistula Treatment

Video-assisted anal fistula treatment (VAAFT) is one of the latest treatment modalities advocated for anal fistula. This technique which is first described by Meinero and Mori, combines the use of a small rigid endoscope inserted through the external opening to follow the tract until the internal opening (Fig. 12.5). This is then followed by electrocautery to fulgurate the fistula tract as the endoscope was slowly withdrawn. The internal opening is then closed either with a local mucosal flap or by stapler technique. One of the purported advantages of the scope includes its ability to exclude secondary fistula tracts or chronic deep abscesses.

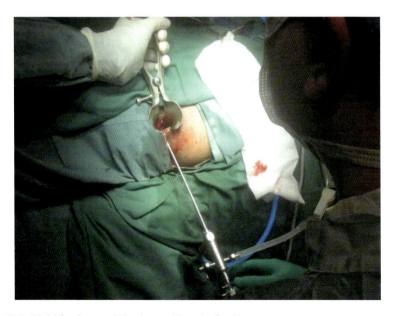

Fig. 12.5 Rigid fistuloscope being inserted into the fistula

12 Integrating Science and Technology to Proctology

This method theoretically discontinues the fistula tract with the anal mucosa and preserves the sphincter continuity by preventing further disruption to the sphincter integrity in high and complex anal fistulas. Meinero's study of 136 patients revealed an 87.1 % healing rate 1 year following the operation (Meinero and Mori 2011). The same study group later included incontinence scoring over a 24-month period for a total of 203 patients and found that none had a change in their continence ability (Meinero et al. 2014).

The promising results of this new technique have made it very attractive, but just like the fibrin glue and fistula plug techniques, this technique needs to be validated by other surgeons from numerous institutions to determine if similar outcomes can be achieved. The cost of the disposables required for this procedure is also a considerable limitation.

12.3.4.4 Fistula Tract Laser Closure

The persistence of the fistula epithelium was deemed to be one of the main reasons for failure in fistula treatment. In recent years, the incorporation of laser technology to ablate the fistula tract has been attempted in the form of fistula tract laser closure (FiLaC).

A laser-emitting diode is threaded through the fistula tract, and the emission of a radial laser from the diode results in contraction of the tract around the laser fibre to induce fibrosis around the fistula tract in an attempt to obliterate it. This procedure is recommended as a follow-up procedure after perianal sepsis is alleviated with draining setons. It can also be combined with another procedure, like a mucosal advancement flap, to seal the internal opening.

Like the VAAFT technique, there are not much available data in the literature due to its novelty. However, from the limited experience with this modality, success rates of 71–82 % have been quoted with minimal adverse effects on incontinence (Giamundo et al. 2014; Wilhelm 2011).

12.3.5 Back to Basics?

Despite the prominence and keen interest in adopting technology and innovation in treating anal fistula, their outcomes have yet to reach levels comparable to conventional treatment modalities. Perhaps, success in fistula surgery may not necessarily lie with continual advancement in technology and innovation.

12.3.5.1 Ligation of Intersphincteric Fistula Tract

A small group of surgeons opted to refocus on the basics of perianal anatomy and the pathological process of anal fistula rather than to continue to apply technology and innovation in this field. Rojanasakul and group described the ligation of intersphincteric fistula tract (LIFT) procedure which puts the emphasis back on the clear delineation of the anatomy and pathology of the anal fistula. It was postulated that the eradication of the infected crypt gland in the intersphincteric space is vital to the LIFT procedure (Fig. 12.6).

Fig. 12.6 Intersphincteric fistula tract

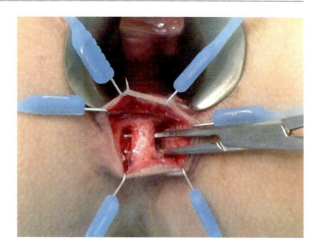

The LIFT procedure became increasingly popular due to its minimal cost and the simplicity of the operation. The initial reported success rate for the LIFT procedure from Rojanasakul et al. was an astonishing 94.4 % (Rojanasakul et al. 2007). Subsequent studies from numerous worldwide institutions have demonstrated more modest success rates from 57 to 82.2 % (Shanwani et al. 2010; Liu et al. 2013; Bleier et al. 2010).

Another purported benefit of this procedure was the conversion of a transsphincteric fistula to an intersphincteric fistula (through the intersphincteric wound) when the procedure fails. This then enables a lay-open fistulotomy to be performed with minimal impact on the anal sphincter function (Yassin et al. 2013). Another controversy of the LIFT procedure was the role of seton prior to the operation. While there were some who advocated inserting a draining seton for 6–8 weeks prior to the LIFT procedure to relieve the sepsis and facilitate identification of the tract, others refute this theory and found that the presence of a seton actually increased the failure rate due to the postulation that the tissues following resolution of inflammation would be more scarred and ischaemic.

Although the initial reports on the LIFT procedure remain promising, we await more long-term data on the effectiveness of the operation before defining its role in the treatment of anal fistula. Some of the other questions that remain unanswered include its true impact of continence and the role of seton prior to the operation (Tan et al. 2011, 2012; Yassin et al. 2013).

12.3.5.2 Combining LIFT with Technological Innovation

As the name implies, the BioLIFT procedure is a combination of the classical LIFT procedure with the placement of a biological material. These can include an anal fistula plug or a bioprosthetic graft in the intersphincteric space in the same setting.

Initial success rate was reported to be between 68.8 and 94.4 % with a recurrence rate of 5.6–31.3 % when coupled with an anal fistula plug (Cui et al. 2012). When LIFT is combined with the insertion of a bioprosthetic graft, initial success rates were reported to be over 90 % (Ellis 2010). However, when this procedure was repeated in Australia, the success rate of the BioLIFT was comparable to the conventional LIFT procedure (Chew et al. 2013; Tan and Lee 2014). The role of biological material in the LIFT procedure remains controversial at this juncture.

12.4 Haemorrhoids

First described by ancient Egyptians on papyruses, the term "haemorrhoids" has been strictly used to describe the normal arteriovenous cushions or plexus in the submucosal layer of the anal canal that are held up by fibromuscular ligaments. However, in clinical practice, the same term is used to describe the condition when patients present with bleeding and/or prolapse.

After over twenty centuries since its first description, the management of haemorrhoidal conditions has surprisingly not changed much since the days of Hippocrates. Despite similar principles of management, technology has come into the fold recently in an attempt to improve the outcomes of haemorrhoidal treatment.

12.5 Treatment of Haemorrhoids: What Has Changed?

From the ancient methods of molten lead, management of haemorrhoid treatment has evolved with the aid of technology. Interestingly, the recurrence and persistence of haemorrhoidal condition have not improved much in spite of introduction of newer techniques. This is probably due to the underlying pathophysiology of the condition. Conservative management, where lifestyle, dietary and defecation habits are modified, still remains the mainstay in treating early haemorrhoidal disease.

12.6 Current "Standard" Procedures

12.6.1 Rubber Band Ligation

Rubber band ligation (RBL) is a convenient, quick and simple office procedure described and refined by Blaisdell and Barron. The main rationale was to strangulate the engorged haemorrhoidal plexus and allow necrosis, sloughing and scar formation to occur (Laisdell 1958). This technique is still frequently performed for grade I, grade II and selected grade III internal haemorrhoids. Studies have shown that up to 70 % of patients remain asymptomatic up to 10 years post RBL for grade II haemorrhoids (Lu et al. 2013). Minimal complications apart from mild to moderate discomfort are experienced.

However, the shortfall of this technique is that it is contraindicated in external haemorrhoids and is not effective in addressing all haemorrhoidal conditions, especially significant prolapse. Add onto the symptom recurrence rate of up to 30 %, other methods of treatment have been gradually introduced.

12.6.2 Excisional Haemorrhoidectomy (Open Milligan-Morgan and Closed Ferguson Techniques)

Haemorrhoidectomy involves the removal of the symptomatic haemorrhoidal tissues. It is said to be the most effective treatment for haemorrhoids that have failed conservative treatment. Patients with grade III or IV haemorrhoids or presenting with acute conditions such as thrombosis have been routinely offered excisional haemorrhoidectomy. In one study comparing excisional haemorrhoidectomy and RBL, excisional haemorrhoidectomy was able to achieve a higher rate of symptom remission than RBL (relative risk [RR] 1.68, 95 % CI 1.00–2.83) with fewer patients requiring retreatment (RR 0.20, 95 % CI 0.09–0.40) albeit with more post-operative pain (RR 1.94, 95 % CI 1.62–2.33) (Shanmugam et al. 2005). The two most commonly described techniques are the open Milligan-Morgan procedure and the closed Ferguson haemorrhoidectomy.

The main difference between the Milligan-Morgan technique and the Ferguson technique lies in the stitching up of the submucosal layer following excision of the haemorrhoidal plexus. The closed Ferguson haemorrhoidectomy technique has better reported outcomes in terms of post-operative incontinence compared to the open Milligan-Morgan technique (Jóhannsson et al. 2006). Differences in the post-operative pain and days taken for symptom remission vary from study to study, with no clear evidence favouring one over the other. Despite a common consensus on that aspect, one cannot ignore the fact that recovery from this technique is still more than 10 days.

12.6.3 Procedure for Prolapsed Haemorrhoids or Stapled Haemorrhoidopexy

Introduced in 1998, this technique involves the use of a circular stapling device used to excise redundant prolapsing or bulging anal mucosal tissue proximal to where the haemorrhoidal tissues are. This results in the tissue overlying the bulging haemorrhoids to be pulled more proximally and thereby reduces the blood flow through the haemorrhoidal plexus. At the same time, the procedure retracts the prolapsed haemorrhoids back into the anal canal.

Some of the reported benefits of this procedure over conventional haemorrhoidectomy include reduced post-operative pain (Senagore et al. 2004; Tjandra and Chan 2007), shorter hospital stay (Nisar et al. 2004; Hetzer et al. 2002), earlier recovery time and reduced operative duration. Some of the common post-operative complications of this procedure include bleeding, acute urinary retention, formation of stricture and fissures. There are also case reports of rectal perforation and chronic pain post stapled haemorrhoidopexy (Pescatori and Gagliardi 2008).

A meta-analysis comparing stapled haemorrhoidopexy to conventional haemorrhoidectomy revealed that even though stapled haemorrhoidopexy allows a shorter hospital stay, the recurrence of haemorrhoidal prolapse (OR 3.60, CI 1.24–10.49) and the need for a second procedure were more common in the

12 Integrating Science and Technology to Proctology

stapled haemorrhoidopexy group (OR 6.78, 95 % CI 2.00–23.00). Complication rates and cost were largely similar for both techniques (Jayaraman et al. 2006; Burch et al. 2009).

12.6.4 Transanal Haemorrhoidal Dearterialisation

In 1995, Morinaga incorporated the understanding of anatomy and pathophysiology of haemorrhoidal disease with the principles of minimally invasive and ultrasound technology to develop a novel non-excisional procedure for haemorrhoidal disease – the transanal haemorrhoidal dearterialisation (THD) (Morinaga et al. 1995). This technique involves the use of an anoscope, specially fitted with an ultrasound probe, to locate the distal rectal arterial branches. These are then ligated with stitches to reduce the blood flow within the haemorrhoidal plexus.

When first described, Morinaga reported that up to 96 % of patients had improvement in pain, 95 % for bleeding and 78 % for prolapse. This potential brought optimism to the advocates of minimally invasive surgery as the results suggest that more can be achieved by doing less, with less damage to the innate anatomy.

A subsequent systemic review of 17 articles involving almost 2000 patients revealed that the post-operative pain was only experienced by 18 % of patients with recurrence rate of between 4.7 and 9.0 % depending on the type of symptoms (Giordano et al. 2009). In view of lack of long-term prospective data, the HubBLe trial, a multicentred randomised control trial, is currently being conducted by a group in Leeds, United Kingdom, to compare the patient-reported symptom recurrence rate and cost-effectiveness between THD and RBL (Vial et al. 2010).

12.6.5 Emerging Technology

With the promising initial short-term data of THD, incorporation of a bipolar device to the anoscope to alleviate the technically more difficult placement of sutures has been attempted using the HET bipolar device (HET Systems, Northvale, NJ, USA). Initial short- and long-term outcomes were presented in 2012 revealing 86.7 % of patients with initial haematochezia from haemorrhoids having resolution of symptoms at 4 weeks and all patients having improvement in haemorrhoidal symptoms at an average follow-up time of 13.1 months (Kantsevoy 2013).

References

Benjelloun EB, Jarrar A, El Rhazi K, Souiki T, Ousadden A, Ait Taleb K (2013) Acute abscess with fistula: long-term results justify drainage and fistulotomy. Updates Surg 65(3):207–211

Bleier JI, Moloo H, Goldberg SM (2010) Ligation of the intersphincteric fistula tract: an effective new technique for complex fistulas. Dis Colon Rectum 53(1):43–46

Blom J, Husberg-Sellberg B, Lindelius A, Gustafsson UM, Carlens S, Oppelstrup H, Bragmark M, Yin L, Nyström PO (2014) Results of collagen plug occlusion of anal fistula: a multicentre study of 126 patients. Colorectal Dis 16(8):626–630

Burch J, Epstein D, Sari AB, Weatherly H, Jayne D, Fox D, Woolacott N (2009) Stapled haemorrhoidopexy for the treatment of haemorrhoids: a systematic review. Colorectal Dis 11:233–243

Cavanaugh M, Hyman N, Osler T (2002) Fecal incontinence severity index after fistulotomy: a predictor of quality of life. Dis Colon Rectum 45(3):349–353

Chew MH, Lee PJ, Koh CE, Chew HE (2013) Appraisal of the LIFT and BIOLIFT procedure: initial experience and short-term outcomes of 33 consecutive patients. Int J Colorectal Dis 28(11):1489–1496

Chung W, Kazemi P, Ko D, Sun C, Brown CJ, Raval M, Phang T (2009) Anal fistula plug and fibrin glue versus conventional treatment in repair of complex anal fistulas. Am J Surg 197(5): 604–608

Cui JJ, Wang ZJ, Zheng Y, Han JG, Yang XQ (2012) Ligation of the intersphincteric fistula tract plus bioprosthetic anal fistula plug (LIFT-plug) in the treatment of transsphincteric perianal fistula. Zhonghua Wei Chang Wai Ke Za Zhi 15(12):1232–1235

Ellis CN (2010) Outcomes with the use of bioprosthetic grafts to reinforce the ligation of the intersphincteric fistula tract (BioLIFT procedure) for the management of complex anal fistulas. Dis Colon Rectum 53(10):1361–1364

Elting AW (1912) The treatment of fistula in ano. Ann Surg 56:744–775

Giamundo P, Geraci M, Tibaldi L, Valente M (2014) Closure of fistula-in-ano with laser – FiLaC™: an effective novel sphincter-saving procedure for complex disease. Colorectal Dis 16(2):110–115

Giordano P, Overton J, Madeddu F, Zaman S, Gravante G (2009) Transanal hemorrhoidal dearterialization: a systematic review. Dis Colon Rectum 52(9):1665–1671

Golub RW, Wise WE Jr, Kerner BA, Khanduja KS, Aguilar PS (1997) Endorectal mucosal advancement flap: the preferred method for complex cryptoglandular fistula-in-ano. J Gastrointest Surg 1(5):487–491

Goodsall DH, Miles WE (1990) Ano-rectal fistula. In: Goodsall DH, Miles WE (eds) Diseases of the anus and rectum. Longmans, Green & Co., London, pp 92–137

Göttgens KW, Vening W, van der Hagen SJ, van Gemert WG, Smeets RR, Stassen LP, Baeten CG, Breukink SO (2014) Long-term results of mucosal advancement flap combined with platelet-rich plasma for high cryptoglandular perianal fistulas. Dis Colon Rectum 57(2):223–227

Hetzer FH, Demartines N, Handschin AE, Clavien PA (2002) Stapled vs excision hemorrhoidectomy: long-term results of a prospective randomized trial. Arch Surg 137(3):337–340

Ho YH, Tan M, Leong AF, Seow-Choen F (1998) Marsupialization of fistulotomy wounds improves healing: a randomized controlled trial. Br J Surg 85(1):105–107

Holzer B, Rosen HR, Urban M, Anzböck W, Schiessel R, Hruby W (2000) Magnetic resonance imaging of perianal fistulas: predictive value for Parks classification and identification of the internal opening. Colorectal Dis 2(6):340–345

Jayaraman S, Colquhoun PH, Malthaner RA (2006) Stapled versus conventional surgery for hemorrhoids. Cochrane Database Syst Rev (4):CD005393

Jóhannsson HO, Påhlman L, Graf W (2006) Randomized clinical trial of the effects on anal function of Milligan-Morgan versus Ferguson haemorrhoidectomy. Br J Surg 93(10):1208–1214

Johnson EK, Gaw JU, Armstrong DN (2006) Efficacy of anal fistula plug vs. fibrin glue in closure of anorectal fistulas. Dis Colon Rectum 49(3):371–376

Kantsevoy SV, Bitner M (2013) Nonsurgical treatment of actively bleeding internal hemorrhoids with a novel endoscopic device (with video). Gastrointest Endosc 78(4):649–653

Kim Y, Park YJ (2009) Three-dimensional endoanal ultrasonographic assessment of an anal fistula with and without H(2)O(2) enhancement. World J Gastroenterol 15(38):4810–4815

Laisdell PC (1958) Prevention of massive hemorrhage secondary to hemorrhoidectomy. Surg Gynecol Obstet 106(4):485–488

Leng Q, Jin HY (2012) Anal fistula plug vs mucosa advancement flap in complex fistula-in-ano: a meta-analysis. World J Gastrointest Surg 4(11):256–261

Liu WY, Aboulian A, Kaji AH, Kumar RR (2013) Long-term results of ligation of intersphincteric fistula tract (LIFT) for fistula-in-ano. Dis Colon Rectum 56(3):343–347

Lu LY, Zhu Y, Sun Q (2013) A retrospective analysis of short and long term efficacy of RBL for hemorrhoids. Eur Rev Med Pharmacol Sci 17(20):2827–2830

McCourtney JS, Finlay IG (1995) Setons in the surgical management of fistula in ano. Br J Surg 82(4):448–452

Meinero P, Mori L (2011) Video-assisted anal fistula treatment (VAAFT): a novel sphincter-saving procedure for treating complex anal fistulas. Tech Coloproctol 15(4):417–422

Meinero P, Mori L, Gasloli G (2014) Video-assisted anal fistula treatment: a new concept of treating anal fistulas. Dis Colon Rectum 57(3):354–359

Memon AA, Murtaza G, Azami R, Zafar H, Chawla T, Laghari AA (2011) Treatment of complex fistula in ano with cable-tie seton: a prospective case series. ISRN Surg 2011:636952

Morinaga K, Hasuda K, Ikeda T (1995) A novel therapy for internal hemorrhoids: ligation of the hemorrhoidal artery with a newly devised instrument (Moricorn) in conjunction with a Doppler flowmeter. Am J Gastroenterol 90(4):610–613

Mylonakis E, Katsios C, Godevenos D, Nousias B, Kappas AM (2001) Quality of life of patients after surgical treatment of anal fistula; the role of anal manometry. Colorectal Dis 3(6):417–421

Nevler A, Beer-Gabel M, Lebedyev A, Soffer A, Gutman M, Carter D, Zbar AP (2013) Transperineal ultrasonography in perianal Crohn's disease and recurrent cryptogenic fistula-in-ano. Colorectal Dis 15(8):1011–1018

Nisar PJ, Acheson AG, Neal KR, Scholefield JH (2004) Stapled hemorrhoidopexy compared with conventional hemorrhoidectomy: systematic review of randomized, controlled trials. Dis Colon Rectum 47(11):1837–1845

Parks AG, Gordon PH, Hardcastle JD (1976) A classification of fistula-in-ano. Br J Surg 63(1):1–12

Pescatori M, Gagliardi G (2008) Postoperative complications after procedure for prolapsed hemorrhoids (PPH) and stapled transanal rectal resection (STARR) procedures. Tech Coloproctol 12(1):7–19

Pu YW, Xing CG, Khan I, Zhao K, Zhu BS, Wu Y (2012) Fistula plug versus conventional surgical treatment for anal fistulas. A system review and meta-analysis. Saudi Med J 33(9):962–966

Ritchie RD, Sackier JM, Hodde JP (2009) Incontinence rates after cutting seton treatment for anal fistula. Colorectal Dis 11(6):564–571

Rojanasakul A, Pattanaarun J, Sahakitrungruang C, Tantiphlachiva K (2007) Total anal sphincter saving technique for fistula-in-ano; the ligation of intersphincteric fistula tract. J Med Assoc Thai 90(3):581–586

Senagore AJ, Singer M, Abcarian H, Fleshman J, Corman M, Wexner S, Nivatvongs S, Procedure for Prolapse and Hemorrhoids (PPH) Multicenter Study Group (2004) A prospective, randomized, controlled multicenter trial comparing stapled hemorrhoidopexy and Ferguson hemorrhoidectomy: perioperative and one-year results. Dis Colon Rectum 47(11):1824–1836

Sentovich SM (2001) Fibrin glue for all anal fistulas. J Gastrointest Surg 5(2):158–161

Shanmugam V, Thaha MA, Rabindranath KS, Campbell KL, Steele RJ, Loudon MA (2005) Systematic review of randomized trials comparing rubber band ligation with excisional haemorrhoidectomy. Br J Surg 92(12):1481–1487

Shanwani A, Nor AM, Amri N (2010) Ligation of the intersphincteric fistula tract (LIFT): a sphincter-saving technique for fistula-in-ano. Dis Colon Rectum 53(1):39–42

Singer M, Cintron J, Nelson R et al (2005) Treatment of fistulas-in-ano with fibrin sealant in combination with intra-adhesive antibiotics and/or surgical closure of the internal fistula opening. Dis Colon Rectum 48:799–808

Stremitzer S, Strobl S, Kure V, Bîrsan T, Puhalla H, Herbst F, Stift A (2011) Treatment of perianal sepsis and long-term outcome of recurrence and continence. Colorectal Dis 13(6):703–707

Swinscoe MT, Ventakasubramaniam AK, Jayne DG (2005) Fibrin glue for fistula-in-ano: the evidence reviewed. Tech Coloproctol 9(2):89–94

Tan KK, Lee PJ (2014) Early experience of reinforcing the ligation of the intersphincteric fistula tract procedure with a bioprosthetic graft (BioLIFT) for anal fistula. ANZ J Surg 84(4):280–283

Tan KK, Tan IJ, Lim FS, Koh DC, Tsang CB (2011) The anatomy of failures following the ligation of intersphincteric tract technique for anal fistula: a review of 93 patients over 4 years. Dis Colon Rectum 54(11):1368–1372

Tan KK, Alsuwaigh R, Tan AM, Tan IJ, Liu X, Koh DC, Tsang CB (2012) To LIFT or to flap? Which surgery to perform following seton insertion for high anal fistula? Dis Colon Rectum 55(12):1273–1277

Tan KK, Kaur G, Byrne CM, Young CJ, Wright C, Solomon MJ (2013) Long-term outcome of the anal fistula plug for anal fistula of cryptoglandular origin. Colorectal Dis 15(12):1510–1514

Tjandra JJ, Chan MK (2007) Systematic review on the procedure for prolapse and hemorrhoids (stapled hemorrhoidopexy). Dis Colon Rectum 50(6):878–892

Vial M, Parés D, Pera M, Grande L (2010) Faecal incontinence after seton treatment for anal fistulae with and without surgical division of internal anal sphincter: a systematic review. Colorectal Dis 12(3):172–178

Wilhelm A (2011) A new technique for sphincter-preserving anal fistula repair using a novel radial emitting laser probe. Tech Coloproctol 15(4):445–449

Yassin NA, Hammond TM, Lunniss PJ, Phillips RK (2013) Ligation of the intersphincteric fistula tract in the management of anal fistula. A systematic review. Colorectal Dis 15(5):527–535

Transdisciplinary Management in Geriatric Oncology

13

Sung W. Sun, Koshy Alexander, and Beatriz Korc-Grodzicki

> **Take-Home Pearls**
> - The number of older adults diagnosed with cancer is projected to increase significantly.
> - Comprehensive Geriatric Assessment is a valuable instrument in the assessment of the older cancer patient that could help tailor an individualized treatment plan.
> - A transdisciplinary team with the knowledge of the principles of geriatrics is essential to provide patient-centered care.
> - As cancer is increasingly taking on the characteristics of chronic diseases, there is a huge need to develop shared care models with a bigger role played by the primary care physician.

13.1 Introduction

As a result of declining fertility and mortality rates, the world is experiencing an aging of its population (Fig. 13.1). According to the UN, the proportion of older adults (60 years and older) comprised 11 % of the world population in 2009 but will represent 22 % by 2050. Due to advances in public health and medicine in just the past 100 years, life expectancy for the average person in Europe, North America, Japan, and other industrialized countries has increased by more than 50 %. Adults in these societies can reasonably count on living into their 80s and 90s. As cancer occurs more commonly in the older adults, this shift is expected to markedly increase the number of cancer diagnoses. Cancer is diagnosed at a higher rate

---

S.W. Sun, MD (✉) • K. Alexander, MD • B. Korc-Grodzicki, MD, PhD
Geriatric Service, Department of Medicine, Memorial Sloan Kettering Cancer Center, 1275 York Avenue, 205, New York, NY 10065, USA

Weill Medical College of Cornell University, New York, NY, USA
e-mail: suns@mskcc.org; korcgrob@mskcc.org

© Springer-Verlag Berlin Heidelberg 2015
K.-Y. Tan (ed.), *Transdisciplinary Perioperative Care in Colorectal Surgery: An Integrative Approach*, DOI 10.1007/978-3-662-44020-9_13

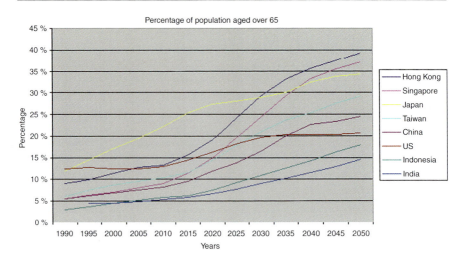

Fig. 13.1 Population projections for the elderly in various countries. Source: US Census Bureau http://www.census.gov/ipc/www/idbnew.html

(53 %), accounts for a higher percentage of survivors (59 %), and results in more deaths among individuals 65 years and older (68 %) compared with younger adults (Hurria et al. 2013). Minorities and older adults represent important population groups that may be particularly vulnerable to suboptimal cancer care, because both groups have been underrepresented in cancer clinical trials (Hutchins et al. 1999) and are also subject to disparities in treatment (Bouchardy et al. 2007; Gross et al. 2008). Colorectal cancer is and will continue to be one of the three leading cancer sites in the year 2030 in both men and women (Smith et al. 2009). Bowel cancer mortality is strongly related to age. In the UK between 2009 and 2011, an average of 57 % of bowel cancer deaths occurred in men and women aged 75 years and over (2014).

In older adults, cancer is often only one of multiple coexisting health conditions. Physical, cognitive, emotional, and social issues add to the complexity of their care needs (Hurria et al. 2013). Older patients often see several providers, a diverse and fragmented group of clinicians with poor communication among them. Older adults are also the biggest consumers of prescription medications, over-the-counter drugs, and nutritional supplements. Nearly one third of community-dwelling adults aged 65 or older take more than five prescription medications (Tinetti et al. 2004). In addition, most hands-on care is provided by family and friends who, despite very little training, play a key role in the health-care infrastructure of the older adult (Hurria et al. 2013).

Just about every aspect of organized medicine follows a disease-by-disease model. This is traditionally how medicine is taught, research is funded, professional societies are formed, journals are published, and medical products are developed. This approach treats the diseases of aging as if they exist in silos, unconnected from one another (Perry 2010). For cancer treatment in older adults to be feasible and successful, there must be effective communication and coordination among multiple providers including not only the oncologist, surgeon, and/or radiation oncologist but also the patient's primary care physician and specialty physicians. A transdisciplinary team with the knowledge of the principles of geriatrics to support the older adults coping with cancer is essential to provide seamless patient-centered care. In a transdisciplinary model, the members of the care team come together from the beginning, exchange ideas, work together, and come up with solutions (Satterfield et al. 2009). Team care improves health care, quality of life, and functional status in older patients while enhancing patient and family understanding of disease and treatment options (Boult et al. 2009).

13.2 Geriatric Assessment

There is a significant heterogeneity among older cancer patients in terms of functional status, comorbidities, physiological reserve, availability of social support, and preference and desire for therapy which will influence patient's ability to tolerate aggressive cancer treatment. An important tool used for the assessment of older cancer patients is the Comprehensive Geriatric Assessment (CGA) designed to identify multiple problems of geriatric patients in order to develop interventions.

13.2.1 What Is CGA?

CGA is a validated holistic approach to evaluate the elderly population. It is a multidisciplinary, multidimensional, and intensive evaluation of a patient who is at significant risk for subsequent functional decline (Reuben et al. 1999). CGA measures aspects such as functional status, comorbid medical conditions, nutritional status, physiological state, social support, and geriatric syndromes involving multidisciplinary interpretation as well as transdisciplinary implementation. Such comprehensive approach reveals information missed by routine history and physical alone (Hurria et al. 2006). Evidence for the value of integrating geriatric evaluation principles into oncology is increasingly being documented in the literature (Extermann et al. 2005).

13.2.2 Role of Geriatric Assessment in Oncology

Evaluation for oncologic treatment consideration routinely includes cancer pathology, staging of the disease, basic functional assessment, functional assessment of several organs, and consideration of comorbid illness. In older cancer patients, this may not be sufficient to predict potentially adverse outcomes such as toxicity, morbidity, disability, and mortality and to properly support clinical decisions. Objectives of performing geriatric assessment in cancer patients are to provide an approximate estimation of life expectancy, help the oncologist understand the potential impact of the patient's cancer during his or her remaining life, identify cancer patients for whom one could expect the greatest benefit from treatment, identify medical and social problems that may decrease the tolerance of cancer treatment and/or be amenable to intervention, formulate appropriate treatment and management strategies, and assist in monitoring clinical and functional outcomes going forward (Hurria and Balducci 2009). A prospective observational cohort study looking at CGA as a predictor of complications in elderly patients after elective surgery for colorectal cancer showed that CGA was able to identify frail patients who have significantly increased risk of severe complications after elective surgery (Kristjansson et al. 2010).

The ultimate goal of CGA is to provide the patient with a holistic view of what to expect in going through cancer treatment and have the patient participate in shared decision-making process of selecting the best treatment option in accordance with the patient's wishes. A recent review on geriatric assessment in the oncology setting showed that it is feasible, and some domains were significantly associated with adverse outcomes. However, they found limited evidence that geriatric assessment impacted treatment decision-making (Puts et al. 2012).

13.2.3 Prediction of Chemotherapy Toxicity

Existing oncology performance status measures (such as Karnofsky performance status [KPS] (Yates et al. 1980) or Eastern Cooperative Oncology Group performance status (Oken et al. 1982)) are applied to adult patients with cancer regardless of age to estimate functional status, assess eligibility for clinical trials, and predict treatment toxicity and survival. However, these tools were validated in younger patients and do not address the heterogeneity in the aging process. There is a need to develop a predictive model that incorporates geriatric and oncologic correlates of vulnerability to chemotherapy toxicity in older adults. The Cancer and Aging Research Group (CARG) study using a pre-chemotherapy geriatric assessment was able to identify risk factors for chemotherapy toxicity in older adults and develop a risk stratification schema. A predictive model for grade 3–5 toxicity was developed. It consisted of geriatric assessment variables, laboratory test values, and patient, tumor, and treatment characteristics. This model had a greater ability to discriminate risk of chemotherapy toxicity than the KPS (Hurria et al. 2011).

The Chemotherapy Risk Assessment Scale for High-Age Patients (CRASH) score is another predictive instrument of chemotoxicity in older adults. Through the assessment of 24 parameters, this study was able to stratify patients into four categories for risk of chemotherapy-related toxicity. The study confirmed that hematological and non-hematological toxicities are associated with different predictors, which may prove important for clinical application and for designing future trials (Extermann et al. 2012).

13.2.4 Preoperative Evaluation of the Older Cancer Patient

The determination of surgical risk for the elderly patient is complex. For these patients, traditional organ system-oriented preoperative assessment has been shown to be lacking in predicting adverse postoperative outcomes. The assessment should encompass multiple domains including underlying functional status, physiologic changes of normal aging, changes related to comorbidities, and the surgical procedure itself. There have been several studies showing that geriatric assessment incorporated into preoperative assessment provides a more accurate picture of what to expect in terms of perioperative morbidity and mortality. In 1991, the Physiological and Operative Severity Score for the enUmeration of Mortality and morbidity (POSSUM) was developed, and since then it has been used in assessing the risk of colorectal surgery (Copeland et al. 1991). By using a validated frailty scoring system which encompasses weight loss, exhaustion, physical activity, walk time, and grip strength, Makary et al. were able to show that frailty independently predicted postoperative complications, length of stay, and discharge to a skilled or assisted living facility in older surgical patients (Makary et al. 2010). Robinson et al. showed that preoperative impaired cognition, low albumin level, history of falls, low hematocrit level, any functional dependency, and a high burden of comorbidities were closely related to 6 months' mortality and postdischarge institutionalization in patients undergoing major thoracic and abdominal operations (Robinson et al. 2009). In the Preoperative Assessment of Cancer in the Elderly (PACE) study, functional dependency, fatigue, and abnormal performance status were associated with a 50 % increase in the relative risk of postoperative complications (Audisio et al. 2008). In patients >65 years of age, lower Mini-mental State Examination score and older age were significantly associated with the development of post-cystectomy delirium, and those who developed delirium were more likely to face readmission and reoperation (Large et al. 2013). In patients undergoing pancreaticoduodenectomy, older age and worse scores *in geriatric assessment* predicted major complications, longer hospital stays, and surgical ICU admissions (Dale et al. 2014).

A validated and brief preoperative evaluation tool that recognizes the unique physiologic vulnerabilities of the geriatric population and accurately predicts outcomes is greatly needed. The Memorial Sloan Kettering Cancer Center (MSKCC) Geriatric Service has incorporated selected elements of the geriatric assessment into its daily clinical practice (Annals of Surgery, accepted for publication). Preoperative assessments are performed by a team that includes a nurse, pharmacist, and geriatrician. Patients are referred to a nutritionist, physical therapist, social worker, and other medical disciplines if needed. The patients have the chance to discuss age-specific concerns and potential geriatric syndromes which may complicate postoperative outcomes.

13.3   Models of Care with Multidisciplinary Teams

Cancer care is undergoing a shift from a disease-focused management to a patient-centered approach in which increasingly more attention is paid to psychosocial aspects, quality of life, patients' rights and empowerment, and survivorship (Borras et al. 2014). Multidisciplinary care is essential to provide for the needs of patients with multiple comorbidities as well as unique social and emotional issues. Support for caregivers of older adults with cancer is also necessary. There is evidence that multidisciplinary care has the potential to significantly increase survival (Junor et al. 1994). The decision-making process by a care team is able to greatly reduce the wide variations in decisions made by professionals acting independently by ensuring that the decisions are consistent with available evidence. In a US study, the initial treatment recommendation for women with breast cancer was changed following a second opinion of a multidisciplinary panel in 43 % of the cases (Chang et al. 2001).

In geriatric oncology, integrated care comprises two broad categories: coordinated health-care delivery and community primary care with support services (Tremblay et al. 2012). *Coordinated health-care delivery* refers to the patterns of interaction between health-care professionals within a multidisciplinary team in order to successfully meet the needs of patients and ensure that health and social services are delivered in tandem and according to a patient's specific needs. Multidisciplinary teamwork is considered the core mechanism to improve both collaboration and care coordination. *Community primary care with support services* includes but is not limited to care delivery through the primary care physician (PCP). Access to social services, mental health services, transportation, and home care services helps limit unnecessary patient hospitalizations.

Teamwork ensures patient-centered care and patients' active role in their own care plan. Delivering an integrated cancer care system requires developing efficient networks between hospitals, primary health-care facilities, human and social services, and the communities. Attention often is focused mainly on the relationship between oncologists and geriatricians and less so on other professionals. This reinforces professional silos and reflects a lack of recognition and understanding of the key positions played by some professionals in accompanying patients on their cancer care pathway (Tremblay et al. 2012). The three most frequently reported needs faced by older adult patients at a cancer center in Pennsylvania during a pilot project to set up a geriatric oncology program were emotional support, caregiver support, and transportation issues (Lynch et al. 2007).

Optimal decision-making in the diagnosis, treatment, and support of cancer patients is being increasingly associated with multidisciplinary teams. Specialized geriatric oncology clinics with multidisciplinary teams, geriatric assessment tools, and other elements tailored to the needs of the older cancer patient have been established in many US cancer centers (McNeil and Caroline 2013). However, the organization and roles they play within their parent institution vary widely. Cancer centers are still exploring several formats. Some serve as the patients' primary base, offering assessment, treatment, and supportive services. Others offer comprehensive care after assessment by the center's geriatric division. Yet others focus primarily on assessment, a critical first step in all geriatric oncology programs, after which they return to their PCP or oncologist for therapy. Some cancer centers offer multidisciplinary clinics where cancer patients can see specialists from various disciplines in one location. Others bring different specialists together to discuss patients' care in a multidisciplinary team meeting. The degree of organization and the type of communication in these meetings have a direct impact on the quality of patient care.

The primary goal of such meetings is to improve the care management for individual patients. One multidisciplinary discussion with all involved specialties is more effective, and the joint decision more accurate than the sum of all individual opinions (Ruhstaller et al. 2006). The team should in general comprise a surgeon, radiotherapist, medical oncologist, and the PCP/geriatrician along with the clinical trial coordinator, a member of the palliative care team, and a specialist nurse. It may include a GNP, primary care nurse, pharmacist, dietician, and social worker depending on the setting (Lynch et al. 2007). The team meeting should maintain an environment that allows all ideas about the patient to be openly discussed. Such a setting is also an ideal learning opportunity for junior doctors and other professionals (Ruhstaller et al. 2006).

13.4 Shared Care Between Specialty Care and Primary Care

The role of the PCP in cancer care has mostly been focused on cancer prevention and screening. Typically they have had the task of identifying and referring patients to specialists in a timely manner, but have stayed on the periphery of cancer care until patients reach the palliative stage. Older patients are likely to have multiple chronic medical conditions and long-term relationships with their PCPs, often see multiple specialists, and take multiple medications. The importance of fluid, accurate, and timely communication among all involved should be top priority in order to avoid fragmentation of care and unintended complications. In addition, the role of the PCP in addressing aging-related issues when caring for older adults in long-term survivorship has not been comprehensively described, and effective collaboration models have not been established.

Shared care across the primary-specialty interface has been defined as the joint participation of PCPs and specialty care physicians in the planned delivery of care, informed by an enhanced information exchange in addition to routine discharge and referral notices (Smith et al. 2007). Within shared care, geriatric oncologists, medical oncologists, PCPs, and other members of the team can bring their own expertise to provide seamless patient-centered care. Shared care is thought to be most important at transition points (e.g., initial diagnosis and staging, recurrence, initiation of and completion of active cancer treatments). It is also important in advanced cancer, as goals shift from more active to palliative treatments and end-of-life care. Communication and coordination could result in improved quality of care in symptom management, decision-making, addressing family burden, and bereavement (Rose et al. 2009).

Existing literature supports the benefit of shared care in the management of chronic diseases such as diabetes mellitus (Smith et al. 2004) and heart failure (McAlister et al. 2004). Cancer has taken on the characteristics of these chronic illnesses with an increasing number of patients with prolonged periods of survival after cancer diagnosis and many dying with their illnesses rather than of it. The PCP is well placed to take on a leading role in improving services for people living with cancer, providing follow-up that addresses patient priorities, and developing more personalized care for cancer survivors. This involves setting up individualized survivorship care plans for the patients (Weller 2008). Dr. Harvey Cohen developed a model for shared care of elderly patients with cancer (Cohen 2009). It proposes a sharing of the patient's care between the oncologist and the PCP. The oncologist takes on a greater role during the initial treatment phase and subsequently if relapses occur. The PCP assumes a greater role during remissions and in survivorship. Throughout the process, palliative care should be part of the team. There may arise more need for palliative care expertise if, at some point, a decision is reached to discontinue cancer-specific treatment and to concentrate on symptom management and comfort. A study of elderly breast cancer survivors revealed that those who continued to see their oncologists were more likely to receive appropriate follow-up mammography for their cancer but those who were monitored by PCPs were more likely to receive all other non-cancer-related preventive services such as influenza vaccine, lipid testing, bone densitometry, and colon and cervical screening. Those who saw both types of practitioners received more of both types of services (Earle 2003).

There are limited data on the feasibility and cost-effectiveness of shared care in oncology and associated improved outcomes. There are several potential barriers to shared care on each side of the primary-oncology interface. Some of these barriers are a lack of certainty over roles and responsibilities, a paucity of formal training in oncology for PCPs that may result in a reluctance to participate actively in the care of oncology patients, and a lack of understanding of the culture of primary care on the part of the oncologists (Owusu and Studenski 2009). A challenge for primary care is to recognize its unrealized potential for promoting survivorship and to develop new models of care that allow it to do so. The general concept here is that care of older patients with cancer may be shared across disciplines over the entire temporal course of the disease, with differing levels of involvement of the particular discipline, depending upon the patient and disease status at any given time. With a transdisciplinary approach, the burden of dealing with the complexities of care for the older cancer patient can thus be eased for the patient, the family, and the professional care provider (Cohen 2009).

13.5 Summary

The care of older adults with cancer is complex. A transdisciplinary approach by a team with the knowledge of the principles of geriatrics is essential to provide seamless patient-centered care. Geriatric assessment is an important tool to identify geriatric syndromes, helping the oncologist and the patient with a holistic view of what to expect in going through cancer treatment. How to provide optimum comprehensive care for older adults with cancer is still being explored. There are multiple models of multidisciplinary and shared care that need further evaluation. However, it is clear that multidisciplinary and/or shared care is essential to provide for the needs of these patients with multiple comorbidities as well as unique social and emotional issues.

References

Audisio RA, Pope D et al (2008) Shall we operate? Preoperative assessment in elderly cancer patients (PACE) can help. A SIOG surgical task force prospective study. Crit Rev Oncol Hematol 65(2):156–163

Borras JM, Albreht T et al (2014) Policy statement on multidisciplinary cancer care. Eur J Cancer 50(3):475–480

Bouchardy C, Rapiti E et al (2007) Older female cancer patients: importance, causes, and consequences of undertreatment. J Clin Oncol 25(14):1858–1869

Boult C, Green AF et al (2009) Successful models of comprehensive care for older adults with chronic conditions: evidence for the Institute of Medicine's "retooling for an aging America" report. J Am Geriatr Soc 57(12):2328–2337

Bowel cancer mortality statistics (2014) From http://www.cancerresearchuk.org/cancer-info/cancerstats/types/bowel/mortality/uk-bowel-cancer-mortality-statistics

Chang JH, Vines E et al (2001) The impact of a multidisciplinary breast cancer center on recommendations for patient management: the University of Pennsylvania experience. Cancer 91(7):1231–1237

Cohen HJ (2009) A model for the shared care of elderly patients with cancer. J Am Geriatr Soc 57(Suppl 2):S300–S302

Copeland GP, Jones D et al (1991) POSSUM: a scoring system for surgical audit. Br J Surg 78(3):355–360

Dale W, Hemmerich J et al (2014) Geriatric assessment improves prediction of surgical outcomes in older adults undergoing pancreaticoduodenectomy: a prospective cohort study. Ann Surg 259(5):960–965

Earle CC (2003) Quality of non-breast cancer health maintenance among elderly breast cancer survivors. J Clin Oncol 21(8):1447–1451

Extermann M, Aapro M et al (2005) Use of comprehensive geriatric assessment in older cancer patients: recommendations from the task force on CGA of the International Society of Geriatric Oncology (SIOG). Crit Rev Oncol Hematol 55(3):241–252

Extermann M, Boler I et al (2012) Predicting the risk of chemotherapy toxicity in older patients: the Chemotherapy Risk Assessment Scale for High-Age Patients (CRASH) score. Cancer 118(13):3377–3386

Gross CP, Smith BD et al (2008) Racial disparities in cancer therapy: did the gap narrow between 1992 and 2002? Cancer 112(4):900–908

Hurria A, Balducci L (2009) Geriatric oncology treatment, assessment and management. Springer Science+Business Media LLC., New York

Hurria A, Lachs MS et al (2006) Geriatric assessment for oncologists: rationale and future directions. Crit Rev Oncol Hematol 59(3):211–217

Hurria A, Togawa K et al (2011) Predicting chemotherapy toxicity in older adults with cancer: a prospective multicenter study. J Clin Oncol 29(25):3457–3465

Hurria A, Naylor M et al (2013) Improving the quality of cancer care in an aging population: recommendations from an IOM report. JAMA 310(17):1795–1796

Hutchins LF, Unger JM et al (1999) Underrepresentation of patients 65 years of age or older in cancer-treatment trials. N Engl J Med 341(27):2061–2067

Junor EJ, Hole DJ et al (1994) Management of ovarian cancer: referral to a multidisciplinary team matters. Br J Cancer 70(2):363–370

Kristjansson SR, Nesbakken A et al (2010) Comprehensive geriatric assessment can predict complications in elderly patients after elective surgery for colorectal cancer: a prospective observational cohort study. Crit Rev Oncol Hematol 76(3):208–217

Large MC, Reichard C et al (2013) Incidence, risk factors, and complications of postoperative delirium in elderly patients undergoing radical cystectomy. Urology 81(1):123–128

Lynch MP, Marcone D et al (2007) Developing a multidisciplinary geriatric oncology program in a community cancer center. Clin J Oncol Nurs 11(6):929–933

Makary MA, Segev DL et al (2010) Frailty as a predictor of surgical outcomes in older patients. J Am Coll Surg 210(6):901–908

McAlister FA, Stewart S et al (2004) Multidisciplinary strategies for the management of heart failure patients at high risk for admission: a systematic review of randomized trials. J Am Coll Cardiol 44(4):810–819

McNeil C, Caroline M (2013) Geriatric oncology clinics on the rise. J Natl Cancer Inst 105(9):585

Oken MM, Creech RH et al (1982) Toxicity and response criteria of the Eastern Cooperative Oncology Group. Am J Clin Oncol 5(6):649–655

Owusu C, Studenski SA (2009) Shared care in geriatric oncology: primary care providers' and medical/oncologist's perspectives. J Am Geriatr Soc 57(Suppl 2):S239–S242

Perry DP (2010) Introduction to aging, cancer, and age-related diseases. Ann N Y Acad Sci 1197: vii–x

Puts MT, Hardt J et al (2012) Use of geriatric assessment for older adults in the oncology setting: a systematic review. J Natl Cancer Inst 104(15):1133–1163

Reuben DB, Frank JC et al (1999) A randomized clinical trial of outpatient comprehensive geriatric assessment coupled with an intervention to increase adherence to recommendations. J Am Geriatr Soc 47(3):269–276

Robinson TN, Eiseman B et al (2009) Redefining geriatric preoperative assessment using frailty, disability and co-morbidity. Ann Surg 250(3):449–455

Rose JH, O'Toole EE et al (2009) Geriatric oncology and primary care: promoting partnerships in practice and research. J Am Geriatr Soc 57(Suppl 2):S235–S238

Ruhstaller T, Roe H et al (2006) The multidisciplinary meeting: an indispensable aid to communication between different specialities. Eur J Cancer 42(15):2459–2462

Satterfield JM, Spring B et al (2009) Toward a transdisciplinary model of evidence-based practice. Milbank Q 87(2):368–390

Smith S, Bury G et al (2004) The North Dublin randomized controlled trial of structured diabetes shared care. Fam Pract 21(1):39–45

Smith SM, Allwright S et al (2007) Effectiveness of shared care across the interface between primary and specialty care in chronic disease management. Cochrane Database Syst Rev (3): CD004910

Smith BD, Smith GL et al (2009) Future of cancer incidence in the United States: burdens upon an aging, changing nation. J Clin Oncol 27(17):2758–2765

Tinetti ME, Bogardus ST Jr et al (2004) Potential pitfalls of disease-specific guidelines for patients with multiple conditions. N Engl J Med 351(27):2870–2874

Tremblay D, Charlebois K et al (2012) Integrated oncogeriatric approach: a systematic review of the literature using concept analysis. BMJ Open 2(6)

Weller DP (2008) Cancer care: what role for the general practitioner? Med J Aust 189(2):59–60

Yates JW, Chalmer B et al (1980) Evaluation of patients with advanced cancer using the Karnofsky performance status. Cancer 45(8):2220–2224

Metastatic Colon and Rectal Cancer: Role of Multidisciplinary Team-Based Management

14

Dedrick Kok-Hong Chan, Tian-Zhi Lim, and Ker-Kan Tan

Take-Home Pearls

- A significant proportion of patients with colorectal cancers present with metastatic disease on diagnosis.
- Clinical, biochemical and radiological tools are utilised to stratify these patients.
- The aim of management for patients with metastatic colon and rectal cancer can range from curative, delay disease progression to palliative measures.
- A multidisciplinary consultative approach is often required to manage these patients with unique situations.

14.1 Introduction

Colorectal cancer is now the number 1 cancer in Singapore and its incidence continues to increase worldwide (GLOBOCAN 2012; Ministry of Health, Health Promotion Board, National Registry of Disease Office 2013). Unfortunately, in spite of widespread availability of healthcare resources and public awareness about the pathology, about 20 % of patients still presents with distant metastasis upon diagnosis of the primary pathology (Siegel et al. 2014).

The three most common sites of distant metastasis excluding lymph node include the liver, lung and peritoneum (Cirocchi et al. 2012; American Cancer Society 2014). Unlike the past, the diagnosis of metastasis may no longer imply incurability (Anwar et al. 2011). The advent of newer and more targeted chemotherapeutic

---

D.K.-H. Chan • T.-Z. Lim • K.-K. Tan (✉)
Division of Colorectal Surgery, Department of Surgery,
National University Health System, University Surgical Cluster,
Singapore, Singapore
e-mail: kerkan@gmail.com

© Springer-Verlag Berlin Heidelberg 2015
K.-Y. Tan (ed.), *Transdisciplinary Perioperative Care in Colorectal Surgery:*
An Integrative Approach, DOI 10.1007/978-3-662-44020-9_14

agents coupled with appropriate surgical interventions to remove the metastasis has brought about a change in the paradigm in these patients with stage IV cancers. However, there remain a sizeable proportion of patients with incurable and extensive metastasis upon diagnosis, whereby chemotherapy and palliative measures are vital to benefit these patients (Damjanov et al. 2009).

The extent of metastases, the presence or possibility of a surgical emergency, the fitness and psychological health of the patients are huge variables that preclude the formation of a set template in the management of these patients. Instead a multidisciplinary team-based approach is strongly advocated in the management of patients with metastatic colon and rectal cancer.

14.2 Presentation

Patients with metastatic colon and rectal cancer can either be diagnosed electively or as a surgical emergency when the patient presents with bowel perforation, obstruction or significant bleeding. These crises can arise from the primary pathology or secondary to the complications of the metastases.

The roles of the radiologists and pathologists are often understated in the management of patients with colorectal cancers. In the American Joint Committee on Cancer (AJCC) 7th edition guidelines, metastatic colorectal cancers can be further subdivided into M1a or M1b (Edge et al. 2010). M1a denotes distant metastasis being confined to 1 organ system while M1b indicates the presence of metastatic deposits in more than 1 site or involvement of the peritoneum. It is hence important to obtain radiological and/or histological confirmations of the extent of metastatic disease.

In the field of radiology, non-invasive scans such as computed tomographic (CT) scan, magnetic resonance imaging (MRI) or a positron emission tomography/computed tomography (PET/CT) are increasingly more widely available for surgeons to evaluate pathologies. A CT scan of the abdomen and pelvis and sometimes the thorax is typically performed to stage the disease when colorectal cancer is first diagnosed (Fig. 14.1). Apart from confirming the location of the primary pathology, the presence of metastatic disease can also be determined. At the same time, these scans are also helpful in monitoring the response to treatment and the detection of tumour recurrences (Vogel et al. 2005).

CT and MRI scans conventionally delineate the anatomical features of a tumour (i.e. shape, size and density). The introduction of PET/CT scans permits for the analysis of not just morphological features but takes into account the metabolic function of the lesion as well (Fig. 14.2). In such circumstances, the use of a radiotracer (i.e. ^{18}F-fluorodeoxyglucose) in a PET/CT scan further enhances the resolution of pathological lesions. The specific indications of radiological scans would be further illustrated in the following subsections.

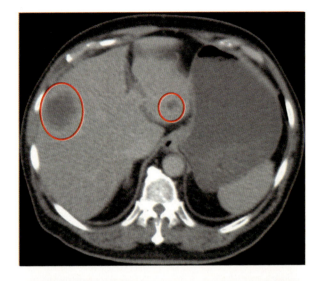

Fig. 14.1 Liver metastasis on CT scan. The *circle* represents the location of liver metastases as seen on CT scan

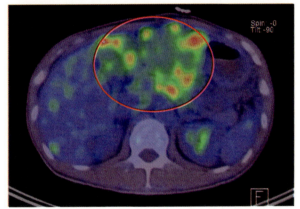

Fig. 14.2 Liver metastasis on PET/CT scan. The *circled* region indicates the location of liver metastases as seen on PET/CT scan

14.3 Primary Colon and Rectal Cancer

Upon diagnosis of stage IV colorectal cancer, it is important to determine if the metastatic disease is potentially resectable or definitely non-resectable. If the metastatic disease is potentially resectable, then a curative resection can be considered if the primary pathology can be removed as well (Anwar et al. 2011).

In these patients, it is imperative to discuss amongst surgical, medical and radiation oncologists whether upfront surgery to remove all apparent disease or to adopt a chemotherapy +/− radiotherapy first approach before re-evaluating the suitability for surgery is preferred.

In patients with unresectable disease, chemotherapy has always been deemed the mainstay of treatment except in emergency situations (Kaufman et al. 2007). However, there remain proponents of surgical resection of the primary pathology (Bacon and Martin 1964; Lockhart-Mummery 1959; Cady et al. 1970; Cook et al. 2005). There appears to be evidence supporting a higher median survival and also reduced future complications from the primary malignancy in the group that underwent surgery for the primary pathology. But a recent Cochrane review (Cirocchi et al. 2012) has established that there is insufficient evidence to advocate surgical resection for asymptomatic patients with stage IV colorectal cancer and the surgery itself does not lead to a reduction in the risk of future complications from occurring.

In addition, surgery itself is not without its own set of perioperative complications (Clements et al. 2009). And the majority of these studies are largely retrospective in nature and lend itself to enormous amount of selection bias. It would not be surprising if the group of patients who underwent surgery for the primary pathology was generally fitter, has lower metastatic load and the primary cancer is easily resected without much morbidity.

14.4 Dealing with Crisis

However, if a patient with metastatic colorectal cancer presents acutely with bowel perforation, obstruction or severe bleeding, these situations may warrant urgent interventions to the primary pathology regardless of the presence or extent of metastatic disease. When the crisis is resolved, the management principles of such patients would be similar to those who present electively.

14.4.1 Perforation

The rate of perforation of colorectal cancer is reported to be around 5–10 % (Ronnekleiv-Kelly and Kennedy 2011). Perforation is itself an indicator of poor prognosis as it is associated with postoperative morbidity and mortality and shorter disease-free survival (RodriGuez-Gonzalez et al. 2013). Perforation can arise from the primary tumour itself or a complication of colonic obstruction.

Conservative measures are often unsuccessful and these patients often require exploratory laparotomy to identify the site of perforation. If technically feasible and the patient fit, a resection of the perforation and the primary pathology should be performed. Otherwise, a proximal stoma to divert the faecal stream can be adopted if the patient is unfit or the tumour is too locally advanced to be operated in the emergency setting. There is also the role of comfort measures in a select group of patients after accounting for their premorbid conditions, fitness for surgery and the extent of metastatic disease.

14.4.2 Obstruction

Large bowel obstruction occurs in 10–30 % of patients with symptomatic metastatic colon and rectal cancer (Clements et al. 2009). These patients often exhibit clinical

Fig. 14.3 Transverse view of an obstructing lesion in descending colon causing intestinal obstruction. The *circled* region shows the location of the obstructing colon lesion

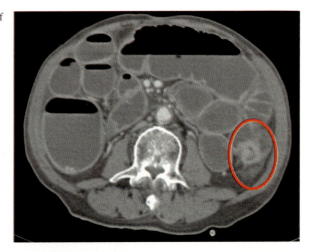

Fig. 14.4 Coronal view of the same obstructing lesion in the descending colon. The *circled* region shows the corresponding lesion as that seen in Fig. 14.3 but on coronal view

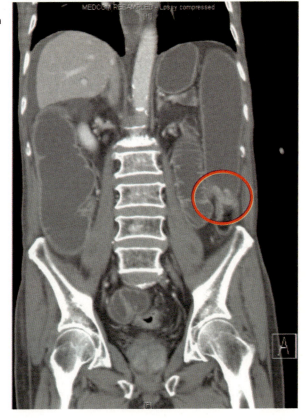

symptoms such as abdominal pain, distension, constipation and vomiting. Radiological findings of proximal bowel dilatation (Figs. 14.3 and 14.4) are commonly seen as the primary pathology is often located in the left colon or rectum (Ruo et al. 2003). Classically, surgical resection of the obstructed segment has been emphasised and the National Comprehensive Cancer Network (NCCN) guidelines

Fig. 14.5 Deployment of an endoscopic colonic stent

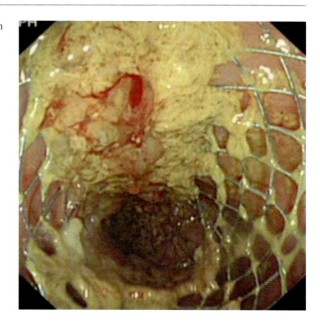

Fig. 14.6 A plain X-ray of the pelvis to confirm position of the stent following endoscopic stenting. The *circled* region shows the location of the stent

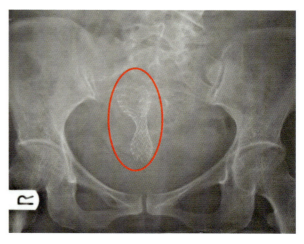

also recommend surgery for patients with metastatic colon and rectal cancer presenting with obstruction. But since the 1980s, Dohmoto has proposed using endoscopic colonic stenting to bypass the obstruction in selected cases (Figs. 14.5 and 14.6) (Dohmoto 1991).

For right-sided lesions, surgical resection with primary anastomosis is still recommended (Baron 2010). Stenting is not recommended as it is technically more challenging and is associated with higher rates of perforation (Baron 2010). Reasons postulated include the longer length of colonoscope inserted into the colon to reach the right-sided pathology which then renders the manipulation of the colonoscope harder. And the further build-up of pressure from the insufflation during the colonoscopy in the presence of a competent ileocaecal valve would only further increase the risk of caecal perforation.

14 Multidisciplinary Management in Metastatic Cancer

Table 14.1 Modalities used for endoscopic treatment of tumour bleeding (Strate and Naumann 2010)

Injection	Mechanical	Thermal
Epinephrine	Clips	Electrocautery: monopolar, bipolar
Ethanol	Detachable loop ligators	Heater probe
Fibrin	Band ligators	Argon plasma coagulation
N-butyl-2-cyanoacrylate		Laser photocoagulation
		Radiofrequency ablation

In left-side-obstructing colorectal cancers, endoscopic stenting has been increasing advocated in recent years. Some of its advantages include the ability to relieve the obstruction, decompress the proximal colon and enables earlier commencement of chemotherapy (Poultsides et al. 2009). Patients also enjoy a shorter hospital stay and reduction in the rates of stoma creation (Vemulapalli et al. 2010). Although reports demonstrated no change in the median survival (McCullough and Engledow 2010), endoscopic colonic stenting is associated with fewer complications when compared to those who underwent upfront surgery (McCullough and Engledow 2010).

As more than 90 % of stents inserted remained patent for more than 6 months following placement (Camúñez et al. 2000), it is a promising option as patients who undergo non-resectional bypass procedures only have a median survival of approximately 7 months (Anwar et al. 2011). However, the availability of the technical capability and resources to perform endoscopic stenting are the major limitations. Another more dire complication is the possibility of perforating the segment of tumour during the procedure which then mandates emergency surgery.

14.4.3 Bleeding

Considerable bleeding from the colorectal cancers often presents with haematochezia with signs and symptoms of anaemia. Blood transfusion to minimise the impact of anaemia is the first step in the management of these patients.

In the presence of metastatic disease, it is imperative to consider the haematological complications of chemotherapeutic agents and also the possibility of further bleeding during the treatment. In the presence of acute emergencies where the patients are bleeding massively, a CT angiography can be performed to localise the bleeding followed by invasive mesenteric embolisation to cease the bleeding temporarily (Martí et al. 2012; Chang et al. 2011; Strate and Naumann 2010). This enables ongoing resuscitation and more definitive plans to address the primary pathology.

While numerous modalities have been described as means to stop the bleeding (Table 14.1), these are often temporary. The mainstays of treatment remain surgical resection and radiotherapy to the malignancy.

14.5 The "Asymptomatic" One

In the majority of patients with metastatic colon and rectal cancer that does not present as a surgical emergency, chemotherapy is key to prolong the overall survival in these patients. As these patients often die from systemic disease due to the massive tumour burden, the aim of treatment should be aimed towards achieving stable disease and to delay tumour progression rather than to primarily induce tumour response. Thus, significant delay in the commencement of chemotherapy could be detrimental (Michel et al. 2004; Muratore et al. 2007; Sarela et al. 2001; Scoggins et al. 1999).

Chemotherapy has not been shown to increase the incidence of complications such as bleeding, perforation or obstruction. These complications following chemotherapy are reported to only occur in less than 10 % of the patients (Nitzkorski et al. 2012). But if the patients are deemed likely to develop any crisis during chemotherapy, surgical resection or other treatment modalities to address these potential crises should be considered so as to allow uninterrupted systemic chemotherapy (Michel et al. 2004; Muratore et al. 2007; Sarela et al. 2001; Scoggins et al. 1999).

Since the 1970s, chemotherapeutic options for colon and rectal cancer are based on 5-flurouracil (5-FU) and leucovorin given as an infusion. Reports of median survival ranged between 10 and 12 months (Glimelius and Cavalli-Bjorkman 2012). Ten years on, the introduction of "doublets", 5-FU/leucovorin plus either irinotecan (FOLFIRI) or oxaliplatin (FOLFOX) extends survival by a further 4 months. However, the FOLFIRI and FOLFOX regimes are associated with complications such as diarrhoea and neurotoxicities, respectively. But unlike the other chemotherapeutic agents, the occurrences of haematological toxicities are relatively uncommon (Fornaro et al. 2010). The onset of neurotoxicity has been the focus for many with the use of oxaliplatin-based chemotherapeutic agents. It was reported in the OPTIMOX trial that the "stop-and-go" approach to administering FOLFOX whereby high dose of FOLFOX was given before maintenance infusion of 5-FU/leucovorin was started and FOLFOX reintroduced when disease progressed reduced occurrence of such toxicities (Tournigand et al. 2006).

Since the mid-1990s, the introduction of the oral chemotherapeutic agent capecitabine (fluoropyrimidine) radically changed the treatment of colon and rectal cancer. Its presence made chemotherapy more convenient and pushed survival towards 18–20 months. Combination "doublets" of capecitabine and irinotecan (CAPIRI) or oxaliplatin (XELOX) were noted to be non-inferior to FOLFIRI and FOLFOX, except in CAPIRI where the severe gastrointestinal toxicities experienced prematurely suspended the trial (Kohne et al. 2008). The triplet form, capecitabine/irinotecan/oxaliplatin (XELOXIRI), also resulted in grade 3–4 diarrhoea. The use of 5-FU/leucovorin plus irinotecan and oxaliplatin (FOLFOXIRI) has resulted in higher radical resection of metastasis and increase in overall survival (Masi et al. 2008). FOLFOXIRI increasingly has become the choice drug in palliative chemotherapy.

The introduction of targeted chemotherapy provided an additional avenue to push survival past the 24-month mark. Tissue samples from the primary tumour and its metastatic site can be obtained via aspiration cytology or tissue block histology. Specific genetic testing (i.e. K-ras mutation) is done routinely on these tissue samples to detect if the drug can bring about specific desired response such as tumour apoptosis. Such targeted therapies seem to be breakthroughs, but we await longer-term data to demonstrate its true efficacy.

14.5.1 Anti-vascular Endothelial Growth Factor (Anti-VEGF)

14.5.1.1 Bevacizumab
Studies show that the addition of Bevacizumab to chemotherapeutic agents allows for longer overall survival (Hurwitz et al. 2004). In the BOND-2 trial (Saltz et al. 2007), longer survival was noted when bevacizumab was added to irinotecan and cetuximab. However, the use of this targeted agent is not without its perils. The high cost involved and occurrence of hypertension question the cost-effectiveness of bevacizumab.

14.5.2 Anti-epidermal Growth Factor Receptor (Anti-EGFR)

14.5.2.1 Cetuximab
The BOND-1 trial (Cunningham et al. 2004) highlighted the use of cetuximab in patients who are resistant to irinotecan-based chemotherapeutic agents. The addition of cetuximab showed that it was possible to overcome this resistance and this therapy was associated with significantly longer progression-free survival. Further analysis with this new antitumour effect showed that having a K-RAS mutation actually hindered the effects of the drug (Van Cutsem et al. 2007; Karapetis et al. 2008). Cetuximab is now used as first line with irinotecan-based agents (Van Cutsem et al. 2009, 2011).

14.5.2.2 Panitumumab
Panitumumab is a fully human monoclonal antibody which is believed to elicit fewer drug-related allergic reactions. We are currently waiting for the results of the ASPECCT trial to determine which is more superior, cetuximab or panitumumab. Through the use of FOLFOX, the addition of panitumumab has also shown to increase progression-free survival.

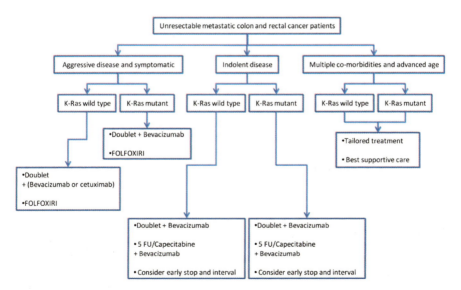

Flowchart 14.1 First-line treatment option for different unresectable metastatic colon and rectal cancer patients based on clinical and molecular factors (Ruo et al. 2003)

14.6 Management of Organ-Specific Metastasis

14.6.1 Hepatic Metastases

The liver is the most common site of colorectal cancer metastases. Unfortunately, less than 25 % of these metastases are potentially resectable upon presentation (Scheele et al. 1995; Bismuth et al. 1996). The 5-year survival amongst patients who have resectable disease is expectedly far better than those who do not. The patients with resectable disease have a median 5-year overall survival of 40–58 % following hepatic resection (Fong et al. 1999; Scheele et al. 1990).

In the modern era, treatments of hepatic colorectal metastases have evolved and include biologic agents, regional hepatic ablative technology and trans-arterial modalities (Saied et al. 2013). These advances have changed the approach in the management of hepatic metastases, such that previously deemed unresectable tumours could become resectable. The ongoing aim is to reduce the number of unresectable lesions and thereby increase the overall survival amongst patients with liver metastases.

14.6.1.1 Detection of Liver Metastases

The importance of obtaining preoperative imaging cannot be understated. Not only is it performed to ascertain the volume, number and location of the metastatic deposits, it is also important to determine the amount of remnant functional liver following liver surgery (Frankel and D'Angelica 2014). There is, however, no one best diagnostic modality to achieve this currently, and the modality adopted is often dependent on facilities and expertise available at individual institution.

The most routinely used imaging modality is the CT scan. This utilises varying contrast enhancement in the arterial and portal venous phases to detect the hepatic lesions. Colorectal cancer metastases to the liver are hypodense compared to the surrounding tissue during the portal venous phase. They also demonstrate rim enhancement which washes out in the delayed phase (Sahani et al. 2004). The disadvantage of the CT is that subcentimetre lesions cannot be accurately characterised.

MRI is another modality that can be used to identify and characterise any hepatic lesions (Braga et al. 2004; Patel et al. 2010). On the MRI scans, colorectal liver metastases appear hypointense on T1 images and hyperintense on T2 and diffusion-weighted series (Frankel and D'Angelica 2014). MRI appears to be superior in the detection of colorectal liver metastases compared to CT. One study showed the sensitivity and specificity of MRI to be 81.1 and 97.2 %, compared to 74.8 and 95.6 %, respectively, in CT scans (Floriani et al. 2010). Another study also demonstrated that MRI had a higher sensitivity than CT in detecting subcentimetre lesions (Niekel et al. 2010). However, MRI does require a significant amount of patient compliance, as the patient needs to be able to tolerate lying still in a closed, confined and noisy environment for an extended period of time.

PET/CT scans have been found to be highly sensitive in the detection of hepatic metastases. It also confers the advantage of also detecting metabolically active metastatic lesions outside the liver. This is especially important in patients who are being considered for hepatic resection for metastases as it would reduce nontherapeutic laparotomy rates considerably. Limited availability and high cost remain its biggest limitations (Frankel and D'Angelica 2014).

14.6.1.2 Role of Hepatic Metastasectomy

Liver resection is a major surgical procedure, and appropriate preoperative considerations must be made prior to surgery. The patient needs to be relatively fit to undergo hepatic resection apart from the resection of the primary. Both hepatic and colonic resection can be performed simultaneously in the same setting, or a liver-first or colon-first approach can also be adopted. When a hepatic resection is considered, apart from the absence of extrahepatic unresectable metastatic deposits, adequate remnant liver function must also be ensured to prevent postoperative liver failure. This is typically achieved through assessment of indocyanine green excretion levels while incorporating serum laboratory values and aggregate scores such as the Model for End-Stage Liver Disease (MELD) score (Schroeder et al. 2006; Uesaka et al. 1996; Imamura et al. 2005). Certain radiological findings are also instrumental to determine the feasibility of liver resection.

The consensus statement on the oncologic and technical criteria for resectability offers guidelines concerning which patients are amenable to resection (Adams et al. 2013). These criteria are summarised in Tables 14.2 and 14.3, which are adapted from the consensus statement article.

In addition, Fong et al. have identified a number of factors that could predict for poorer overall survival following hepatic resection for colorectal metastatic deposits. These include a positive hepatic resection margin, presence of

Table 14.2 Oncologic criteria for resection

Oncologic criteria for resectability
1. Pretreatment radiological staging is required to assess for metastatic disease
2. If patients have extrahepatic disease, these should be amenable to surgical resection before hepatic metastases resection is considered
3. Patients should be able to have disease manageable by adjuvant therapies and should be expected to achieve long-term disease control
4. Patients on preoperative chemotherapy who are not able to achieve control of metastatic disease should have surgical resection deferred

Table 14.3 Technical criteria for resection

Technical criteria for resectability
1. A margin negative resection must be achievable
2. Two contiguous segments of the liver must be preserved
3. Adequate vascular inflow, outflow and biliary drainage must be achieved
4. Post-resection liver volume should be at least 20 % in normal liver and 30 % in pretreated liver with chemotherapy
5. Liver function post-resection must be preserved

extrahepatic disease, number and size of tumours, high preoperative CEA, lymph node-positive primary and short disease-free interval (Fong et al. 1999). Patients with a poor score were found to have a median survival of only 22 months compared to 74 months in better-scoring individuals.

14.6.1.3 Surgical Points

The goal of surgical therapy is to achieve negative resection margins. While formal hepatic resections such as hemihepatectomies or tri-sectionectomies were previously performed, newer studies have suggested that limited nonanatomical hepatic resection can achieve similar oncological benefits while preserving maximal hepatic volume and function as long as negative margins are attained (Zorzi et al. 2006; Gold et al. 2008; Kokudo et al. 2001).

14.6.1.4 Regional Hepatic Therapies

Apart from surgery, regional hepatic therapies can also be considered in patients who have initially unresectable disease. These treatment modalities can broadly be classified into either ablative, arterial or non-arterial modalities (Saied et al. 2013).

Ablative methods, such as radiofrequency ablation (RFA) which is already commonly used in primary hepatic tumours, achieve tumour necrosis by inciting high temperatures. RFA is suitable for lesions up to about 5 cm, owing to the size of current probes. RFA for hepatic metastatic lesions has been associated with a recurrence rate of about 9–20 % (Gillams and Lees 2000; De Baere et al. 2000). RFA in combination with systemic chemotherapy has also been proven in the EORTC 40004 randomised controlled trial to have superior progression-free survival rates at 3 years of 27.6 % compared to 10 % in the systemic chemotherapy-only group (Ruers et al. 2012).

Radiation-based therapies can be administered intra-arterial or extra-arterial. Intra-arterial strategies include the use of yttrium 90. This agent is administered into the hepatic artery and emits beta rays. Pre-therapy planning is critical. The presence of hepatopulmonary shunting and reflux into the gastrointestinal arcades needs to be excluded as the yttrium 90 which enters these circulations can have severe consequences (Saied et al. 2013). Yttrium 90 has been associated with longer median survival rates of 70, 46 and 46 % at 6, 12 and 18 months, respectively (Stubbs and Wickremesekera 2004).

Non-arterial therapy is an evolving treatment modality which has recently entered the treatment armamentarium. A phase II trial using intensity-modulated radiation therapy with image-guided radiation therapy has been attempted. The trial reported a local tumour control at 1 year of 54 % and progression-free survival and overall survival of 14 and 78 %, respectively (Engels et al. 2012).

14.6.1.5 Outcomes

The resection of colon and rectal metastases to the liver can offer considerable hope of a chance of cure to the patient. With adequate patient selection, 5-year survival rates have approached 50 %, and 10-year survival rates ranging from 20 to 30 % have been reported (Wei et al. 2006; Giuliante et al. 2009). As mentioned

Table 14.4 Criteria as described by Alexander and Haight (Alexander and Haight 1947)

Criteria for surgical intervention in pulmonary metastases
1. Control of primary tumour
2. Absence of other metastatic sites
3. Sufficient pulmonary reserve

above, the advent of increasing regional and systemic therapies has added to the arsenal of treatment modalities used in tackling even non-resectable disease. A multidisciplinary approach involving hepatobiliary and colorectal surgeons, medical and radiation oncologists, radiologists and pathologists must be adopted to achieve the best possible outcomes.

14.6.2 Pulmonary Metastases

14.6.2.1 Introduction

Between 10 and 30 % of patients diagnosed with colorectal cancer have pulmonary metastases on presentation (Jemal et al. 2006; Mitry et al. 2010). The lung can be the only site of distant spread in 2–10 % of patients.

The surgical management of pulmonary metastasis was first proposed by Alexander and Haight in an article published in 1947 (Alexander and Haight 1947). They proposed the aggressive surgical management of pulmonary metastasectomies and laid the foundation for surgical intervention in the form of a set of criteria (Table 14.4). Since then, further refinements of these criteria have taken down but it remained remarkably similar to the original guidelines.

Encouraging outcomes following complete resection of pulmonary metastases with 5-year survival ranging from 40 to 60 % have been reported in the literature (Pfannschmidt et al. 2007).

14.6.2.2 Pathophysiology

Metastasis from colorectal cancer to the lungs occurs primarily via the vascular and lymphatic routes (Zisis et al. 2013). Cancer cells can enter via the pulmonary vasculature and disperse in alveolar capillaries. These few tumour cells which adhere to the capillary endothelium within the lungs subsequently localise to the pulmonary parenchyma where they form discrete nodules. They may then extend locally to invade the surrounding structures.

Tumour cells which reach the lungs via the lymphatic route do so through spread from regional lymph nodes towards the lymphatics of the lung. It is believed that retrograde extension proceeds from the lymphatics towards the pulmonary parenchyma. Spread to mediastinal lymph nodes via this manner is not only encountered in colon cancer but also in melanomas, breast and kidney cancers (Quiros and Scott 2008).

14.6.2.3 Detection of Pulmonary Metastases in Pulmonary Staging

The diagnosis of pulmonary metastasis can be achieved using chest X-ray (CXR), CT thorax and PET-CT thorax. CXR was evaluated as a staging modality in two

Fig. 14.7 This patient has a right thoracic lung lesion (*circled*). He was referred to the thoracic surgeon for removal of the lesion

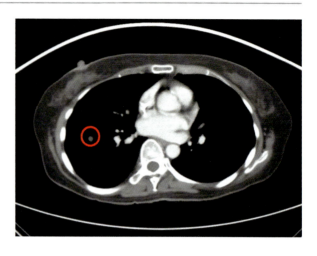

Table 14.5 Comparison of pulmonary staging modality

Author	Number of patients	Staging modality	Pulmonary lesions detected
McIntosh et al. 2005	38	CXR	4
		CT thorax/abdomen	17
Kronawitter et al. 1999	202	CXR	0
		CT thorax	71
Povoski et al. 1998	100	CXR	0
		CT thorax	14

studies (Gielen et al. 2009; Griffiths et al. 2005). These studies highlighted the low detection rate (2–4 %) of pulmonary lesions in patients with colorectal carcinoma. Even when detected, the final management of the patient did not always change. These findings led the authors to doubt the efficacy of CXR as a routine staging modality.

CT thorax (Fig. 14.7) was noted to be more sensitive in the detection of pulmonary metastases than CXR. In three studies which evaluated the use of CT thorax compared with CXR only, a greater number of patients with pulmonary lesions were detected (Table 14.5).

The greater sensitivity of CT thorax is balanced by its low specificity. A large number of lesions detected on CT thorax is defined as "clinically indeterminate lesions", with many being <10 mm in size. In fact, the incidence of CILs can approach 25 % in lung cancer screening studies even amongst a healthy population (Henschke et al. 1999). The additional functional aspect of the PET/CT thorax has also not added much to the improved characterisation of these lesions, due to the similar resolution between CTs and PET/CTs at the current technological level.

Perhaps the strongest indication for CT thorax as a surveillance modality lies in patients deemed at highest risk for pulmonary metastases. Two studies have reported the increased incidence of pulmonary metastases in rectal cancer compared with colon cancer, suggesting that patients with rectal cancer constitute a high-risk group which may benefit most from CT thorax (Grossmann et al. 2010; Tan et al. 2009).

Isolated pulmonary metastases in patients with rectal cancer constituted 10–20 % of the patients, whereas such metastases were present in only 5–6 % of colon cancer patients. It is likely that in view of the higher risk of pulmonary metastases in rectal cancer patients, they would benefit greatest from screening using such a highly sensitive mechanism.

Ultimately, in resolving these difficulties associated with the various imaging modalities, Parnaby et al. suggested that no clear guideline on the superiority of one imaging modality over another can be drawn based on current evidence and should best follow local institution guidelines in deciding the most appropriate imaging modality, taking into account current knowledge on the limitations of each (Parnaby et al. 2012).

14.6.2.4 Selection Criteria for Surgery

The sole aim of pulmonary metastasectomy is for a potentially curative operation (Pfannschmidt et al. 2007). But prior to surgery, it is important to confirm the fitness for operation in these patients. A good pulmonary function is integral before consideration for surgery (Kick et al. 2005). Spirometry, or lung function test, is an important evaluative tool, allowing for measurements of forced vital capacity (FVC), forced expiratory volume (FEV1), maximum midexpiratory flow (MMEF) and maximum voluntary ventilation (MVV) (Zisis et al. 2013).

14.6.2.5 Surgical Points

Surgical access to the pulmonary metastases is usually approached either via the lateral or posterolateral approach. The median sternotomy incision is another option which allows for good visualisation of bilateral pulmonary lesions (Zisis et al. 2013). Minimally invasive approaches such as video-assisted thoracoscopic surgery (VATS) have also been increasingly attempted to reduce postoperative pain, length of stay as well as better cosmesis (Zisis et al. 2013).

Adjuncts in surgery include the use of guidewires placed during preoperative CT thorax, marking with methylene blue, and intraoperative ultrasound (Daniel 2005). The standard procedure is the atypical open wedge resection together with lymphadenectomy of the mediastinal lymph nodes, with larger lesions requiring anatomic resections such as lobectomy (Pfannschmidt et al. 2012). The extent of surgical resection must bear in mind the possibility of further resections in case of relapse, as well as for the preservation of pulmonary function (Zisis et al. 2013).

Complications are reported in up to 10 % of patients (Roth et al. 1986). The common complications include atelectasis and pneumonia, arrhythmias and bronchopleural fistulas. Factors increasing the risk of morbidity have been found to include the patient's premorbid condition, surgical approach and the extent of resection (Vogt-Moykopf et al. 1994; Welter et al. 2007).

14.6.2.6 Outcomes

Based on current guidelines, the 5-year survival of patients who underwent pulmonary metastasectomy approaches 60 %. Even amongst patients who undergo repeated pulmonary resection of metastases, survival ranges between 30 and 50 %

Table 14.6 Prognostic factors for long-term outcome (Kanemitsu et al. 2004)

Prognostic factors
1. Primary histology
2. Hilar or mediastinal lymph node involvement
3. Number of metastases
4. Preoperative carcinoembryonic antigen level
5. Extrathoracic disease

(Kim et al. 2008; Kanemitsu et al. 2004). Kanemitsu et al. identified five prognostic factors for favourable long-term outcomes (Table 14.6).

The above results prove that when in suitable patients, resection of pulmonary metastases can have a large clinical impact on this group of patients.

14.6.3 Peritoneal Metastases

14.6.3.1 Introduction

Peritoneal metastasis is present in 5–10 % of patients at the time of diagnosis of the primary cancer (Segelman et al. 2012; Jayne et al. 2002). The detection of peritoneal carcinomatosis has traditionally been regarded as a terminal event, and commencement of palliative therapy was the norm in this group of patients. These patients often have poor overall and progression-free survivals (Franko et al. 2012). The medial survival time of patients with peritoneal carcinomatosis on a background of colorectal cancer ranges from 5 to 12 months. And this is in spite of modern chemotherapy and biologic regimes such as FOLFOX/FOLFIRI with bevacixumab (Franko et al. 2012; Verwaal et al. 2003; Sadahiro et al. 2009; Klaver et al. 2012). This might be due to the relative avascularity of peritoneal metastases and the limited penetration of systemic chemotherapeutic agents to these peritoneal metastatic deposits (Schroeder et al. 2006).

Because of the above findings and postulations, cytoreductive surgery (CRS) and hyperthermic intraperitoneal chemotherapy (HIPEC) became increasingly considered in carefully selected cases. However, the high rates of morbidity and mortality still prevent widespread adoption of this procedure outside specialised units.

14.6.3.2 Detection of Peritoneal Metastases

Imaging of the abdomen is important in identifying the presence of peritoneal metastases in the colorectal cancer patient. CT scans (Fig. 14.8) tend to underestimate the extent of peritoneal disease due to its poor accuracy at detecting lesions <5 mm in size (Koh et al. 2009; De Bree et al. 2004). The use of PET/CT has been shown to increase the detection of carcinomatosis peritonei. MRI can also be used to assess bulky mesenteric tumours and lesions involving the bladder (Pfannenberg et al. 2009; Riss et al. 2013).

In the case of carcinomatosis peritonei, the best diagnostic tool is actually diagnostic laparoscopy that is performed just prior to commencement of the intended surgical resection. This enables direct visualisation of the peritoneum. The detection of any peritoneal deposits has been shown to improve the completeness of

Fig. 14.8 This patient has left lateral wall peritoneal thickening (*circled*)

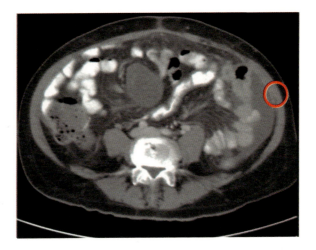

resection during eventual CRS (Iversen et al. 2013). When disease is more extensive than previously highlighted on imaging, such that it contraindicates further surgery, diagnostic laparoscopy can help to reduce the incidence of unnecessary intervention and hence is a crucial step prior to CRS and HIPEC (Riss et al. 2013).

14.6.3.3 Patient Selection

CRS and HIPEC is a procedure associated with high morbidity and mortality, and best results require careful evaluation of the patient for suitability of surgery. The performance status of the patient should be assessed to ascertain if the patient is fit enough to undergo surgery (Jacquet and Sugarbaker 1996). As with any major surgical intervention, the cardiovascular and respiratory function of the patient need to be optimised to reduce perioperative morbidity and mortality.

A number of prognostic scoring indices have been developed to assist the surgeon is selecting the patients for whom CRS and HIPEC are suitable. The most widely used prognostic indicator is the Peritoneal Carcinomatosis Index (PCI) developed by Sugarbaker (Fig. 14.9) (Carmignani et al. 2003).

The PCI requires assessment of nine areas of the abdominal cavity and four regions of the bowel. A score from 0 to 3 based on the lesion size score is accorded to each of these areas based on the size of tumour. The maximum possible PCI score is 39. The abdominal cavity may be assessed intraoperatively via a laparoscopy. Carmignani et al. reported a 1-year survival of 50 % when the PCI was 20 or less and 0 % when the score was greater than 20. Elias et al. (2010) reported 4-year survival rates of 44, 22 and 7 % when the PCI score was <6, 7–12 and >19, respectively. Generally, CRS and HIPEC are not recommended when the PCI score is greater than 20.

The Peritoneal Surface Disease and Severity Score (PSDSS) (Fig. 14.10) is another instrument which can be used to select and prognosticate patient survival following CRS and HIPEC.

The PSDSS requires the summation of arbitrary scores assigned to clinical symptomatology, PCI score and histology. The summation of these values accords

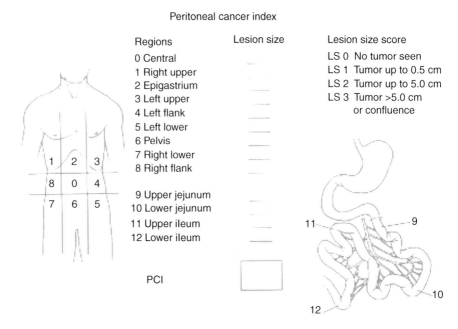

Fig. 14.9 Peritoneal cancer index (Carmignani et al. 2003)

Clinical	PCI	Histology	
No symptoms	<10	Well-differentiated Moderately differentiated/No	
	0 points	1 point	1 point
Mild symptoms	10–20	Moderately differentiated/N1 or N2	
	1 point	3 points	3 points
Severe symptoms	>20	Every poorly differentiated Every signet ring	
	6 points	7 points	9 points

Mild symptoms: Weight loss <10 % body weight mild abdominal pain, or asymptomatic ascites

Severe symptoms: Weight loss >10 % body weight, unremitting pain, bowel obstruction, or symptomatic ascites

PCI: Peritoneal CarcinomatosisIndex (0–39)

Fig. 14.10 Peritoneal Surface Disease and Severity Score (PSDSS) (Pelz et al. 2010)

a stage from I to IV to the disease. Low PSDS scores (PSDS I to III) have been shown to have better 1- and 2-year outcomes than high PSDS (PSDS IV) scores. At 1 year, survival for PSDS I, II, III and IV was 100, 80, 80 and 8 %, respectively (Pelz et al. 2010). At 2 years, survival was 100, 80, 80 and 0 %, respectively (Pelz et al. 2010). The PSDSS score has been shown to be an independent predictor for survival in multivariate analysis (Pelz et al. 2009; Shimizu et al. 2013).

14.6.3.4 Surgical Points

Cytoreductive surgery aims to remove all peritoneal deposits and proceeds in a quadrant by quadrant systematic fashion to ensure total removal. All obviously visible tumours should be removed. Peritonectomy of the upper right quadrant proceeds by taking down the falciform ligament and proceeding superiorly to reach the bare area of the liver. The tendinous portion of the diaphragm is then removed. Stripping of peritoneum in the left upper quadrant exposes the left adrenal gland, distal pancreas and perinephric fat. A splenectomy and greater omentectomy are also performed. Towards the pelvis, the peritoneum overlying the bladder as well as resection of the rectosigmoid colon and its mesenteries up to the root of the inferior mesenteric artery completes a total peritonectomy.

Following a complete peritonectomy, HIPEC can begin. This involves hyperthermia which increases the dose intensity to the exposed surfaces. Chemotherapy together with hyperthermia enhances the cytotoxicity of the chemotherapeutic agents and increases tissue penetration amongst cancerous versus normal tissue (Carmignani et al. 2003). At the moment, there is no consensus on the specific chemotherapeutic agent used, although one recent phase I study of a combination of mitomycin C, 5-fluorouracil and oxaliplatin was shown to result in marked growth inhibition amongst colorectal cells in vitro (Shimizu et al. 2013).

14.6.3.5 Outcomes
One study reported a 5-year overall survival of 35 % with disease-free survival at 16 % following CRS and HIPEC. This was compared to only a 5-year overall survival rate of 4.1 % in patients with peritoneal carcinomatosis who had only undergone palliative chemotherapy (Goéré et al. 2013).

Verwaal et al. compared outcomes of patients randomly assigned to either CRS or chemotherapy and showed that median survival of patients after a median follow-up of 8 years was 12.6 months in the group who had chemotherapy, versus 22.2 months in the group which underwent CRS and HIPEC (Verwaal et al. 2008).

CRS and HIPEC are now regarded as a treatment option in selected patients with peritoneal carcinomatosis from colorectal cancer. But the survival rates quoted above need to be considered with the caveat that patients need to be carefully selected and that, ultimately, less than one-third of patients presenting with peritoneal metastases are candidates for surgical management (Goéré et al. 2013).

14.7 Palliative Care

In metastatic oncological diseases, palliative care plays a crucial role in enabling smooth transition from the diagnosis of poor prognosis till the patient's demise. Apart from appropriate pain relief, the psychological and social stressors experienced by the patient and the family are immense. These psychological issues can often be overlooked by oncologists (Bonito et al. 2013). These symptoms can actually arise at the various stages of the treatment of their disease (at diagnosis, before and after operation, during surveillance of their conditions and side effects of treatment).

The magnitude of psychosocial needs and support in cancer patients has been reported to be as high as 40 % (Derogatis et al. 1983). Psychosocial issues have been noted to commonly manifest as adjustment disorders, major depressive disorder, anxiety disorders, insomnia and pain where intervention can be appropriately instituted at an early stage (Bonito et al. 2013; Derogatis et al. 1983; Garland et al. 2013; Krok and Baker 2013). Such needs can be intervened through early education, cognitive behavioural therapy, relaxation techniques and peer support (Kilbourn et al. 2013).

Caregivers are an invaluable source of comfort to cancer patients and they devote their time to take care of their loved ones. Multiple studies have proven the positive effects of good care giving leading to better outcomes for patients (Wu et al. 2013).

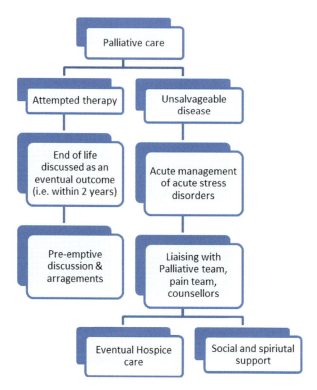

Flowchart 14.2 Overview of palliative approaches to provide care to patients

Pain is perhaps one of the most important factors in the management of the palliative patient. Pain is commonly experienced amongst patients with advanced cancers, with studies reporting up to 80 % of patients with advanced cancer experiencing severe pain (Breivik et al. 2009; Teunissen et al. 2007; Van den Beuken-van Everdingen et al. 2007; Goudas et al. 2005; Larue et al. 1995). The

14 Multidisciplinary Management in Metastatic Cancer

Table 14.7 Hospices in Singapore

Metta Hospice Care (MHC)
Agape Methodist Hospice (AMH)
Singapore Cancer Society (SCS)
St. Joseph's Home & Hospice (SJH)
Assisi Hospice (AH)
Bright Vision Hospital (BVH)
Dover Park Hospice (DPH)
HCA Hospice Care (HCA)

causes of pain in colorectal patients can originate from tumour infiltration of nerves, bowel obstruction and distension of Glisson's capsule (Fisher et al. 2013). Cancer pain management utilises the World Health Organization analgesic ladder, in which opioids occupy the second and third steps of this ladder, and these are typically recommended for moderate to severe pain. The use of opioids allows for patients to undergo a peaceful death and reduce the anxiety amongst family members as they go through the final stages of their loved one's life. Even at this stage when the primary surgeon's role in terms of surgical care is limited, being aware of optimising pain control and prescribing the right dose and type of opioids is critical not just for the patient but also for the patient's relatives. Involvement of a pain specialist or a palliative physician in the overall care of the patient is prudent at this stage of disease.

Singapore Hospice Council (2014) is one such local organisation which looks into improving the quality of life of patients at the tail end of terminal disease. Its goal is to "alleviate suffering and maximise quality of life for patients and their loved ones". The Singapore Hospice Council is the umbrella body which coordinates the services rendered by various hospices found in Singapore (Table 14.7).

Hospices provide a wide range of services available to the patient and caregivers. This ranges from the loaning of medical equipment to religious support. Recreational activities are also organised to drive home the important point that the end of life is not a period of desolation and despair, but merely an extension of our human condition. A fullness of life can be lived close to death, just as with any other period of that person's life.

Conclusion

Metastatic colorectal cancers pose numerous challenges for the individual, family and the attending physician. Each obstacle should be individually tackled while considering the patients' premorbid condition, extent of the primary cancer and the metastatic disease. However, it is important to have a broader picture in mind, and incorporating the inputs from various specialists in this multidisciplinary approach is instrumental to ensuring the best possible outcomes in these patients.

References

Adams RB et al; Americas Hepato-Pancreato-Biliary Association; Society of Surgical Oncology; Society for Surgery of the Alimentary Tract (2013) Selection for hepatic resection of colorectal liver metastases: expert consensus statement. HPB (Oxford) 15(2):91–103

Alexander J, Haight C (1947) Pulmonary resection for solitary metastatic sarcomas and carcinomas. Surg Gynecol Obstet 85:129–146

American Cancer Society. Colorectal cancer facts and figures 2011–2013. Accessed Apr 2014 http://www.cancer.org/acs/groups/content/@epidemiologysurveilance/documents/document/acspc-028312.pdf

Anwar S et al (2011) Palliative excisional surgery for primary colorectal cancer in patients with incurable metastatic disease. Is there a survival benefit? A systematic review. Colorectal Dis 14:920–930

Singapore Hospice Council. available from http://www.singaporehospice.org.sg/. Assessed 5 Apr 2014

Bacon HE, Martin PV (1964) The rationale of palliative resection for primary cancer of the colon and rectum complicated by liver and lung metastasis. Dis Colon Rectum 7:211–217

Baron TH (2010) Colonic stenting: a palliative measure only or a bridge to surgery? Endoscopy 42:163–168

Bismuth H et al (1996) Resection of nonresectable liver metastases from colorectal cancer after neoadjuvant chemotherapy. Ann Surg 224(4):509–520

Bonito A et al (2013) Do healthcare professionals discuss the emotional impact of cancer with patients? Psychooncology 22:2046–2050

Braga L et al (2004) Modern hepatic imaging. Surg Clin North Am 84(2):375–400

Breivik H et al (2009) Cancer-related pain: a pan-European survey of prevalence, treatment, and patient attitudes. Ann Oncol 20(8):1420–1433

Cady B et al (1970) Survival of patients after colonic resection for carcinoma with simultaneous liver metastases. Surg Gynecol Obstet 131:697–700

Camúñez F et al (2000) Malignant colorectal obstruction treated by means of self-expanding metallic stents: effectiveness before surgery and in palliation. Radiology 216:492–497

Carmignani CP et al (2003) Cytoreductive surgery and intraperitoneal chemotherapy for the treatment of peritoneal surface malignancy. Rev Oncol 5(4):192–198

Chang WC et al (2011) Intra-arterial treatment in patients with acute massive gastrointestinal bleeding after endoscopic failure: comparisons between positive versus negative contrast extravasation groups. Korean J Radiol 12(5):568–578

Cirocchi R et al (2012) Non-resection versus resection for an asymptomatic primary tumour in patients with unresectable stage IV colorectal cancer. Cochrane Database Syst Rev (8):CD008997

Clements D et al (2009) Management of the asymptomatic primary in the palliative treatment of metastatic colorectal cancer. Colorectal Dis 11:845–848

Cook AD et al (2005) Surgical resection of primary tumour in patients who present with stage IV colorectal cancer: an analysis of Surveillance, epidemiology and end results data, 1988–2000. Ann Surg Oncol 12:637–645

Cunningham D et al (2004) Cetuximab monotherapy and cetuximab plus Irinotecan in Irinotecan-refractory metastatic colorectal cancer. N Engl J Med 351:337–345

Damjanov N et al (2009) Resection of the primary colorectal cancer is not necessary in nonobstructed patients with metastatic disease. Oncologist 14:963–969

Daniel TM (2005) A proposed diagnostic approach to the patient with the subcentimeter pulmonary nodule: techniques that facilitate video-assisted thoracic surgery excision. Semin Thorac Cardiovasc Surg 17:115–122

De Baere T et al (2000) Radiofrequency ablation of 100 hepatic metastases with a mean follow-up of more than 1 year. AJR Am J Roentgenol 175(6):1619–1625

De Bree E et al (2004) Peritoneal carcinomatosis from colorectal or appendiceal origin: correlation of preoperative CT with intraoperative findings and evaluation of interobserver agreement. J Surg Oncol 86(2):64–73

Derogatis LR et al (1983) The prevalence of psychiatric disorders among cancer patients. JAMA 249(6):751–757

Dohmoto M (1991) New method. Endoscopic implantation of rectal stent in palliative treatment of colorectal neoplastic obstructions. Endosc Dig 3:1507–1512

Edge S et al (2010) AJCC cancer staging manual, 7th edn. Springer, New York, XV, 649

Elias D et al (2010) Peritoneal colorectal carcinomatosis treated with surgery and perioperative intraperitoneal chemotherapy: retrospective analysis of 523 patients from a multicentric French study. J Clin Oncol 28(1):63–68

Engels B et al (2012) Phase II study of helical tomotherapy in the multidisciplinary treatment of oligometastatic colorectal cancer. Radiat Oncol 7:34

Fisher J et al (2013) Use of opioid analgesics among older persons with colorectal cancer in two health districts with palliative care programs. J Pain Symptom Manage 46(1):20–29

Floriani I et al (2010) Performance of imaging modalities in diagnosis of liver metastases from colorectal cancer: a systematic review and meta-analysis. J Magn Reson Imaging 31(1):19–31

Fong Y et al (1999) Clinical score for predicting recurrence after hepatic resection for metastatic colorectal cancer: analysis of 1001 consecutive cases. Ann Surg 230(3):309–318

Fornaro L et al (2010) Palliative treatment of unresectable metastatic colorectal cancer. Expert Opin Pharmacother 11(1):63–77

Frankel TL, D'Angelica MI (2014) Hepatic resection for colorectal metastases. J Surg Oncol 109(1):2–7

Franko J et al (2012) Treatment of colorectal peritoneal carcinomatosis with systemic chemotherapy: a pooled analysis of north central cancer treatment group phase III trials N9741 and N9841. J Clin Oncol 30(3):263–267

Garland SN et al. (2013) Dispositional mindfulness, insomnia, sleep quality and dysfunctional sleep beliefs in post-treatment cancer patients. Pers Individ Dif 55(3):306–311

Gielen C et al (2009) Staging chest radiography is not useful in patients with colorectal cancer. Eur J Surg Oncol 35:1174–1178

Gillams AR, Lees WR (2000) Survival after percutaneous, image-guided, thermal ablation of hepatic metastases from colorectal cancer. Dis Colon Rectum 43(5):656–661

Giuliante F et al (2009) Role of the surgeon as a variable in long-term survival after liver resection for colorectal metastases. J Surg Oncol 100(7):538–545

Glimelius B, Cavalli-Bjorkman N (2012) Metastatic colorectal cancer: current treatment and future options for improved survival medical approach – present status. Scand J Gastroenterol 47:296–314

GLOBOCAN 2012: estimate cancer incidence, mortality and prevalence worldwide in 2012. http://globocan.iarc.fr/Pages/fact_sheets_cancer.aspx. Accessed Mar 2014

Goéré D et al (2013) Is there a possibility of a cure in patients with colorectal peritoneal carcinomatosis amenable to complete cytoreductive surgery and intraperitoneal chemotherapy? Ann Surg 257(6):1065–1071

Gold JS et al (2008) Increased use of parenchymal-sparing surgery for bilateral liver metastases from colorectal cancer is associated with improved mortality without change in oncologic outcome: trends in treatment over time in 440 patients. Ann Surg 247(1):109–117

Goudas LC et al (2005) The epidemiology of cancer pain. Cancer Invest 23(2):182–190

Griffiths EA et al (2005) Evaluation of a pre-operative staging protocol in the management of colorectal carcinoma. Colorectal Dis 7:35–42

Grossmann I et al (2010) Preoperative staging with chest CT in patients with colorectal carcinoma: not as a routine procedure. Ann Surg Oncol 17(8):2045–2050

Henschke CI et al (1999) Early lung cancer action project: overall design and findings from baseline screening. Lancet 354:99–105

Hurwitz H et al (2004) Bevacizumab plus irinotecan, fluorouracil, and leucovorin for metastatic colorectal cancer. N Engl J Med 350:2335–2342

Imamura H et al (2005) Assessment of hepatic reserve for indication of hepatic resection: decision tree incorporating indocyanine green test. J Hepatobiliary Pancreat Surg 12(1):16–22

Iversen LH et al (2013) Value of laparoscopy before cytoreductive surgery and hyperthermic intraperitoneal chemotherapy for peritoneal carcinomatosis. Br J Surg 100(2):285–292

Jacquet P, Sugarbaker PH (1996) Clinical research methodologies in diagnosis and staging of patients with peritoneal carcinomatosis. Cancer Treat Res 82:359–374

Jayne DG et al (2002) Peritoneal carcinomatosis from colorectal cancer. Br J Surg 89: 1545–1550

Jemal A et al (2006) Cancer statistics, 2006. CA Cancer J Clin 56:106–130

Kanemitsu Y et al (2004) Preoperative probability model for predicting overall survival after resection of pulmonary metastases from colorectal cancer. Br J Surg 91(1):112–120

Karapetis CS et al (2008) K-ras mutations and benefit from cetuximab in advanced colorectal cancer. N Engl J Med 359:1757–1765

Kaufman MS et al (2007) Influence of palliative surgical resection on overall survival in patients with advanced colorectal cancer: a retrospective single institutional study. Colorectal Dis 10:498–502

Kick J et al (2005) Resection of lung metastases – risk or chance? Zentralbl Chir 130:534–538

Kilbourn KM et al (2013) Feasibility of EASE: a psychosocial program to improve symptom management in head and neck cancer patients. Support Care Cancer 21:191–200

Kim AW et al (2008) Repeat pulmonary resection for metachronous colorectal carcinoma is beneficial. Surgery 144(4):712–717

Klaver YL et al (2012) Outcomes of colorectal cancer patients with peritoneal carcinomatosis treated with chemotherapy with and without targeted therapy. Eur J Surg Oncol 38(7): 617–623

Koh JL, Yan TD, Glenn D, Morris DL (2009) Evaluation of preoperative computed tomography in estimating peritoneal cancer index in colorectal peritoneal carcinomatosis. Ann Surg Oncol 16(2):327–333

Kohne CH et al (2008) Irinotecan combined with infusional 5-fluorouracil/folinic acid or capecitabine plus celecoxib or placebo in the first-line treatment of patients with metastatic colorectal cancer. EORTC study 40015. Ann Oncol 19:920–926

Kokudo N et al (2001) Anatomical major resection versus nonanatomical limited resection for liver metastases from colorectal carcinoma. Am J Surg 181(2):153–159

Krok JL, Baker TA (2013) The influence of personality on reported pain and self-efficacy for pain management in older cancer patients. J Health Psychol;1–10

Kronawitter U et al (1999) Evaluation of chest computed tomography in the staging of patients with potentially resectable liver metastases from colorectal carcinoma. Cancer 86: 229–235

Larue F et al (1995) Multicentre study of cancer pain and its treatment in France. BMJ 310(6986):1034–1037

Lockhart-Mummery HE (1959) Surgery in patients with advanced carcinoma of the colon and rectum. Dis Colon Rectum 2:36–39

Martí M, Artigas JM et al (2012) Acute lower intestinal bleeding: feasibility and diagnostic performance of CT angiography. Radiology 262(1):109–116

Masi G et al (2008) Triplet combination of fluoropyrimidines, oxaliplatin, and irinotecan in the first-line treatment of metastatic colorectal cancer. Clin Colorectal Cancer 7:7–14

McCullough JA, Engledow AH (2010) Overview: treatment options in obstructed left-sided colonic cancer. Clin Oncol 22:764–770

McIntosh J et al (2005) Pulmonary staging in colorectal cancer – is computerised tomography the answer? Ann R Coll Surg Engl 87:331–333

Michel P et al (2004) Colorectal cancer with non-resectable synchronous metastases: should the primary tumor be resected? Gastroenterol Clin Biol 28:434–437

Ministry of Health, Health Promotion Board, National Registry of Disease Office. Singapore Cancer Registry Interim Annual Registry Report, trends in cancer incidence in Singapore, 2008–2012. Accessed Mar 2013

Mitry E et al (2010) Epidemiology, management and prognosis of colorectal cancer with lung metastases: a 30-year population based study. Gut 59:1383–1388

Muratore A et al (2007) Asymptomatic colorectal cancer with un-resectable liver metastases: immediate colorectal resection or up-front systemic chemotherapy? Ann Surg Oncol 14:766–770

14 Multidisciplinary Management in Metastatic Cancer

Niekel MC et al (2010) Diagnostic imaging of colorectal liver metastases with CT, MR imaging, FDG PET, and/or FDG PET/CT: a meta-analysis of prospective studies including patients who have not previously undergone treatment. Radiology 257(3):674

Nitzkorski JR et al (2012) Outcome and natural history of patients with stage IV colorectal cancer receiving chemotherapy without primary tumor resection. Ann Surg Oncol 19:379–383

Parnaby CN et al (2012) Pulmonary staging in colorectal cancer: a review. Colorectal Dis 14(6):660–670

Patel J et al (2010) Diagnosis of cirrhosis with intravoxel incoherent motion diffusion MRI and dynamic contrast-enhanced MRI alone and in combination: preliminary experience. J Magn Reson Imaging 31(3):589–600

Pelz JO et al (2009) Evaluation of a peritoneal surface disease severity score in patients with colon cancer with peritoneal carcinomatosis. J Surg Oncol 99(1):9–15

Pelz JO et al (2010) Evaluation of best supportive care and systemic chemotherapy as treatment stratified according to the retrospective peritoneal surface disease severity score (PSDSS) for peritoneal carcinomatosis of colorectal origin. BMC Cancer 10:689

Pfannenberg C et al (2009) (18)F-FDG-PET/CT to select patients with peritoneal carcinomatosis for cytoreductive surgery and hyperthermic intraperitoneal chemotherapy. Ann Surg Oncol 16(5):1295–1303

Pfannschmidt J et al (2007) Surgical resection of pulmonary metastases from colorectal cancer: a systematic review of published series. Ann Thorac Surg 84:324–338

Pfannschmidt J et al (2012) Surgical intervention in pulmonary metastases. Dtsch Arztebl Int 109(40):645–651

Poultsides GA et al (2009) Outcome of primary tumor in patients with synchronous stage IV colorectal cancer receiving combination chemotherapy without surgery as initial treatment. J Clin Oncol 27:3379–3384

Povoski SP et al (1998) Role of chest CT in patients with negative chest x-rays referred for hepatic colorectal metastases. Ann Surg Oncol 5:9–15

Quiros RM, Scott WJ (2008) Surgical treatment of metastatic disease to the lung. Semin Oncol 35:134–146

Riss S et al (2013) Peritoneal metastases from colorectal cancer: patient selection for cytoreductive surgery and hyperthermic intraperitoneal chemotherapy. Eur J Surg Oncol 39(9):931–937

RodriGuez-Gonzalez D et al (2013) Metastatic lymph nodes and lymph node ratio as predictive factors of survival in perforated and Non-perforated T4 colorectal tumors. J Surg Oncol 108:176–181

Ronnekleiv-Kelly SM, Kennedy GD (2011) Management of stage IV rectal cancer: palliative options. World J Gastroenterol 17(7):835–847

Roth JA et al (1986) Comparison of median sternotomy and thoracotomy for resection of pulmonary metastases in patients with adult soft-tissue sarcomas. Ann Thorac Surg 42(2):134–138

Ruers T et al; EORTC Gastro-Intestinal Tract Cancer Group, Arbeitsgruppe Lebermetastasen und—tumoren in der Chirurgischen Arbeitsgemeinschaft Onkologie (ALM-CAO) and the National Cancer Research Institute Colorectal Clinical Study Group (NCRI CCSG) (2012) Radiofrequency ablation combined with systemic treatment versus systemic treatment alone in patients with non-resectable colorectal liver metastases: a randomized EORTC Intergroup phase II study (EORTC 40004). Ann Oncol 23(10):2619–2626

Ruo L et al (2003) Elective bowel resection for incurable stage IV colorectal cancer: prognostic variables for asymptomatic patients. J Am Coll Surg 196:722–728

Sadahiro S et al (2009) Prognostic factors in patients with synchronous peritoneal carcinomatosis (PC) caused by a primary cancer of the colon. J Gastrointest Surg 13(9):1593–1598

Sahani DV et al (2004) Intraoperative US in patients undergoing surgery for liver neoplasms: comparison with MR imaging. Radiology 232(3):810–814

Saied A et al (2013) Regional hepatic therapies: an important component in the management of colorectal cancer liver metastases. Hepatobiliary Surg Nutr 2(2):97–107

Saltz LB et al (2007) Randomized phase II trial of cetuximab, Bevacizumab, and irinotecan compared with cetuximab and bevacizumab alone in irinotecan-refractory colorectal cancer: the BOND-2 study. J Clin Oncol 25(29):4557–4561

Sarela AI et al (2001) Non-operative management of the primary tumour in patients with incurable stage IV colorectal cancer. Br J Surg 88:1352–1356

Scheele J et al (1990) Hepatic metastases from colorectal carcinoma: impact of surgical resection on the natural history. Br J Surg 77(11):1241–1246

Scheele J et al (1995) Resection of colorectal liver metastases. World J Surg 19(1):59–71

Schroeder RA et al (2006) Predictive indices of morbidity and mortality after liver resection. Ann Surg 243(3):373–379

Scoggins CR et al (1999) Nonoperative management of primary colorectal cancer in patients with stage IV disease. Ann Surg Oncol 6:651–657

Segelman J et al (2012) Incidence, prevalence and risk factors for peritoneal carcinomatosis from colorectal cancer. Br J Surg 99:699–705

Shimizu T et al (2013) Hyperthermic Intraperitoneal chemotherapy using a combination of mitomycin C,5-fluorouracil, and oxaliplatin in patients at high risk of colorectal peritoneal metastasis: a phase I clinical study. Eur J Surg Oncol 13:943–948

Siegel R et al (2014) Cancer statistics. CA Cancer J Clin 64(1):9

Strate LL, Naumann CR (2010) The role of colonoscopy and radiological procedures in the management of acute lower intestinal bleeding. Clin Gastroenterol Hepatol 8(4):333–343

Stubbs RS, Wickremesekera SK (2004) Selective internal radiation therapy (SIRT): a new modality for treating patients with colorectal liver metastases. HPB (Oxford) 6(3):133–139

Tan KK et al (2009) How uncommon are isolated lung metastases in colorectal cancer? A review from database of 754 patients over 4 years. J Gastrointest Surg 13(4):642–648

Teunissen SC et al (2007) Symptom prevalence in patients with incurable cancer: a systematic review. J Pain Symptom Manage 34(1):94–104

Tournigand C et al (2006) OPTIMOX1: a randomized study of FOLFOX4 or FOLFOX7 with Oxaliplatin in a stop-and-go fashion in advanced colorectal cancer: a GERCOR study. J Clin Oncol 24:394–400

Uesaka K et al (1996) Changes in hepatic lobar function after right portal vein embolization. An appraisal by biliary indocyanine green excretion. Ann Surg 223(1):77–83

Van Cutsem E et al (2007) Open-label phase III trial of panitumumab plus best supportive care compared with best supportive care alone in patients with chemotherapy-refractory metastatic colorectal cancer. J Clin Oncol 25:1658–1664

Van Cutsem E et al (2009) Cetuximab and chemotherapy as initial treatment for metastatic colorectal cancer. N Engl J Med 360:1408–1417

Van Cutsem E et al (2011) Cetuximab plus irinotecan, fluorouracil, and leucovorin as first-line treatment for metastatic colorectal cancer: updated analysis of overall survival according to tumor kras and braf mutation status. J Clin Oncol 29:2011–2019

Van den Beuken-van Everdingen MH et al (2007) Prevalence of pain in patients with cancer: a systematic review of the past 40 years. Ann Oncol 18(9):1437–1449

Vemulapalli R et al (2010) A comparison of palliative stenting or emergent surgery for obstructing incurable colon cancer. Dig Dis Sci 55:1732–1737

Verwaal VJ et al (2003) Randomized trial of cytoreduction and hyperthermic intraperitoneal chemotherapy versus systemic chemotherapy and palliative surgery in patients with peritoneal carcinomatosis of colorectal cancer. J Clin Oncol 21(20):3737–3743

Verwaal VJ et al (2008) 8-year follow-up of randomized trial: cytoreduction and hyperthermic intraperitoneal chemotherapy versus systemic chemotherapy in patients with peritoneal carcinomatosis of colorectal cancer. Ann Surg Oncol 15(9):2426–2432

Vogel WV et al (2005) Colorectal cancer: the role of PET/CT in recurrence. Cancer Imaging 5:143–148

Vogt-Moykopf I et al (1994) Surgery for pulmonary metastases. The Heidelberg experience. Chest Surg Clin N Am 4(1):85–112

Wei AC et al (2006) Survival after hepatic resection for colorectal metastases: a 10-year experience. Ann Surg Oncol 13(5):668–676

14 Multidisciplinary Management in Metastatic Cancer

Welter S et al (2007) Long-term survival after repeated resection of pulmonary metastases from colorectal cancer. Ann Thorac Surg 84(1):203–210

Wu LM et al (2013) Patient and spouse illness beliefs and quality of life in prostate cancer. Psychol Health 28(4):355–368

Zisis C et al (2013) The management of the advanced metastatic colorectal cancer: management of the pulmonary metastases. J Thorac Dis 5(S4):S383–S388

Zorzi D et al (2006) Comparison between hepatic wedge resection and anatomic resection for colorectal liver metastases. J Gastrointest Surg 10(1):86–94

Transdisciplinary Stoma Care

15

Yu-Jing Ong, Choo-Eng Ong, Lay-Choo Chee, and Gregory K.E. Heng

---

Take-Home Pearls

- Each member of the healthcare team plays a vital role in delivering comprehensive stoma care through a transdisciplinary approach.
- Stoma care begins preoperatively and continues postoperatively and after discharge in the rehabilitation phase.
- Common objectives shared by patients and the transdisciplinary team improve recovery outcomes and increase acceptance of the stoma.

15.1 Introduction

Stoma, a Greek word also known as 'ostomy', is an artificial opening in the skin of an individual created surgically to allow fluid withdrawal. Stomas are fashioned in different ways depending on their indications. Table 15.1 summarises the classification of stoma and type of procedures. Creating a stoma may be temporary or permanent, and the diversion of intra-abdominal fluids aims to improve quality of life or aid in recovery from the disease process. Table 15.2 illustrates the type of stoma and description of output consistency.

The need for a stoma is often regarded as a drastic changing event which can be traumatising for patients both psychologically and physically (Gesaro 2012). An ostomist's journey is apprehensive with many difficulties to face, requiring

---

Y.-J. Ong (✉) • L.-C. Chee
Nursing Administration, Khoo Teck Puat Hospital, Singapore, Singapore
e-mail: ong.yu.jing@alexandrahealth.com.sg; chee.lay.choo@alexandrahealth.com.sg

C.-E. Ong
Nursing Administration, Singapore General Hospital, Singapore, Singapore
e-mail: ong.choo.eng@sgh.com.sg

G.K.E. Heng
Department of General Surgery, Khoo Teck Puat Hospital, Singapore, Singapore

© Springer-Verlag Berlin Heidelberg 2015
K.-Y. Tan (ed.), *Transdisciplinary Perioperative Care in Colorectal Surgery: An Integrative Approach*, DOI 10.1007/978-3-662-44020-9_15

Table 15.1 Classification of stoma and procedures

Type of procedures	Ileostomy	Colostomy	Urostomy
Abdominoperineal resection (APR)		√	
Hartmann's		√	
Low anterior resection	√		
Ultra-low anterior resection	√		
Proctocolectomy	√		
Cystectomy			√

Table 15.2 Type of stoma and description of output consistency

Type of stoma	Ileostomy	Colostomy	Urostomy
Description of output	Watery to loose faecal matter	Formed faecal matter	Urine
End			
Loop			
Double-barrel			

significant adaptation. Challenges encountered have an impact on all aspects of an ostomist's life, including psychosocial, spiritual, physical and sexual health and cultural and religious beliefs. Thus, a transdisciplinary approach in the delivery of stoma care would provide much benefit in dealing with these challenges.

Transdisciplinary stoma care encompasses the collaborative input from various healthcare professionals' different specialties for holistic care. This team comprises a colorectal nurse specialist, surgeon, oncologist, social worker, dietician, pharmacist, caregiver and the patient (Fig. 15.1). Each member of the team plays an important role with the common goals of improving an ostomist's outcome, rehabilitation to the premorbid status and achieving self-care. Effective communication between the

Fig. 15.1 Transdisciplinary stoma team

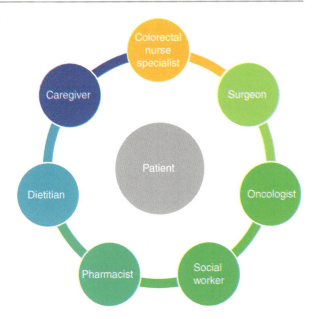

healthcare team and the patient or caregiver is crucial to ensure continual and holistic stoma care, enhancing each dedicated role in the team for holistic stoma care. In this chapter, the delivery of stoma care in a transdisciplinary approach will be discussed.

15.2 Roles of Healthcare Professionals

Many aspects of healthcare involve a collaboration between doctors and allied healthcare professionals. In transdisciplinary stoma care, each member of the team plays a vital role in the provision of comprehensive stoma care.

15.2.1 Medical Professionals

The surgeon is traditionally seen as the team leader and primary decision maker for the surgical patient. In a transdisciplinary team, the surgeon continues to manage the surgical aspects of patient care but takes a step back and actively listens and incorporates the input from the other members of the team.

The decision for a stoma is ultimately a surgical decision. The need for a stoma may be required given the nature of the surgery but may also be an intraoperative decision. If there is a possible or definite need for a stoma, the surgeon would counsel the patient appropriately but should also highlight this to the transdisciplinary team, allowing for various members of the team to initiate contact with the patient preoperatively. This will aid in the patient's subsequent acceptance of the stoma and accelerate their ability to provide self-care.

15.2.2 Medical Social Worker (MSW)

The medical social worker plays an important role in patients who have financial, caregiver or social issues and if psychosocial support is required. Elderly patients may require step-down facilities for rehabilitation postoperatively, and the MSW is required for the consideration of step-down options, for instance, community hospital or day rehabilitation services. For patients who stay alone, the MSW could arrange an interim caretaker for a few weeks to help boost the patient's confidence in self-care.

The MSW can provide counselling and psychosocial support for patients and family, for both stoma care and especially in patients with terminal disease. The MSW can provide a listening ear while spending time with the patient and may link the patient up with an appropriate support group. Financial assistance for stoma care can also be arranged. In our local setting, an application can be made for the provision of stoma supplies from a charitable organisation – Singapore Cancer Society. Thus, the MSW works together with the colorectal nurse specialist, ensuring that appropriate appliances can be provided to patients with support from respective institution as required.

15.2.3 Dietician

The dietician serves the role of providing dietary advice and dietary guide for stoma patients. In our institution, the dietician counsels for small frequent meals with low fibre during the initial postoperative period for colonic resections. In patients with high ileostomy output, the dietician and pharmacist work together to provide education on usage of oral rehydration salt (ORS) as salt replacement and on appropriate fluid intake. Specific dietary plans may be required in patients with premorbid medical issues such as end-stage renal failure or heart failure. Supplements may be introduced to patients who are malnourished with the aim to increase caloric intake.

15.2.4 Pharmacists

In patients with high ileostomy output, education to the patient and caregiver by the pharmacist on the use of ORS (6 sachets in 1 l of water) is required. The surgeon may also initiate antidiarrhoeal medications such as loperamide. The pharmacist is required to provide counselling on the titration of loperamide to the patient and caregiver to prevent overdosing. Alternatively, the pharmacist should educate the patient to drink isotonic water to replace the electrolytes lost from the ileostomy output. Involvement from stoma care nurses includes educating patients to measure their output and titrate their medication accordingly after discharge.

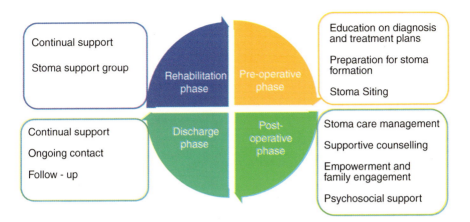

Fig. 15.2 Role of the colorectal nurse specialist (Adapted from Borwell 2009)

Elderly patients with multiple medical issues may have numerous medications and supplements. Medication reconstitution is done by pharmacists to help them identify medications which are stopped and in the introduction of new medications. Furthermore, a medication pillbox is a useful aid for elderly patients to ensure compliance to their long-term medications. Advices on the effect of specific medications on the colour of stools should be provided to the patient and caregiver to allay anxiety and prevent unnecessary readmissions.

15.2.5 Colorectal Nurse Specialist

The colorectal nurse specialist plays the role of the facilitator and ensures smooth collaboration between team members for the care of the ostomist from preoperative to postoperative phases. Moreover, the provision of care does not end upon discharge from the hospital. The continuation of stoma care with follow-up after discharge by the nurse is fundamental in ensuring all needs are taken care of (Borwell 2009). Figure 15.2 illustrates the role of the colorectal nurse specialist in different phases of an ostomist's preparation to a life with stoma. The nurse serves as a coordinator ensuring that the team provides the delivery of holistic care for ostomists.

Case Study We present the journey of Mr. J., a 28-year-old gentleman with familial adenomatous polyposis (FAP) and anal cancer, to illustrate the role of transdisciplinary team. Mr. J. underwent neoadjuvant chemotherapy prior to surgery, with the aim of curative resection through a total proctocolectomy with an end ileostomy. Through the different phases of preparation, he completed the journey to become an ostomist with the transdisciplinary team.

15.3 Preoperative Phase

The preoperative phase marks the commencement of an ostomist's journey towards living with a stoma. The goal for preoperative care is to prepare patients to cope with stoma physically and psychologically, allowing them to anticipate the subsequent phases. This also increases acceptance of a stoma and reduces the impact on body image (Slater 2010).

15.3.1 Preoperative Counselling Session

Prior to an elective surgery, a planned session between the patient and the colorectal nurse specialist serves as a valuable platform to build rapport and establish the foundation for a smooth-sailing transition to living with a stoma (Slater 2010). Not only does it provides an opportunity for the patient to raise concerns or difficulties, but also aids in maintaining ownership of health (Borwell 2009). Furthermore, it allows the nurse to perform an initial assessment which encompasses biological, physical and psychosocial aspects and to gain an understanding of the patient's expectation.

The initial assessment is important as every individual differs in their concerns, needs and expectations. During preoperative counselling and consultation, the colorectal nurse specialist will bring the patient through the diagnosis and proposed treatment plan such as surgery, chemotherapy and need for the creation of stoma. Details on the management of stoma and expectation of postoperative changes will also be further discussed with the patient. Table 15.3 states the components of preoperative counselling. The use of multimedia such as brochures, flip charts and video or the showcasing of stoma pouches is used to engage the patient. Provision of detailed information will allow the patient to have a better understanding of the effects of surgery and stoma. Moreover, it offers better awareness and allays anxiety.

A preoperative counselling session was arranged with the surgeon, colorectal nurse specialist and Mr. J. present. The surgeon discussed the operation including the creation of a stoma and its potential complications with the aid of illustrations for better understanding. The colorectal nurse specialist explored his understanding of the operation and stoma creation and clarified doubts. Moreover, the colorectal nurse specialist provided him an alternative date for a second preoperative counselling session to prevent information overload and allow him time to think through and process the information.

Table 15.3 Components of preoperative counselling

Diagnosis and prognosis
Preparation for life with stoma
Type and effects of surgery
Communication
Psychological/sexual awareness
Future care (chemotherapy)
Stoma siting

15.3.2 Placement of Stoma and Its Consideration

Stoma siting is a crucial step in preoperative care as suboptimal stoma placement will lead to problems and issues with acceptance. Cooperation from the patient is essential; hence, the process is explained in advance. The appropriate placement of stoma needs to take into account the patient's background, occupation and body habitus contours. Siting of stoma starts with the identification of the patient's waistline and rectus muscle shift. The rectus muscle extends from the midline to one-third the distance from the midline to the iliac crest. Sitting the patient up off the edge of the bed aids in the recognition of skin folds and creases which need to be avoided. Siting away from areas where working adults need to wear belts or pouches is important to prevent external pressure from the belt or pouch on the stoma.

In contrast, an elderly lady with abdominal skin folds and pendulous breasts will require stoma siting away from her breasts and at the 'peak' of the abdomen to avoid the skin creases. Stoma siting aids the surgeon intraoperatively, preventing difficulties related to improper siting.

15.3.3 Fears and Concerns

Undergoing a major surgery is already a stressful event for patients. The creation of stoma will only add on more sorrow and burden. The patient will naturally be concerned about changes in his or her lifestyle with a stoma and the impact on occupation, society's perception and even interpersonal relationships. The recognition of these areas of concerns allows ample time for the nurse and patient to address them.

During each consultation with Mr. J., the colorectal nurse specialist took time to explore his feelings and thoughts about stoma creation. Understanding his situation and establishing rapport allowed the nurse to minimise the patient's fears and concerns. Mr. J. expressed fears of losing his job and concerns regarding the acceptance of stoma. Identifying his worries helped the colorectal nurse specialist to provide him with solutions to counter them. Table 15.4 summarises the fears and concerns of an ostomist.

Table 15.4 Fears and concerns of an ostomist	Psychological impact (body image and sexuality)
	Independence in self-care
	Security of stoma appliance
	Odour and cleanliness
	Employment
	Financial issue
	Cultural and religious beliefs
	Adapted from Borwell (2009), *British Journal of Community Nursing*

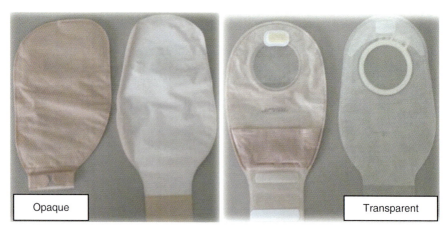

Fig. 15.3 Opaque and transparent pouch

Fig. 15.4 Dummy stoma

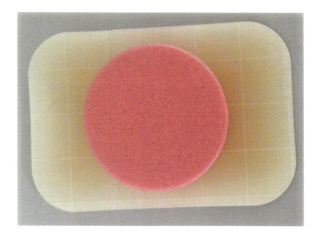

15.3.4 Body Image

Stoma is often perceived as a dirty foreign object on one's body and this affects the patient's psychological self-image. 'Embarrassment', 'weird feeling having something popping out' or 'having "poo" outside of my body' are thoughts running through one's mind when requiring a stoma (Williams 2012b). These thoughts were shared by Mr. J., resulting in him delaying his surgery for weeks.

The colorectal nurse specialist assisted him in his acceptance of stoma by instilling a positive self-perception of himself with a stoma by displaying opaque stoma products which remove the visibility of faeces (Fig. 15.3). Furthermore, the nurse provided him with a trial usage of a dummy stoma which was applied over the proposed site with water placed in the pouch to provide a realistic experience and stimulate psychological and physical adjustments for having a stoma (Fig. 15.4). During this period of time, he became accustomed to the proposed

15 Transdisciplinary Stoma Care

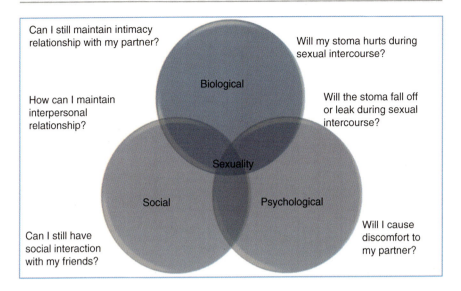

Fig. 15.5 Aspects of sexuality

position and was pleased with its discreet lie under his clothing (Slater 2010). This also provided reassurance on the security and durability of the stoma appliance.

15.3.5 Sexuality and Relationship

Sexuality is a sensitive topic which patients often have concerns about but is often neglected by healthcare professionals. Maslow's hierarchy of needs (1954) illustrated that sex is one of the basic human physiological needs in life, with sexuality encompassing biological, psychological and social aspects. Figure 15.5 illustrates the aspects of sexuality. It does not just involves the physical aspect but includes the whole wellbeing of a human – security, comfort, intimacy and interpersonal relationship (Williams 2012b).

Sexual dysfunction after surgery may occur in both men and women. In women, dyspareunia is often being reported (Sprunk and Alteneder 2000). After surgery, tightness and dryness over the vaginal area occur due to the formation of scar tissues and lack of natural lubrication. During preoperative counselling, patients need to be informed of this to prepare themselves mentally that they may experience pain during sexual intercourse (Williams 2006).

On the other hand, males are at risk for impotence, infertility or retrograde ejaculation as a result of injury to the nerves that control ejaculation or erection (Williams 2012b). For Mr. J., this was a major concern as he was planning to get married with his fiancée. Preoperative care for him will need to take maintenance of hygiene and an intimate relationship with his spouse into consideration. Due to the

Fig. 15.6 Small pouch

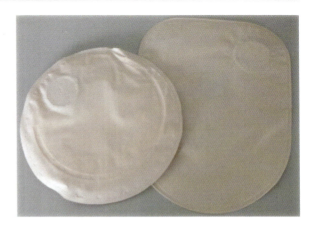

possibility of infertility, storage of sperm in a sperm bank was considered. Thus, referral to the KK in vitro fertilisation (KKIVF) centre at KK Women's and Children's Hospital was made for sperm storage prior to surgery.

Additionally, encouraging him to engage in open communication with his fiancée was essential in conserving their relationship. This enabled the development of trust as part of a healing process for him. The following is a list of advices provided for an ostomist to promote a positive relationship with his or her partner:

- Letting the patient know that it is okay to feel sensitive about the alteration in his or her body.
- Sharing feelings with his or her partner and responding to each other's concerns.
- Informing his or her partner that sexual intercourse will not hurt the stoma.
- Wearing a small pouch or specially designed underwear, lingerie or pouch cover for a pleasant appearance (Fig. 15.6).
- Emptying pouch prior to sexual intercourse will ease the feeling of uneasiness.
- Be assured that as long as the appliance is placed properly, any position should not affect or dislodge it.
- During sexual activity, bowels are relaxed; hence, it is unlikely that stools or gas will enter the stoma.

With mutual understanding and a positive attitude, a constructive relationship can be developed.

15.3.6 Independence in Self-care

Stoma self-care is a vital goal in the patient's journey. Empowering every ostomist to learn a new skill in caring for a stoma is a challenge to the patient and nurse (Gesaro 2012). Preoperative education on stoma plays an important role as patients tend to absorb more information prior to surgery without the effect of postoperative drugs.

Fig. 15.7 Stoma template

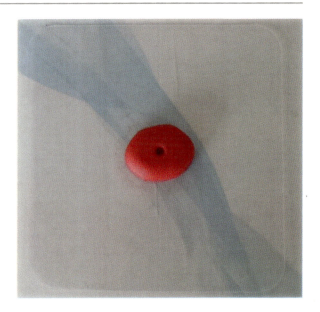

The usage of stoma templates for the practice of stoma care serves as a stimulation tool for competency in caring of stoma (Fig. 15.7). In order to establish fruitful rehabilitation in stoma care, continuity in stoma education until the postoperative period and after discharge is essential (Gesaro 2012).

Regaining independence in self-care for stoma was essential for Mr. J. At a young age, he will still need to work and play like any adult. Empowering him in taking care of his stoma by himself is one of the goals to be achieved.

15.3.7 Society Acceptance

Lending a pair of listening ears and paying attention to the patient's fears, concerns, needs and expectations after surgery serves as a helping hand to them and lightens their worries. If the patient is still anxious or wants to speak to someone with experience, there is the option of an introduction to a patient ambassador to allay their anxiety. In addition, this aids in providing the patient with a positive perception that he or she is not alone.

Mr. J. was fearful of what would happen after surgery, afraid of not being accepted by his peers and afraid of losing his job due to his employer's inability to accept the stoma. Arrangement for an ostomist to meet Mr. J. was organised with both parties' consent. This meeting helped him to recognise that 'he was not alone in the society'. He felt much better after speaking to another ostomist who had a shared experience. The perspective of a colorectal nurse specialist with vast experience in stoma care differs from that of a layman with true life experience on stoma. A layman's words would be heartfelt and aid in allaying the fear and anxiety of a new ostomist. This also enhances social interaction and provides a message to ostomists that they are accepted by society, helping to boost their confidence level in having a stoma.

15.3.8 Employment and Travelling

Job security is a top priority in life. Undergoing surgery and having a stoma having a stoma is an added contributing factor to a new ostomist's fear of being jobless. Once a confident professional, the patient might now be fearful of being discriminated by colleagues and afraid of losing his or her job. Regaining one's confidence is challenging and requires an individual to stay optimistic. Helping a new ostomist regain confidence is essential. Encouragement from family or the nurse to go back to work or return to a patient's usual activities, for example, running, swimming or cycling, helps to increase a patient's confidence level. However, reinforcement on information such as the avoidance of heavy object lifting and rough contact exercises such as rugby, wrestling or boxing is important.

Mr. J. is an all-rounded event coordinator. Having a stoma might limit his capability in performing his usual physical tasks. Encouraging him to communicate with his employer to develop a common understanding would strengthen the employer-employee relationship. He managed to have an open conversation with his employer and is currently working on an ad hoc basis, taking his health into consideration.

Travelling locally or abroad should be encouraged to promote social interaction and decrease the perception of society discrimination for an ostomist. Making a checklist before taking off is encouraged to promote pleasant and hassle-free travelling (Fig. 15.8).

15.3.9 Financial Issue

Permanent ostomists require long-term usage of stoma products which might be taxing to the family and patient financially, amounting to over 100 dollars per month. Ostomists faced with frequent change of stoma products due to multiple factors may face further financial difficulty. Factors affecting the frequency of change of stoma products need to be investigated as follows:

- Inadequate understanding of stoma care by family and patient
- Knowledge deficiency in stoma care by family and patient
- Skin irritation or excoriation
- Product allergy
- Stoma complications

Understanding the financial background of the patient and the subsequent engagement of the medical social worker for social support or financial aid is important.

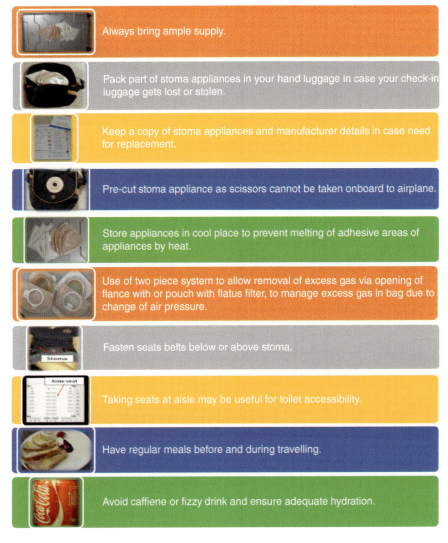

Fig. 15.8 Checklist for travel

15.3.10 Cultural and Religious Beliefs

In a multiracial society with diverse cultures, respecting and meeting the needs of each culture and religion is challenging. Concerns from different ethnic groups cannot be neglected. Ostomists can often continue their religious activities such as praying or special diet restrictions despite having a stoma. Table 15.5 provides pointers to note as regards the assorted religions of patients.

Table 15.5 Pointers to note for the assorted religions of patients

Muslim
Must take fresh ablutions before each prayer interval
Emptying of pouch prior to prayer time to prevent leakage during prayer time
Stoma siting may need to be discussed with the patient as he or she may prefer the site to be above the umbilical area
During the Ramadan period may not be advisable in fear of dehydration and disruption of output with diarrhoea and constipation
Judaism
Dietician input for dietary advice as Jews have strict diet restrictions
In anticipation of Jewish Shabbat day with limited supplies of electricity and papers, a reminder for early preparation is required
Christianity
Religious symbols and items such as rosary and cross may need to be kept with the patient at all times
Sikhism
Dietician input as many Sikhs are vegetarians
Avoid medication prescription of animal-based gelatine medications
Hinduism
Proper cleansing of stoma pouch prior to prayer
Avoiding of 'hot' and 'cold' food

15.4 Postoperative Phase

Undergoing a major surgery is a major stress factor, while having a stoma adds on an image burden to an individual. The provision of transdisciplinary support needs to continue postoperatively. Input from various healthcare professionals makes holistic care possible.

15.4.1 Psychological Support

During the immediate postoperative period, a patient rouses in an unfamiliar situation and tends to be fearful of what to expect. Preoperative counselling helps in managing expectations especially with regard to the presence of lines, tubes, stoma and pain. Encouraging caregivers to stay at the bedside or the presence of familiar objects by the bedside aids in reducing postoperative delirium in the elderly patient. The patient will feel safer with the presence of caregivers who will aid him or her in the event that the nursing responses to his or her calls are not readily available. The provision of psychological support to patients is important, as is letting them know they are not alone, this helps to reduce the psychological barriers to recovery and self-care. Engaging family members in caregiver training helps boost patients' self-esteem and sense of security.

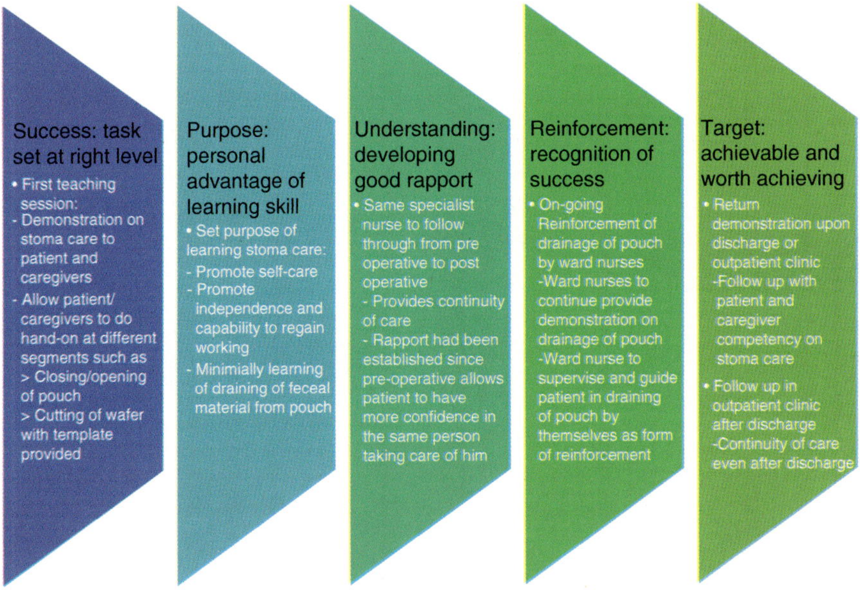

Fig. 15.9 SPURT model (Adapted from Williams 2012a)

15.4.2 Caregiver and Self-care Training

To facilitate early discharge, clearance from the surgeon on when to proceed with stoma caregiver training can be obtained from the second or third postoperative day. Engaging the patient's caregiver who may be a spouse, maid or parent provides encouragement and support during the process of learning. Demonstration of stoma care by the colorectal nurse specialist and ongoing guidance from ward nurses on draining of output into the pouch with return demonstrations by the patient or caregiver will commence during the admission and continue upon discharge on an outpatient basis till competence is achieved. Stoma nurses often use innovative methods to hold a patient or caregiver's attention and concentration through the use of brochures, stoma kit, dummy stoma, actual stoma or videos. The first teaching session usually entails cleansing, drying and application of stoma appliances.

Adopting Williams' (2012b) SPURT model, developed from Petty's (2004) SPERT model, helps to shorten the learning curve with promotion of self-belief and motivation in stoma care. SPURT model provides an individualised stoma teaching plan for every patient. Stoma nurses break down stoma care into different segments for patient to understand and attain the goals successfully. Reinforcement by ward nurses is essential to boost the patient's confidence and adaptation of new skills learnt. Realistic goals are set in collaboration with the patient to achieve the goal of independent self-care. Figure 15.9 demonstrates how stoma care teaching is carried out with the use of the SPURT model.

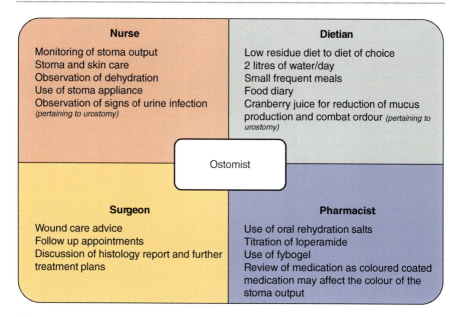

Fig. 15.10 Education on stoma care by the transdisciplinary team

Education on skin care, dietary advice and management of high ileostomy output need to be provided. Input from the dietician on dietary advice and pharmacists on titration of loperamide is required. Figure 15.10 illustrates how a transdisciplinary team approaches ostomists for stoma care.

15.5 Discharge Phase

Planning for early discharge begins from the first postoperative day and involves the transdisciplinary team, patients and family. Assessment of the need for step-down care support such as home nursing foundation or community hospital needs to be initiated early to facilitate early discharge. Information and advice to be given to the patient and caregivers include the following:

- Provide sufficient stoma appliance for at least 1 month upon discharge (approximately a box of 10 sets).
- Provide stoma starter kit and brochures (Fig. 15.11).
- Inform about the venue for purchase of stoma appliance – only hospital-based pharmacy. It should be reinforced that they should not wait until stock runs low in fear of a shortage of products in the pharmacy.
- Provide information on the availability of external support such as home visits from stoma appliance vendors.

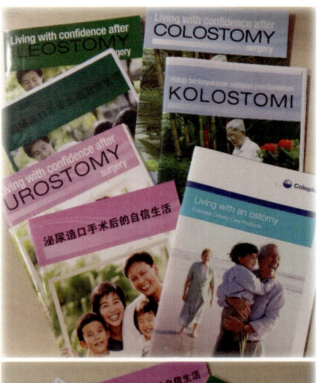
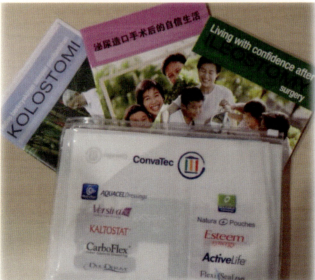

Fig. 15.11 Stoma starter kits and brochures

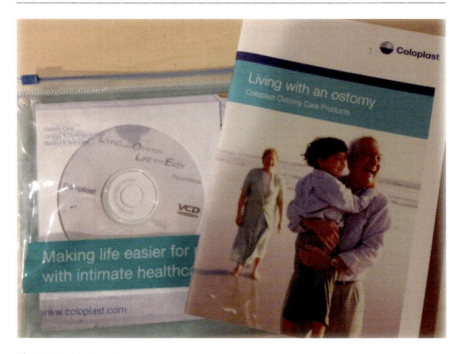

Fig. 15.11 (continued)

- Arrange for outpatient clinic visit after discharge for follow-up of:
  - Wound
  - Removal of stoma rod
  - Ileostomy output
  - Coping of patient and family at home
- Arrange for follow-up appointment for stoma care until patient and caregiver are competent.

Reinforcement of advice on stoma care prior to discharge allows patients and caregivers to remember important points to note. Education from dietician and pharmacist needs to be provided as well. The surgeon's appointment needs to be arranged for follow-up visits, investigations or further oncological treatment. Furthermore, the provision of contact numbers of colorectal nurse specialists/stoma nurses provides a fall-back plan and a sense of security.

15.6 Rehabilitation Phase

The care of the patient does not stop at discharge but continues after. The patient may encounter problems after they start chemotherapy or radiotherapy. Peristomal hernias or other possible stoma complications may develop and result in the disturbance of daily activities. Help from colorectal nurse specialists/stoma nurses will come in handy with constant continuity of care even after discharge.

15 Transdisciplinary Stoma Care

Introducing stoma support group to patients and encouraging them to join serves the objective of letting them know that they are not alone and that there are others who suffer the same condition as them. The older ostomists can share their experiences with a new member during the meeting. The support group also provides education programmes to educate them on common stoma complications and on management that may be required while living with the stoma. The support group serves as a platform for them to mingle and learn from each other. Subsequently, the cycle of care can continue, and the new ostomist can then be given the opportunity to become an ambassador to other patients who are planning for surgery with stoma.

Conclusion

In a transdisciplinary team, every member of the team plays an important and dedicated role to ensure that holistic care is provided to a patient undergoing surgery with stoma creation. Everyone in the team enhances their role with the knowledge of each other's roles and flags out suggestions best for the patient. Each member contributes to ensure that seamless and continuous care is provided from the preoperative phase until after discharge. Having each healthcare professional's input paves the way for a new ostomist to achieve early recovery and independence in stoma self-care.

References

Borwell B (2009) Continuity of care for the stoma patient: psychological considerations. Br J Community Nurs 14(8):326–331

Gesaro AD (2012) Self-care and patient empowerment in stoma management. Gastrointest Nurs 10(2):19–23

Slater RC (2010) Managing quality of life in the older person with a stoma. Br J Community Nurs 15(10):480–485

Sprunk E, Alteneder RR (2000) The impact of an ostomy on sexuality. Clin J Oncol Nurs 4(2):85–88

William J (2006) Sexual health: case study of patient who has undergone stoma formation. Br J Nurs 15(14):760–763

Williams J (2012a) Patient stoma care: educational theory in practice. Br J Nurs 21(13):786–794

Williams J (2012b) Stoma care: intimacy and body image issues. Pract Nurs 23(2):91–93

Healing and Psychosocial Issues Surrounding Surgery

16

Mary Rockwood Lane and Michael Samuels

Take-Home Pearls
- Psychosocial techniques speed recovery.
- Guided imagery speeds recovery.
- Art making promotes spiritual healing.
- Preoperative education speeds healing.

16.1 Introduction

Recent psychosocial advances in colorectal surgery have greatly reduced hospital stay and anxiety and improved postsurgical recovery. The advances have put together education, preoperative care, postoperative care, pain control, mobility, and postsurgical attitude education. This chapter addresses the psychosocial aspects of colorectal surgery care to optimize the experience and healing of patients.

Research studies have shown that preoperative education greatly improves results. Showing patients a video or using teaching tools to show what will happen reduces fear and anxiety and improves healing. The mechanisms for this are now becoming clear. Education reduces anxiety, shifts patients to autonomic parasympathetic relaxation response, and promotes endorphins and immune system modulators.

For example, research has shown that education is more effective if undertaken in the preoperative setting. It results in shorter times to stoma proficiency and earlier

---

M.R. Lane, PhD, RN (✉)
University of Florida College of Nursing, Gainesville, FL, USA
e-mail: maryrockwoodlane@gmail.com

M. Samuels, MD
John F. Kennedy University, College of Holistic Medicine,
Pleasant Hill, CA 94523, USA

© Springer-Verlag Berlin Heidelberg 2015
K.-Y. Tan (ed.), *Transdisciplinary Perioperative Care in Colorectal Surgery:*
An Integrative Approach, DOI 10.1007/978-3-662-44020-9_16

discharge from the hospital. It also reduces stoma-related interventions in the community and has no adverse effects on patient well-being.

Since the beginning of enhanced recovery programs more than a decade ago, programs have become widely used following colorectal surgery. Most of the parts of these programs come from solid evidence and are derived from peer-reviewed trials. These programs use different tools to reduce the stress of surgery with the aim of improving outcomes and speeding up recovery post surgery. The most important factors before surgery are teaching correct expectations and optimizing any associated diseases. During the surgery, the use of short-acting anesthetics, the maintenance of normal body temperature, and the increased use of minimal access surgery all help.

Postsurgical care can be optimized with good pain control, early mobilization, and early feeding. This way of treating patients reduces hospital stay to 2–4 days. There is evidence that the results from the implementation of an enhanced recovery program do not cause deterioration in quality of life or costs more to implement. It is clear that education builds confidence and improves overall outcome of many variables.

16.2 Jean Watson's 10 Caritas Steps to Caring, Loving, and Compassion

Jean Watson, at the Watson Caring Science Institute, has created 10 processes to guide us in implementing caring science in healthcare systems and hospitals. These processes are constantly changing – organic and experiential. They provide us with the ability to articulate and create a language to shift our way of being. They are derived from the essential nature of nursing as proposed by Florence Nightingale a hundred years ago. They are from the clinical essence of what nurses are actually doing but don't often describe. They make the invisible become visible. In this chapter, the 10 Caritas steps will be our guide to creating psychosocial care to optimize healing and recover. This chapter will take you through the steps in a practical, concrete, direct way to help you create optimal psychosocial care.

Using Jean Watson's 10 Caritas processes to implement psychosocial care for colorectal patients

1. Cultivating loving kindness, compassion, and equanimity with self and others. This process is basic to psychosocial care. When the caregiver has all acts come from loving kindness, the patients relax, go into the physiology of healing, and have less side effects and heal better.
2. Being authentically present, enabling the belief system and subjective world of self and others. This step validates each person's world and honors their fears, loves, and wishes for healing.
3. Cultivating your own spiritual practices beyond ego and self to authentic transpersonal presence. This process allows the spirit to heal, not you. It is crucial to optimal healing.

16 Healing and Psychosocial Issues Surrounding Surgery

4. Sustaining loving trusting caring relationships.
5. Allowing the expression of feelings and authentically listening and holding another person's story for them. This process relieves anxiety and fear and allows optimum communication with caregivers.
6. Creative solution seeking through the caring process. Full use of self with all ways of knowing/doing/being. Engaging in human caring practices and modalities. This process encourages creativity in problem solving which will result in different caring modalities for each person.
7. Authentic teaching and learning – staying within the other's frame of reference, shifting towards a health coaching model. This process is necessary to educate patients about colorectal issues.
8. Creating a healing environment – physical and nonphysical, a subtle environment of energy, consciousness, wholeness, beauty, and dignity.
9. Reverently respecting basic needs, intentional caring consciousness by touching the embodied spirit of another as a sacred practice, working with life force of another – honoring the mystery of life and death. This process is crucial after surgery with body issues of pain, discomfort, and fear.
10. Opening and attending to the spiritual and mysterious, unknown, and existential dimensions of all vicissitudes of life, death, suffering, pain, joy, transitions, and life change – allowing for a miracle. This process builds hope.

As you can see, the steps do not depend on your belief in a religion, psychological method but come from the spiritual part of you within. The techniques are based on the steps Jean Watson uses to teach nurses loving and caring in hospitals; they come from many of the world's wisdom traditions and from modern practices of psychology and conflict resolution. This model results in a total change of care and caregiving to create a psychosocial model of care as opposed to a mechanical dogmatic model.

This chapter will focus on two advanced therapeutic techniques for surgery optimization, guided imagery and art interventions. These new techniques have been shown to advance care. They are examples of newer techniques of psychosocial care that changes colorectal care with enhanced recovery and comfort.

16.3 Guided Imagery

Patients undergoing surgery often experience a loss of control and can feel more like victims than patients. Anxiety, fear of the unknown, fear of pain, dependency, uncertainty, and helplessness are common feelings which can make pain worse. Stress can also add to prolonged postoperative recovery and suppress the patient's immune system. To help gain an enhanced feeling of control, patients can learn psychosocial skills including guided imagery, relaxation, and positive outcome expectations.

Guided imagery is a technique that draws on the images in the brain to change psychological and physiological states. The patient listens to mp3 or CD and holds l image that help focus concentration. This state of consciousness produces relaxation and a sense of well-being. Patients can use guided imagery to deal with anxiety, depression, and stressful situations. Guided imagery has also been shown to strengthen the immune system and enhance healing. Guided imagery can help promote relaxation, clear the mind, and change the body's physiological and psychologically state

Diane Tusek, Department of Colorectal Surgery, the Cleveland Clinic Foundation, Ohio, has demonstrated that guided imagery provides a significant advance in the care of patients undergoing elective colorectal surgery.

Tusek states that guided imagery uses images in the mind as thoughts to influence psychological and physiological states. Research studies have shown that guided imagery can decrease anxiety, analgesic requirements, and length of stay for surgical patients. She performed a study to determine whether guided imagery in the perioperative period could improve the outcome of colorectal surgery patients.

She conducted a prospective, randomized trial of patients undergoing their first elective colorectal surgery at a tertiary care center (Tusek et al. 1997). Patients were randomly assigned into one of two groups. Group 1 received standard perioperative care, and group 2 listened to a guided imagery tape 3 days preoperatively; a music-only tape during induction, during surgery, and postoperatively in the recovery room; a guided imagery tape during each of the first six postoperative days. Both groups had postoperative patient-controlled analgesia. All patients rated their levels of pain and anxiety daily, on a linear analog scale of 0–100. Total narcotic consumption, time of first bowel movement, length of stay, and number of patients with complications were also recorded.

Virtually all of the guided imagery patients reported that they appreciated using the tapes and attributed benefits including improved quality of sleep, speeded recovery, and reduced anxiety and pain after surgery. Most believed that all patients having major abdominal surgery should have the opportunity to use the guided imagery tapes.

The conclusion of her study was that guided imagery significantly reduced postoperative anxiety, pain, and narcotic requirements of colorectal surgery and increased patient satisfaction. Thus, guided imagery is a simple and low-cost adjunct in the care of patients undergoing elective colorectal surgery that can easily be implemented into cancer care in any center with dramatic results.

Patients who undergo surgery usually experience fear and apprehension about their surgical procedures. Dealing with this is a crucial and basic psychosocial preparation for surgery.

Eric Gonzales at the Wilford Hall Medical Center, Lackland Air Force Base, San Antonio, Texas, USA, did research to evaluate the effects of guided imagery on postoperative outcomes in patients undergoing same-day surgical procedures (Gonzales et al. 2010). Forty-four adults scheduled for head and neck procedures were randomly assigned into two groups for this single-blind investigation. Anxiety and baseline pain levels were documented preoperatively. Both groups received 28 min of privacy, during which subjects in the experimental group listened to a guided imagery compact disk (CD), but control group patients received no intervention. Data were collected on pain and narcotic consumption at 1- and 2-h postoperative intervals. In addition, discharge times from the postoperative anesthesia care unit (PACU) and the ambulatory procedure unit and patient satisfaction scores were collected.

He found that the change in anxiety levels decreased significantly in the guided imagery group. At 2 h, the guided imagery group reported significantly less pain. In addition, length of stay in PACU in the guided imagery group was an average of 9 min less than in the control group. The use of guided imagery can significantly reduce preoperative anxiety, which can result in less postoperative pain and earlier PACU discharge times.

16.3.1 Seeing with the Mind's Eye, How to Do Guided Imagery

Thus, research has shown that guided imagery is a basic psychosocial tool in healing. In ancient times this tool was not called guided imagery; it was called ecstatic journeying, seeing into the spiritual world, prayer, and trance. In terms of modern psychology, altered states of consciousness, prayer, meditation, hypnosis, and guided imagery are all ways patients can see into their intuitive inner world and heal. They all change people's body's physiology to produce a healing state. Patients can easily learn to do guided imagery; this tool is part of their way of being already. We all do guided imagery. You do guided imagery already when you picture something in your mind's eye to remember, to make plans, to practice a sport, or get a creative idea. Many people do it daily as part of yoga, sports, and creativity.

Guided imagery is a basic life skill like riding a bicycle. Once people learn it in their body, it's easy and they don't forget it. Guided imagery is extremely useful for healing, achieving goals, doing sports, and enhancing spiritual life. There are no absolutes, no right way, no one way to do guided imagery.

Guided imagery is a visualization, a meditation technique which uses the mind to change consciousness (Fig. 16.1). It is ancient and comes from and is still part of religions all over the world, from Egypt, Sumer and Greece, from Tibetan Buddhism, Christian/Judaic/Moslem, prayer and from Hinduism. It is used to deepen the experience of prayer and ceremony. Guided imagery exercises are now used in hospitals, cancer centers, and surgery units worldwide to help healing. It is used to help you see into your inner world, into your visionary space, and to moving healing energy in your body.

The way guided imagery is used today in healing centers is useful for any patient in the postsurgical cafe. Doing guided imagery is easier than writing about it or reading about it. Many people who use guided imagery divide the process into these parts:

1. The first part is abdominal breathing.
2. The second relaxation.
3. The third deepening.
4. The fourth is the subject of the imagery, the intent, and the content.
5. The fifth is the return and grounding.
6. The final step is an instruction for carrying something forward into your life.

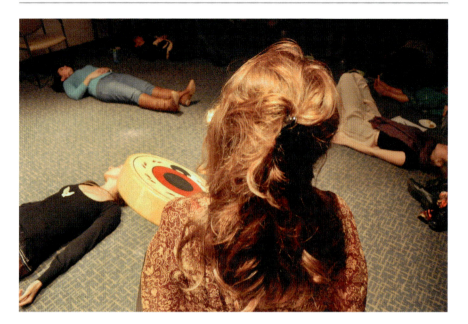

Fig. 16.1 Mary Rockwood Lane doing guided imagery with nursing students at University of Florida College of Nursing

Guided imagery is also used to create heart coherence. The authors teach patients to imagine the heart and gratitude in many guided imageries. Each part is important; as patients get better and better, they can shorten the introductions and closing somewhat if they wish. The relaxation takes place instantly after many practices.

16.3.2 Research Findings on Health Benefits of Guided Imagery

- Helps physical symptoms
- Promotes relaxation
- Helps stress reduction
- Decreases anxiety in preop and cancer situations
- Decreases cortisol (stress hormone) levels
- Increases positive outlook/mood
- Improves depression
- Relieves fatigue
- Decreases pain, post-op and in chronic illnesses
- Decreases the need for post-op analgesics
- Enhances immune function
- Improves comfort during radiotherapy for cancer patients
- Makes the chemotherapy experience significantly more positive
- Decreases symptoms of post-traumatic stress disorder for veterans
- Improves abstinence rates for smoking cessation
- Increases feelings of spiritual connectedness

16.4 How to Be an Artist for Psychosocial Healing

The second tool for psychosocial improvement of colorectal surgery is art. Art and healing is an advanced therapeutic method to enhance psychosocial healing. There are simple steps to making art for healing. Any patient can do it; they do it already. This advice about making art for psychosocial healing is derived from work with creativity, spirituality, and healthcare at University of Florida College of Nursing and College of Medicine (Fig. 16.2). As cofounder and codirector of Arts In Medicine University of Florida, the author developed ways to use creativity to heal patients with life-threatening illness (Fig. 16.3). These methods were the subject of peer-reviewed research. The process of making art to heal applies to psychosocial methods for colorectal care.

The arts offer accessible, nonverbal, and universal tools for facilitating mind-body health, and they are easy to implement in medical, educational, and recreational settings. While the arts themselves are healing, even greater value can be obtained from the arts when a therapeutic dimension is added. Those who use the arts as therapy work through metaphor by focusing on the process of expression and the self that is revealed through it (Figs. 16.4 and 16.5). By reflecting on unconscious themes that emerge, the arts can heighten self-awareness, which allows for behavior change.

The wide-range health value of the arts and the creative arts therapies is supported by a growing body of well-done scientific studies, a larger body of case studies, and observations by experts. For example, the arts have been used to

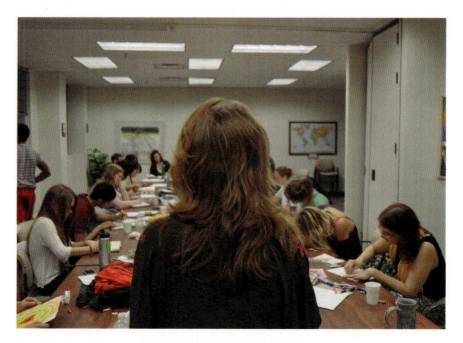

Fig. 16.2 Mary Rockwood Lane teaching nursing students how to make art with patients

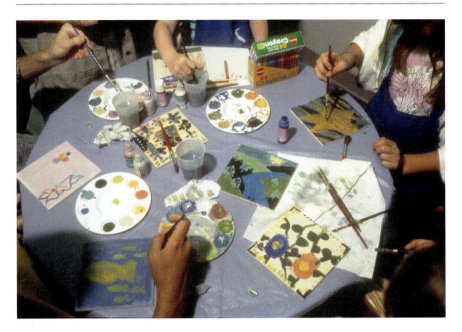

Fig. 16.3 Cancer patients painting tiles in a studio

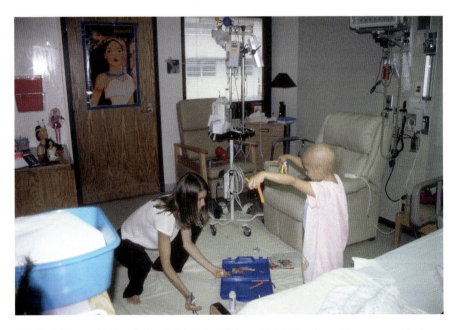

Fig. 16.4 Dancer in Shands Arts in Medicine, Gainesville Fl., dancing with a cancer patient

improve recovery from injury, mental dysfunction, pain, depression, stress, self-esteem, quality of life during hospice care, anxiety in normal medical care and medical procedures, substance abuse, child and adolescent behavior and development, immune function, emotional trauma, and future risk of violence.

16 Healing and Psychosocial Issues Surrounding Surgery

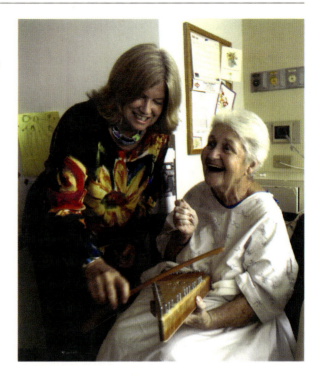

Fig. 16.5 Musician in residence at Shands Arts in Medicine, Gainesville Fl., playing music with a patient

Since the inception of arts and healing programs in hospitals, many new publications have emerged that include rigorous randomized, controlled trials; review articles that summarize studies on a specific subject; and meta-analytic studies that draw conclusions by analyzing the combined findings of similar studies.

16.4.1 Steps to Art Healing

There are three steps to using art to heal:

- Reclaiming the inner artist
  - Realize you want to be an artist to heal.
  - Let go of insecurities. Anyone can do it, we are all artists.
  - Let go of fear and your inner critic.
  - Say to yourself, "I am an artist to heal."
  - Broaden your artistry to include your whole life.
  - Realize that being an artist is a natural human ability.
- Making your life your studio
  - Create space in your busy life for creativity.
  - Make a commitment to make art for healing.
  - Regard art as an important thing you do to heal.
  - Begin with yourself as the focus of your healing process.
  - Make your studio beautiful.
  - Put in personal things to make it deeply yours.

- Make it convenient and accessible.
- Create a routine to make art every day.
- Give yourself attention and listen to yourself.
- Create a boundary around yourself.
- Create sacred space with a prayer or altar.
- Choosing a media
  - Don't worry about which media you choose.
  - Remember a time when you were most creative as a child. Which media did you use then? Let go of voices from your childhood of criticism, you can do it.
  - Which media resonates with your flow of energy?
  - Which material comes to your mind first?
  - Which process comes to your mind first?
  - What is your secret desire?
  - Allow yourself to experiment.
  - Be open to choices ahead.
  - Now, choose one and begin.

Patients can use art to produce psychosocial healing on all levels. Art has been used for surgery, PTSD, and trauma and is routinely used in cancer centers worldwide as advanced therapeutics. Because art and healing changes your body's physiology, it is effective in physical healing. There is a comprehensive research report in the *Journal of Public Health* that looked at all the recent research and described proven ways art healed (Stuckey and Nobel 2010). The results showed that art helped many parameters that promote healing and quality of life.

In many research studies, art and healing has been shown to:

- Enhance social support
- Enhance psychological strength
- Help people gain new insights about their illness experience
- Lessen social dysfunction
- Express complex emotions (anxiety, isolation, fear)
- Cope with trauma
- Experience joy
- Connect with the spirit
- Help depression
- Uplift the spirit
- Enhance spirituality
- Reduce stress, depression, and anger
- Increase immune function
- Increase endorphins
- Alter perception of pain
- Induce mind-body changes

It is clear that art and healing is a valuable tool for promoting psychosocial support in colorectal patients. Combined with guided imagery and education before

16 Healing and Psychosocial Issues Surrounding Surgery

and after surgery, the patients can lessen anxiety, lessen pain medication use, reduce hospital stay, and increase quality of life and promote more rapid healing. Psychosocial care is a necessary and basic part to modern advanced healing.

Conclusion

Psychosocial aspects are important to consider in promoting healing after surgery. These aspects cannot be ignored by the caregiver and surgical team. Guided imagery and the use of art are important tools in this process.

References

Gonzales EA, Ledesma RJ, McAllister DJ, Perry SM, Dyer CA, Maye JP (2010) Effects of guided imagery on postoperative outcomes in patients undergoing same-day surgical procedures: a randomized, single-blind study. AANA J 78(3):181–188

Stuckey HL, Nobel J (2010) The connection between Art, healing, and public health: a review of current literature. Am J Public Health 100(2):254–263

Tusek DL, Church JM, Strong SA, Grass JA, Fazio VW (1997) Guided imagery: a significant advance in the care of patients undergoing elective colorectal surgery. Dis Colon Rectum 40(2):172–178

Index

A
Academy of Nutrition and Dietetics, malnutrition, 43
Access-related sepsis, 69–70
ACTH level, laparoscopic surgery, 122, 123
Activities of daily living (ADLs), elderly patient, 17–18
Acute postoperative phase, rehabilitation, 111–112
Ageing. *See also* Elderly surgical patients
   biological, 14
   changes to respiratory system, 14
   and medication, 93–94
   process of, 13
American Society for Parenteral and Enteral Nutrition (ASPEN)
   diagnostic characteristics, 43
   routine radiograph, 69
   SGA, 46
American Society of Anesthesiologists (ASA) scores, 123–124
Amsterdam criteria II, 141, 142
Anaesthetic care
   antimicrobial prophylaxis, 81
   management, 81, 89–90
   perioperative fluid management, 82–83
   PONV prevention, 81–82
   shared vision and goal, 5
   thromboembolism prophylaxis, 80–81
Anal endosonography. *See* Endoanal ultrasound (EAUS)
Anal fistula, 171–172
   fibrin glue, 176–177
   FiLaC, 179
   fistula plug, 177–178
   LIFT, 179–181
   preoperative assessment, 172–174
   surgical management
      fistulotomy, 174–175
      mucosal advancement flap, 176

seton, 175
   VAAFT, 178–179
Analgesia
   in critical care, 99
   epidural, 6, 81, 82, 86, 88
   opioids for, 96
   postoperative, 84–85
Anesthesia
   and aspiration, 49
   immediate oral intake, 58
   laparoscopic colorectal surgery, 127–128
Anorexia, ageing, 16–17
Anticoagulation effects, 96
Anti-epidermal growth factor receptor (Anti-EGFR), 205
Antihypertensive medications, 94–97
Antimicrobial prophylaxis, 81
Anti-vascular endothelial growth factor (Anti-VEGF), 205
Arginine, 60
Art healing
   for psychosocial improvement, 251–253
   steps to, 253–255
ASA scores. *See* American Society of Anesthesiologists (ASA) scores
ASPECCT trial, panitumumab, 205

B
Barthel scale, 17
Basic activities of daily living, elderly patient, 17
Bethesda criteria, 141, 142
Bevacizumab, anti-VEGF, 205
Bilateral transversus abdominis plane block, 85, 90
Biofeedback
   fecal incontinence, 164
   PFMT and, 166

© Springer-Verlag Berlin Heidelberg 2015
K.-Y. Tan (ed.), *Transdisciplinary Perioperative Care in Colorectal Surgery: An Integrative Approach*, DOI 10.1007/978-3-662-44020-9

Index

Bleeding
  hypotension, 96
  laparoscopic colectomy, 122
  metastatic colon, 203
Body image, stoma care, 232–233
Bolus feeding, 61
BOND-2 trial, bevacizumab, 205
BOND-1 trial, cetuximab, 205
Bowel incontinence
  in elderly, 165–166
  pathophysiology and types, 159–160
Bowel manipulation, in laparoscopic surgery,
    122
Bowel movement, in critical care, 100
Bowel obstruction, PJS, 152
Bowel preparation, 80

C
Calcium, requirement, 51
Cancer and Aging Research Group (CARG)
    study, 190
Capecitabine and irinotecan (CAPIRI), 204
Capsule endoscopy, PJS, 152
Carbohydrate
  loading, preoperative factors, 80
  and PN, 66
Carcinomatosis peritonei, 212
Caregiver
  appointments for patients, 116
  encouraging, 238
  palliative care, 216
  rehabilitation, 79
  stoma care, 31, 239–240
Care planning, elderly surgical patients,
    23–24
CARG study. *See* Cancer and Aging Research
    Group (CARG) study
Catheter-related sepsis, 69–70
Central PN (CPN), 61–63
Central venous catheter (CVC), 63
Central venous pressure (CVP), 63
Cetuximab, anti-EGFR, 205
CGA. *See* Comprehensive Geriatric
    Assessment (CGA)
Charlson weighted comorbidity index, 124
Chemotherapy
  colon and rectal cancer, 200, 203–204
  with hyperthermia, 215
  toxicity, prediction, 190
Chemotherapy Risk Assessment Scale
    for High-Age Patients (CRASH)
    score, 190
Chest X-ray (CXR), 209–210

Chromium, requirement, 52
Cleveland Clinic Florida Fecal Incontinence
    Score (CCF-FIS), 160
Cochrane review
  metastatic colon and rectal cancer, 200
  postoperative factors, 86
Cognitive impairment, ADL, 18
Colectomy
  FAP, 147
  with ileorectal anastomosis, 143
  vs. IRA and RPC, 146
Colonoscopy, 143–145
Colorectal Adenoma/Carcinoma Prevention
    Programme 2 (CAPP2), 143
Colorectal nurse specialist
  body image, 232
  counselling session, 230
  fears and concerns, 231
  rehabilitation phase, 242
  role in stoma care, 229
  society acceptance, 235
Colorectal surgeon, FI, 159, 168
Communication
  effective, 5–6
  between healthcare team and patient,
    226–227
  heightened, 21
  in multidisciplinary nursing, 31
  problems, fecal incontinence, 166
  role enrichment, 34
  tools, 10
  in transdisciplinary nursing, 33
Community nursing, 114
Community primary care with support
    services, 192
Comprehensive Geriatric
    Assessment (CGA), 189, 190
Computed tomographic (CT) scan
  bleeding, 203
  disadvantage of, 206
  metastatic colon and rectal cancer,
    198, 199
  preoperative workup, 132
Continuous infusion, 61
Coordinated health-care
    delivery, 192
Copper, requirement, 52
Counselling
  inadequate, 144
  MSW providing, 228
  patients on side effects, 98
  postoperative tools, 5
  preoperative, 79, 230, 238
CPN. *See* Central PN (CPN)

CRASH score. *See* Chemotherapy Risk Assessment Scale for High-Age Patients (CRASH) score
CR-POSSUM score, 124
Cryptoglandular theory, 171, 172
Crystalline amino acids, PN, 66
CT thorax, 209–211
Cultural and religious beliefs, stoma care, 237–238
Cumulative summation (CUSUM) methodology, 37, 38
CVC. *See* Central venous catheter (CVC)
CVP. *See* Central venous pressure (CVP)
CXR. *See* Chest X-ray (CXR)
Cytokine response, 122
Cytoreductive surgery (CRS)
    outcomes, 215
    patient selection, 213
    peritoneal metastases, 212
    PSDSS, 214
Cytotoxic chemotherapy agents, 143

D

Decision-making process
    by care team, 192
    for elderly surgical patients, 23–24
    patients profile, 3
    PE surgery, 133
Decompression
    of colon proximal, 124–126
    nasogastric, 58
Defecography, fecal incontinence, 164
Dehydration
    perioperative fluid management, 82
    renal function, 14
Dementia
    and ageing, 15
    poor appetite, 16
Desmoid disease, FAP, 150
Dextrose, and PN, 66
Diabetics, preoperative considerations, 96
Dietician
    in FI, 168
    in stoma care, 228
Digestive system, and ageing, 15
Discharge phase, stoma care, 240–242
Disease-by-disease model, 188
Drug-drug interactions
    concurrent issues, 98
    probability of, 94, 95
Drug interactions, postoperative care, 96
Dumping syndrome, 61
Duodenal disease, FAP, 149

E

Early mobilisation, 86, 87
    physiotherapy clinical experience, 116
    postsurgical rehabilitation, 112
Eastern Cooperative Oncology Group, 190
EAUS. *See* Endoanal ultrasound (EAUS)
Edentulism, elderly patient, 17
Education
    in clinical nutrition, 45–46
    and healing, 245
    on stoma care, 240
Elderly surgical patients
    activities of daily living, 17–18
    approach to, 94–95
    care planning, 23–24
    complexities of, 13–14
    decision-making, 23–24
    family engagement, 24
    frailty and geriatric syndromes, 15–16
    Khoo Teck Puat Hospital Geriatric Surgery Service (*see* Khoo Teck Puat Hospital Geriatric Surgery Service)
    laparoscopic colorectal surgery in, 126–127
    nutritional aspects, 16–17
    physiological changes, 14–15
    prehabilitation in, 127
    psychosocial aspects, 18
    transdisciplinary approach in, 18–19
Electrolytes
    abnormalities, 67–68
    and PN, 66–67
    requirements, function and deficiency, 50–51
Employment, stoma care, 236
EN. *See* Enteral nutrition (EN)
Endoanal ultrasound (EAUS)
    anal fistula, 173
    fecal incontinence, 163
Endoscopic management, duodenal disease, 149
Energy expenditure equations, 49
Enhanced Recovery After Surgery (ERAS)
    laparoscopic colorectal surgery, 128–129
    transdisciplinary management, 114
Enhanced recovery program, 77–78
    anaesthetic factors, 80–83
    intraoperative factors, 83–84
    postoperative factors, 84–86
    postsurgical care, 246
    preoperative factors, 79–80
    success/failure, 86, 88–89
Enteral feeding, PN, 69

Index

Enteral nutrition (EN)
  access-or catheter-related complications, 69–70
  enteral formulas, 62
  metabolic complications, 67–69
  postoperative nutrition therapy, 58–59
  practical approach to, 61
  preoperative nutrition therapy, 57, 58
Epidural analgesia, 6, 81, 82, 86, 88
ERAS. *See* Enhanced Recovery After Surgery (ERAS)
Esmolol, postoperative care, 97
European Society for Clinical Nutrition and Metabolism (ESPEN)
  energy requirements, 49
  immunonutrition therapy, 61
  preoperative nutritional support, 57
Evidence-based treatment, 2
Exercise, prehabilitation patients
  frequency/intensity, 108
  supervised *vs.* non-supervised setting, 108, 111
  time/duration, 108

F

Familial adenomatous polyposis (FAP)
  desmoid disease, 150
  diagnosis, 144–145
  duodenal disease, 149
  genetics, 144
  multidisciplinary surgical decision-making, 148
  mutations, 145
  risk stratification for, 140
  surgical intervention, 145
  surgical options, 146–147
  surveillance, 145
Familial colorectal cancer (CRC), 139–140
  evaluating risk, 140–141
  FAP (*see* Familial adenomatous polyposis (FAP))
  juvenile polyposis, 152
  Lynch syndrome, 141–143
  MAP, 150–151
  PJS, 151–152
  serrated polyposis, 152
  type X, 143
FAP. *See* Familial adenomatous polyposis (FAP)
"FASTHUGS" mnemonic, 98
Fasting
  preoperative factors, 80
  before surgery, 57

Fast-track pathways, 77, 78, 89
  perioperative care, 128–129
Fears and concerns, stoma care, 231
Fecal incontinence (FI)
  assessment, initial management, and referral, 160–163
  awareness and role of education, 159
  in elderly, 165–166
  etiology, 162
  evaluation and specialist management, 163–165
  pathophysiology, 159–160
  prevalence, risk factors, and economics, 158
  transdisciplinary team role, 166–168
  traumatic vaginal delivery, 159
Feeding, in critical care, 99
Ferguson technique, 182
FI. *See* Fecal incontinence (FI)
Fibrin glue, anal fistula, 176–177
FiLaC. *See* Fistula tract laser closure (FiLaC)
Financial issue, stoma care, 236–237
Fistula plug, anal fistula, 177–178
Fistula tract laser closure (FiLaC), 179
Fistulotomy, anal fistula, 174–175
Fluids
  balance in critical care, 100
  management, 82–83
  overloading, 84
  and PN, 66–67
5-Flurouracil (5-FU), colon/rectal cancer, 204
FOLFIRI
  with bevacixumab, 212
  metastatic colon, 204
FOLFOX
  with bevacixumab, 212
  metastatic colon, 204
  panitumumab, 205
FOLFOXIRI, metastatic colon, 204
Folic acid, requirement, 56
Frailty
  laparoscopic surgery, 124
  syndromes, elderly patient, 15–16

G

Gastric feeding, 61
Gastrointestinal (GI) endoscopy, FAP, 144
Genetic testing, 204
Geriatric assessment
  CGA, 189
  chemotherapy toxicity, 190
  life expectancy, 187–189
  multidisciplinary teams, 191–193

in oncology, 189–190
preoperative evaluation, 190–191
specialty care and primary care, 193–194
Geriatric physician, FI, 168
Geriatric Surgery Service (GSS)
of Alexandra Health, 37–38
medication reconciliation, 94
Geriatric syndromes, elderly patient, 15–16
Glucose, in critical care, 100
Glutamine, 60
Goal-directed haemodynamic management, 82
Goodsall rule, anal fistula, 172
Guided imagery, 247–249
ecstatic journeying, 249
health benefits of, 250
process, 249–250

H
Haemorrhoidopexy, stapled, 182–183
Haemorrhoids
emerging technology, 183
excisional, 182
prolapsed, 182–183
RBL, 181
THD, 183
treatment of, 181
Healing, 245
art healing, 251–255
enhanced recovery programs, 246
guided imagery, 247–250
Jean Watson's 10 Caritas processes,
246–247
Healthcare
caring science in, 246–247
infrastructure, complexities, 4
professionals role in stoma care, 227–229
Heart, and ageing, 14
Helicobacter pylori infection, 17
Heparin-induced thrombocytopaenia, 80
Hepatic metastasectomy, 207–208
Hepatic metastases
hepatic metastasectomy, 207–208
liver metastases detection, 206–207
outcomes, 208–209
regional hepatic therapies, 208
surgical therapy, 208
Hereditary non-polyposis colorectal cancer
(HNPCC). *See* Lynch syndrome
HET bipolar device, 183
Heterogeneity, in patient characteristics, 105
Holistic care, surgical patients, 3
Home therapy, transdisciplinary
management, 114

Hormone response, laparoscopic
colorectal surgery, 122
HubBLe trial, THD, 183
Hydralazine, postoperative care, 97
Hyperalimentation, PN, 68
Hyperlipidaemia, 35–40
Hyperplastic polyposis. *See* Serrated
polyposis
Hypertension
case study, 35–40
postoperative, 96
Hyperthermic intraperitoneal chemotherapy
(HIPEC), 212
outcomes, 215
patient selection, 213
Hypothermia prevention, 83

I
Ileorectal anastomosis (IRA)
vs. colectomy and RPC, 146
colectomy with, 143
FAP, 147
Immediate postoperative period, 114
Immediate preoperative management,
49, 57
Immune response, laparoscopic colorectal
surgery, 122
Immunonutrition, 59–61
Implanted port CVC, 63
Incontinence nurse, FI, 168
Instrumental activities of daily living, 17–18
Integumentary system, and ageing, 15
Interdisciplinary care, 7–8
International Continence Society, fecal
incontinence, 159
Interpersonal skill, role enrichment, 34
Interprofessional competency, 9–10
Intraoperative factors
hypothermia prevention, 83
intraperitoneal drains avoidance, 84
management, 89
nasogastric tubes avoidance, 83
surgical factors, 83
Intraperitoneal drains, avoidance, 84
Intravenous antihypertensive medications, 97
Iron, requirement, 53
'I'-shaped personnel, 30

J
Jean Watson's 10 Caritas processes, 246–247
Journal of Public Health, art healing, 254
Juvenile polyposis, 152

K

Karnofsky performance status (KPS), 190
Katz ADL scale, 17
Khoo Teck Puat Hospital Geriatric Surgery
    Service, 19–20
  case study of MdmGKK, 24–26
  coordination of care, 21, 22
  goal-setting identification, 20
  heightened communication, 21
  patient involvement, 20, 21
  physiotherapy clinical experience,
    115–116
  post discharge care, 22–23
  role enhancements, 22
KK in vitro fertilisation (KKIVF) centre, 234
KPS. *See* Karnofsky performance
    status (KPS)
K-RAS mutation, 204, 205

L

Labetalol, postoperative care, 97
Laparoscopic colorectal surgery, 119
  anesthesia, 127–128
  in elderly patients, 126–127
  ERAS, 128–129
  immune, cytokine, and hormone response,
    122
  less invasive nature, 121–122
  penetration rate of, 121
  stenosis caused by tumor, 124–126
  surgical risks evaluation, 122–124
  take-up rate of, 120
Laparoscopic fast track (LAFA), 128, 129
Large bowel obstruction, 200
LCT. *See* Long-chain triglycerides (LCT)
Leucovorin, colon/rectal cancer, 204
Life expectancy, geriatric oncology, 187–188
Ligation of intersphincteric fistula tract
    (LIFT), 179–181
Lipid, and PN, 65, 66
Liver
  dysfunction, 68
  metastases, 206–207
  resection, 207
LMWH, thromboembolism
    prophylaxis, 80
Long-chain triglycerides (LCT), 66
Lynch syndrome
  diagnosis, 141–142
  genetics, 141
  medical intervention, 143
  surgical intervention, 143
  surveillance, 143

M

M1a, 198
Magnesium, requirement, 50
Magnetic resonance imaging (MRI)
  anal fistula, 173–174
  fecal incontinence, 163–164
  hepatic lesions, 206
  metastatic colon and rectal
    cancer, 198, 199
  PE surgery, 133
Malnourished patients
  postoperative nutrition therapy
    for, 58–59
  preoperative nutrition therapy for, 57–58
Malnutrition
  definition of, 44
  elderly surgical patients, 16
  influence on surgical outcomes, 43–45
  nutrition risk screening, 46–48
  transdisciplinary clinical nutrition
    education, 45–49
Malnutrition Universal Screening Tool
    (MUST), 46
Manganese, requirement, 52
M1b, 198
MCT. *See* Medium-chain triglycerides (MCT)
Medical professionals, stoma care, 227
Medical social worker (MSW),
    stoma care, 228
Medication
  ageing and, 93–94
  in critical care, 99–100
Medication reconciliation (MR), 94, 152
Medium-chain triglycerides (MCT), 66
Memorial Sloan Kettering Cancer Center
    (MSKCC) Geriatric Service, 191
Metastatic colon, 197–198
  Anti-EGFR, 205
  Anti-VEGF, 205
  bleeding, 203
  chemotherapy, 203–204
  obstruction, 200–203
  organ-specific metastasis
    (*see* Organ-specific metastasis)
  palliative care, 215–217
  perforation, 200
  presentation, 198–199
  primary colon, 199–200
Mid-thoracic epidural, 84, 90
Milligan-Morgan technique, 182
Mini Nutritional Assessment (MNA), 46
Mismatch repair (MMR) genes, 141–142
MNA. *See* Mini Nutritional
    Assessment (MNA)

Index

Model for End-Stage Liver Disease (MELD) score, 207
MR. *See* Medication reconciliation (MR)
MRI. *See* Magnetic resonance imaging (MRI)
MSW. *See* Medical social worker (MSW)
Mucosal advancement flap, 176
Multicentred randomised control trial, 183
Multidisciplinary care
    availability of, 19
    drawback in, 166
    fast-paced, 6
    nurse specialists in, 30–31
    pitfalls
        completion and follow-through, 6–7
        effective communication, 5–6
        planning and coordination, 5
        shared vision and goal, 4–5
        team understanding, 6
    surgical decision-making, 148
    with teams, 191–193
    vs. transdisciplinary and interdisciplinary, 7–8
Multidisciplinary nursing, 30–32
Multimodal surgical approach, 89, 90
MUST. *See* Malnutrition Universal Screening Tool (MUST)
MUTYH-associated polyposis (MAP), 150–151

N
Nasogastric tubes
    avoidance, intraoperative factors, 83
    decompression, 58
Nervous system, and ageing, 15
Nitroglycerin, postoperative care, 97
Non-arterial therapy, 208
Nonsteroidal anti-inflammatory drugs (NSAIDs), 98
Non-tunneled CVC, 63
NST. *See* Nutrition support team (NST)
Nucleotides, 60
Nursing care
    integration of, 24–26
    multidisciplinary nursing, 30–32
    outcomes of, 37
    transdisciplinary nursing, 32–33
Nutrition
    elderly surgical patients, 16–18
    postoperative management of, 58–59
    preoperative management of, 49, 57–58

requirements
    calculating, 48–49
    electrolytes, 50–51
    trace element, 52–53
    vitamin, 54–56
risk screening, 46–48
Nutritional care, postoperative factors, 85–86
Nutrition support team (NST), 45–46

O
Obstruction
    metastatic colon, 200–203
    by tumor, 124–126
Omega-3 fatty acids, 60
Ondansetron, 82
OPTIMOX trial, 204
Oral rehydration salt (ORS), stoma care, 228
Organ-specific metastasis
    hepatic metastases, 206–209
    peritoneal metastases, 212–215
    pulmonary metastases, 209–212
Overfeeding, PN/EN, 68

P
PACE study. *See* Preoperative Assessment of Cancer in the Elderly (PACE) study
Pain, palliative care, 216–217
Palliative care, 215–217
Panitumumab, 205
Parenteral nutrition (PN)
    access-or catheter-related complications, 69–70
    central access, 63
    cessation of, 69
    constituents, 65–67
    CPN, 61–62
    customization, 65
    metabolic complications, 67–69
    peripheral access, 63–65
    postoperative nutrition therapy, 59
    PPN, 62–63
    preoperative nutrition therapy, 57, 58
    ready-to-use formulas, 65
    venous access for, 63–65
Parks classification
    anal fistula, 172
    fecal incontinence, 160
Patient recovery, transdisciplinary management, 113–114
PCP. *See* Primary care physician (PCP)

Pelvic exenteration (PE) surgery
  planning preoperatively, 132–134
  postoperative care and quality of life,
    136–137
  reconstruction, 136
  sacrectomy, 134–135
  vascular resection and reconstruction,
    135–136
Pelvic floor muscle training (PFMT), 162
Perforation, 200
Perioperative care planning, 24
Perioperative fluid management, 82–83
Peripheral intravenous cannula, PN, 70
Peripherally inserted central catheter (PICC),
    63
Peripheral PN (PPN), 62–65
Peritoneal Carcinomatosis Index (PCI), 213,
    214
Peritoneal metastases
  detection of, 212–213
  outcomes, 215
  patient selection, 213–214
  surgical points, 214–215
Peritoneal Surface Disease and Severity Score
    (PSDSS), 213–214
Peritonectomy, 215
PE surgery. See Pelvic exenteration (PE)
    surgery
PET scans. See Positron emission tomography
    (PET) scans
Peutz-Jeghers syndrome (PJS), 151–152
PFMT. See Pelvic floor muscle training
    (PFMT)
Pharmacists
  ageing and medication, 93–94
  elderly surgical patient, approach to, 94–95
  in FI, 168
  postoperative care, 96–100
  preoperative considerations, 95–96
  roles, 98, 101
  in stoma care, 228–229
Phosphate, requirement, 51
Physiological and Operative Severity Score for
    the enUmeration of Mortality and
    morbidity (POSSUM), 191
Physiological changes, elderly surgical
    patients, 14–15
Physiotherapists, 104
  fecal incontinence, 166
  role in FI, 168
Physiotherapy, 104
  acute postoperative phase, 111–112
  clinical experience, 115–116
  prehabilitation (see Prehabilitation)
  rehabilitation (see Rehabilitation)

requirement for colorectal surgery,
    104–106
  subacute postoperative phase, 112
PICC. See Peripherally inserted central
    catheter (PICC)
PN. See Parenteral nutrition (PN)
Polypharmacy, 93
PONV. See Postoperative nausea and vomiting
    (PONV)
Poor appetite, ageing, 16–17
Poor dentition, elderly patient, 17
Positron emission tomography/computed
    tomography (PET/CT)
  hepatic metastases, 206–207
  metastatic colon and rectal cancer, 198,
    199
Positron emission tomography (PET) scans,
    133–134
POSSUM score, laparoscopic surgery, 124
Postoperative anesthesia care unit (PACU),
    249
Postoperative care, 96–98
  analgesia, 84–85
  audit, 86
  complications, 96
  early mobilization, 86, 87
  management
    of nutrition, 58–59
    satisfactory, 90
  nutritional care, 85–86
  physiotherapy, 106
  postoperative ileus prevention, 84
  rehabilitation, 104
  stoma
    caregiver and self-care training,
      239–240
    psychological support, 238
  symptoms and signs during second 12-h,
    89
Postoperative fluid therapy, 82
Postoperative ileus, prevention, 84
Postoperative nausea and vomiting (PONV),
    81–82
Post-op medication management, 96
Post-pyloric feeding, 61
Postsurgical outcomes, prehabilitation
    improving, 107–108
Potassium, requirement, 50
PPN. See Peripheral PN (PPN)
Practice-based learning, 34
Pre-anaesthetic medication, 81
Prehabilitation
  designing, 108–111
  duration of, 108
  in elderly patients, 127

Index 267

improving postsurgical outcomes, 107–108
integration of, 24–26
perioperative care, 24
preoperative factors, 79
protocols summary, 109–110
transdisciplinary management, 114
Preoperative Assessment of Cancer in the
Elderly (PACE) study, 191
Preoperative care
bowel preparation, 80
carbohydrate loading, 80
considerations, 95–96
counselling, 79
evaluation
older cancer patient, 190–191
and optimization, 79
fasting, 80
management of nutrition, 49, 57–58
stoma
body image, 232–233
counselling session, 230
cultural and religious beliefs, 237–238
employment and travelling, 236
fears and concerns, 231
financial issue, 236–237
independence in self-care, 234–235
placement, 231
sexuality and relationship, 233–234
society acceptance, 235–236
Primary care physician (PCP), 192–194
Primary colon, 199–200
Proctocolectomy, FAP, 145
Prophylactic colectomy, FAP, 145
Prophylactic surgery, Lynch syndrome, 143
Protein, and PN, 66
Psychological support, stoma care, 238
Psychosocial aspects, elderly surgical patients,
18
Pudendal nerve terminal motor latency
(PNTML), 163
Pulmonary metastases
outcomes, 211–212
pathophysiology, 209
in pulmonary staging, 209–211
selection criteria for surgery, 211
surgical points, 211
Pulmonary staging, pulmonary metastases,
209–211

R
Radiation-based therapies, 208
Radiofrequency ablation (RFA), 208
Radiologist, FI, 168
RBL. *See* Rubber band ligation (RBL)

RCTs
bowel preparation, 80
cochrane review of, 83
postoperative nutritional care, 85
Ready-to-use formulas, PN, 65
Rectal cancer
and metastatic colon (*see* Metastatic colon)
primary colon and, 199–200
surgical management for, 131
Refeeding syndrome, PN, 68
Regional hepatic therapies, 208
Rehabilitation
acute postoperative phase, 111–112
high-risk patients, 105–106
integration of, 24–26
low-risk patients, 105
measuring progress and success, 113
mobility and functional, 104
perioperative care, 24
postoperative, 104
stoma care, 242–243
subacute postoperative phase, 112
Rehabilitative hospitals, infrastructure, 4
Renal function
and ageing, 14–15
determine, 95
Respiratory function
and ageing, 14
management, 104
Restorative proctocolectomy (RPC)
vs. colectomy and IRA, 146
FAP, 147
multidisciplinary surgical decision-making,
148
Role enrichment
interpersonal and communication skill, 34
transdisciplinary care, 8–9
transdisciplinary nursing, 33
Role expansion
transdisciplinary care, 9
transdisciplinary nursing, 33
Role extension, 8
Role release
transdisciplinary care, 9
transdisciplinary nursing, 32
Role support, 9
RPC. *See* Restorative proctocolectomy (RPC)
Rubber band ligation (RBL), 181

S
Sacral nerve stimulation (SNS), 164–165
Sacrectomy, 134–135
Sandwich Generation, 3
Selenium, requirement, 53

Self-care training, stoma care, 239–240
Sepsis
  catheter-related complications, 69
  caudal spread of, 171–172
Serotonin receptor antagonists, 82
Serrated polyposis, 152
Serum electrolytes, in critical care, 100
Seton, anal fistula, 175
Sexuality
  aspects of, 233
  and relationship, stoma care, 233–234
SGA. *See* Subjective Global Assessment
    (SGA)
Sigmoidoscopy, FAP, 145
Silver tsunami, surgical care, 2
Singapore Hospice Council, palliative
    care, 217
SNS. *See* Sacral nerve stimulation (SNS)
Society acceptance, stoma care, 235–236
Sodium
  nitroprusside, 97
  requirement, 50
Specialty care, 193–194
Splenectomy, 215
SPURT model, 239
Stapled haemorrhoidopexy, 182–183
Stenosis, 124–126
Stenting, 202
Stoma care
  classification, 226
  colorectal nurse specialist role in, 229
  dietician role in, 228
  discharge phase, 240–242
  dummy stoma, 232
  education on, 240
  medical professionals role in, 227
  MSW role in, 228
  pharmacists role in, 228–229
  postoperative phase
    caregiver and self-care training,
      239–240
    psychological support, 238
  preoperative phase
    body image, 232–233
    counselling session, 230
    cultural and religious beliefs,
      237–238
    employment and travelling, 236
    fears and concerns, 231
    financial issue, 236–237
    independence in self-care,
      234–235
    placement, 231
    sexuality and relationship, 233–234
    society acceptance, 235–236

  rehabilitation phase, 242–243
  starter kits and brochures, 240–242
  type, 226
Stress, postoperative recovery, 247
Subjective Global Assessment (SGA), 46, 47
Surgical management
  anal fistula
    fistulotomy, 174–175
    mucosal advancement flap, 176
    seton, 175
  changing profile
    of patients, 3
    of society, 3
  information abundance, 2
Surgical stress response, 78
Swiss Cheese model, 32

T
Team-based approach, clinical finding, 23–24
Team-based integrative care, 131–132
  PE surgery (*see* Pelvic exenteration (PE)
      surgery)
  planning preoperatively, 132–134
  postoperative care and quality of life,
      136–137
THD. *See* Transanal haemorrhoidal
    dearterialisation (THD)
Thromboembolism prophylaxis, 80–81
Total knee replacements (TKRs), 107
Total proctocolectomy (TPC), FAP, 145, 146
TPUS. *See* Transperineal ultrasound (TPUS)
Trace elements
  and PN, 67
  requirements, function and deficiency,
      52–53
Transanal decompression tube, 126
Transanal haemorrhoidal dearterialisation
    (THD), 183
Transdisciplinary care
  Alexandra Health, 33
  clinical nutrition education, 45–46
  communication tools, 10
  documentation and follow-up, 10
  in elderly surgical patients, 18–19
  fecal incontinence (*see* Fecal incontinence
      (FI))
  fundamentals of, 8–9
  implementation of, 9–10
  vs. interdisciplinary and multidisciplinary,
      7–8
  management
    challenges of, 115
    patient recovery in, 113–114
  stoma care (*see* Stoma care)

Transdisciplinary Geriatric Surgery Service, 34
Transdisciplinary nurse, 33–35
  case study, 35–40
Transdisciplinary nursing, 32–33
  nursing failures, 39
  post-operative role of nurse, 36
  preoperative role of nurse, 35
Transdisciplinary team, FI, 166–168
Transperineal ultrasound (TPUS), 163
Traumatic vaginal delivery, fecal incontinence, 159
Travelling
  checklist for, 237
  stoma care, 236
Trimodal prehabilitation program, 127
'T'-shaped transdisciplinary nurse, 32–34, 39
Tumour bleeding, endoscopic treatment, 203
Tunneled CVC, 63

U
Ureter
  obstruction, 150
  reconstruction, 136
Urologist, FI, 168

V
VAAFT. *See* Video-assisted anal fistula treatment (VAAFT)
Vascular access devices, PN, 70

Vascular resection and reconstruction, 135–136
VATS. *See* Video-assisted thoracoscopic surgery (VATS)
Venous access, PN
  central access, 63
  peripheral access, 63–65
Venous thromboembolic (VTE), 98, 99
Video-assisted anal fistula treatment (VAAFT), 178–179
Video-assisted thoracoscopic surgery (VATS), 211
Vitals, in critical care, 100
Vitamin
  and PN, 67
  requirements, function and deficiency, 54–56
VTE. *See* Venous thromboembolic (VTE)

X
XELOX, 204
XELOXIRI, 204

Z
Zinc, requirement, 53

Printed by Printforce, the Netherlands